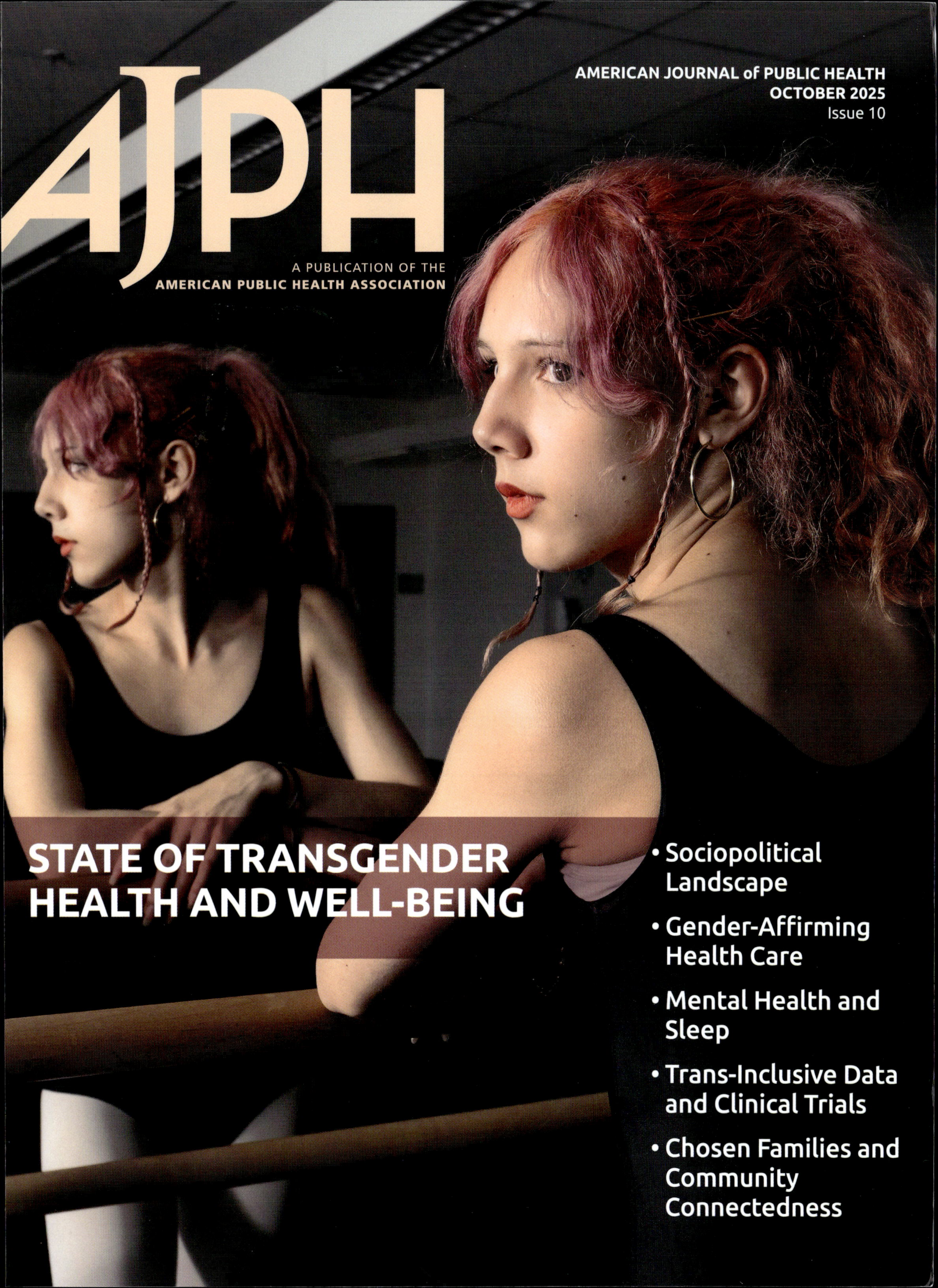

AJPH

AMERICAN JOURNAL of PUBLIC HEALTH
OCTOBER 2025
Issue 10

A PUBLICATION OF THE
AMERICAN PUBLIC HEALTH ASSOCIATION

STATE OF TRANSGENDER HEALTH AND WELL-BEING

- Sociopolitical Landscape
- Gender-Affirming Health Care
- Mental Health and Sleep
- Trans-Inclusive Data and Clinical Trials
- Chosen Families and Community Connectedness

APHA
AMERICAN PUBLIC HEALTH ASSOCIATION
For science. For action. For health.

AJPH®, published monthly, is the official Journal of the American Public Health Association®, 800 I St NW, Washington, DC 20001-3710; (202) 777- APHA; TDD (202) 777-2500. APHA is a nongovernmental professional society founded in 1872, representing all disciplines and specialties in public health.

The *American Journal of Public Health*® (*AJPH*) (print ISSN: 0090-0036; electronic ISSN: 1541- 0048), first published in 1911, is the official journal of the American Public Health Association® (APHA). The oldest and largest organization of public health professionals in the world, APHA represents approximately 30 000 members from more than 50 occupations of public health.

Submissions: Visit www.editorialmanager.com/ajph or ajph.edmgr.com for online manuscript preparation and submission guidelines. Contributions of original unpublished research, social science analyses, scholarly essays, critical commentaries, departments, and letters to the editor are welcome. Questions? Write ajph.submissions@apha.org or call APHA at (202) 777-2469.

Print plus online subscriptions: Institutional price (print copy with online access for a single institution and all authorized users, regardless of geographic location) varies by size of organization and ranges from $993–$1445 for US organizations, and $1073–$1526 for international organizations (air delivery); multiple campuses not permitted without special arrangement. Details of the tiered pricing system at https://subscriptionoffice.com/pages/apha-landing-page. To order, write apha.subscriptions@apha.org.

Online-only subscriptions: Institutional price for one institution and its authorized users (regardless of geographic location) is $878–$1307. To order, write apha.subscriptions@apha.org. For academic consortia or multisite corporate subscriptions, contact apha.subscriptions@apha.org.

Print-only subscriptions: Institutional price is US $701, $782 international.

Back print issues: A limited number of print issues are for sale. Single copies are US $65, $75 international (air delivery). Shipping included; prepay only. To order, write apha.subscriptions@apha.org.

Reprints: For prices and ordering information on 50 or more reprints, check the Reprints section at www.ajph.org. To order smaller quantities of reprints (rush delivery), use the "Purchase Article" link on the article site itself.

Electronic access: Online articles more than 10 years old are available free for personal use at www.ajph.org. Recent articles are available through pay-per-view: single PDF article for $24, single issue access for 24 hours for $33, or entire site access for 24 hours for $38.

Postal information: Periodicals postage paid at Washington, DC, and additional mailing offices. Postmaster: Send address changes to American Journal of Public Health, 800 I St NW, Washington, DC 20001-3710.

Address changes: Send to AJPH, Membership Department (members) or AJPH Subscriptions (subscribers), APHA, 800 I St NW, Washington, DC 20001-3710. Or write to membership.mail@apha.org (members) or apha.subscriptions@apha.org (subscribers).

Advertising: For pricing and other information, see www.ajph.org. Please write to brian.selzer@apha.org or call (202) 777-2470 for other advertising opportunities. Ask about special exhibit packages and sponsorships. Acceptance of advertising by the *Journal* does not imply endorsement of products.

Indexes: Publications that index or abstract articles from *AJPH* include the following: Ageline, Assia (Applied Social Science Index and Abstracts), Biological Abstracts, Chemical Abstracts, CINAHL, Criminal Justice Abstracts, EMBASE, EMCare, Environmental Abstracts, e-psyche, ERIC, ETOH (Alcohol and Alcohol Problems Science Database), Excerpta Medica, Food Science and Technology, General Science Index, Grateful Med, Hospital Literature Index, Human Resources Abstracts, International Pharmaceutical Abstracts (IPA), Medline, Physical Education Index, Pollution Abstracts, Psychological Abstracts, PsychINFO, Safety Science Abstracts, Sage Family Studies Abstracts, Sage Human Resources Abstracts, Science Citation Index, SCOPUS, SIIC Data Bases, Social Work Research and Abstracts, and Statistical Reference Index (SRI)/LexisNexis.

Medscape Publishers' Circle

AJPH

A PUBLICATION OF THE
AMERICAN PUBLIC HEALTH ASSOCIATION

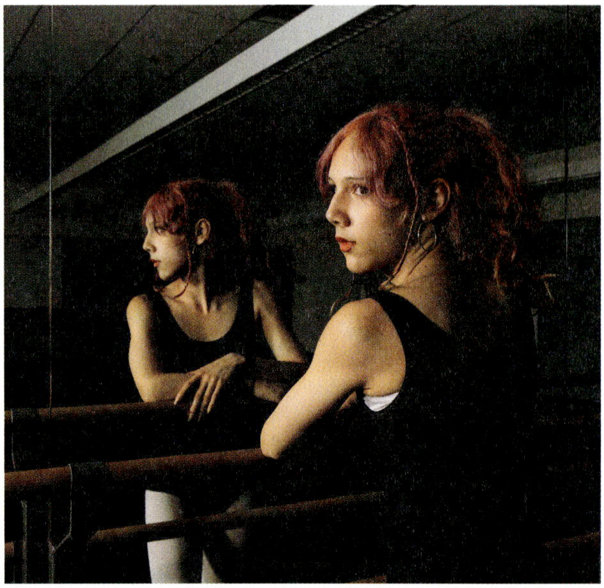

COVER: Evan in her high school ballet studio in Los Angeles, California in May 2023. Evan said she knew she was transgender from a very young age. She said ballet is one of the many ways she is in touch with her identity. "I'm really self-assured—like I'm really, really secure," she said. "I know who I am."

Cover caption and selection by Aleisha Kropf. Photograph by Em Monforte/EHM Studio, LLC. Printed with permission.

APHA
AMERICAN PUBLIC HEALTH ASSOCIATION
For science. For action. For health.

Promoting public health research, policy, practice, and education is the *AJPH* mission. As we widen our scope to embrace global issues, we also sharpen our focus to support the needs of public health practitioners. We invite contributions of original unpublished research, opinion and commentary, and letters to the editor.

The *Journal* is printed on acid-free recycled paper.

OPEN ACCESS · ONLINE ONLY · PODCAST · DATA SUPPLEMENT AVAILABLE

EDITOR'S CHOICE

1550 Unprecedented Times Lead to Unprecedented Young Researchers
K. M. Anderson

OPINIONS, IDEAS, & PRACTICE

EDITORIALS

1551 From Race and Ethnicity as Proxy Variables to Measuring What It Means: The Next Evolution of Health Equity Research
J. K. Kaholokula

1554 Reassessing the Heuristic of the "Healthy Immigrant" in an Era of Turmoil
J. S. Guadamuz

1557 A Case for Welcoming Refugees, Asylees, and Groups of Special Humanitarian Concern to the United States
C. Payton

1561 Healthy Food at Retail: Supplemental Nutrition Assistance Program Cuts or Food Quality
J. L. Pomeranz

1564 Abortion Bans Do Not End Abortion, but Rather Delay and Complicate Necessary Health Care
K. Hansen and B. G. Darney

1567 Mobilizing Public Health to Promote Equitable Access to High-Quality, Life-Enhancing Sex Education in the United States
E. S. Goldfarb and L. D. Lieberman

1570 MAHA's Hallucinations
A. A. Eyler, J. K. Harris, and K. J. Johnson

1572 Can War Help in Better Understanding of Burnout?
J. Owoc, M. Mańczak, R. Olszewski, O. Shevchuk, S. Zaporozhan, and M. Korda

PERSPECTIVES

1575 The Changing Landscape of Maternal Health Care in the United States: A Call to Action
P. Xaverius, S. M. Harvey, M. Kiely, and P. Factor-Litvak

NOTES FROM THE FIELD

1579 Public Health Education and Training in Sex, Gender, and Transgender Health: A Course to Advance Health at a US School of Public Health
S. L. Reisner and K. P. Todd

1584 Implementation of Doxy-PEP in a Diverse Sexual Health Program in Northern Manhattan: The Doxy-Care Study
S. Huang, C. Carnevale, N. Neu, J. Klein, D. Quigee, E. Perez, L. Burrell, K. Meyers, J. McLean, M. E. Sobieszczyk, D. Castor, and J. Zucker

1589 Ending the HIV Epidemic: Development and Evaluation of CyberGIS-HIV, a Web-Based Prediction Application
M. S. Chan, B. Fayaz-Farkhad, S. Y. Han, J. Park, S. Wang, and D. Albarracin

LGBTQ+ TRANSGENDER HEALTH

1594 Transgender Public Health Today
B. E. Coston

1598 Understanding Provider Treatment Approaches for the Provision of Gender-Affirming Hormones in the Current US Political Climate
N. E. Stetten, P. J. A. Kelly, T. I. Shireman, E. Balkan, G. Babbs, A. B. Alpert, H. L. Wolfe, D. J. Meyers, and J. M. W. Hughto

1602 Public Health's Defense of Pediatric Gender-Affirming Care
R. P. O'Brien

1605 Challenges and Best Practices Using Claims Data to Study Gender-Affirming Surgery in Transgender and Gender-Diverse Populations
G. Babbs, D. Dai, E. R. Boskey, E. Balkan, and J. M. W. Hughto

1611 Beyond Prevention: How Gender-Affirming Care Can Transform HIV Outcomes for Transgender and Gender-Diverse Populations
M. O. de la Paz and H. Barbee

1616 Aging Amidst Anti-Trans Legislation: Strategies for Safeguarding the Mental Health of Transgender Older Adults
N. M. Lampe and J. E. Sumerau

RESEARCH & ANALYSIS

LGBTQ+ TRANSGENDER HEALTH

1621 Addressing Transgender Erasure in HIV Clinical Trials: The Scorecard for Transgender and Gender-Diverse Inclusion
B. Minalga and C. Feuer

1631 Community Connectedness as a Source of Adherence to HIV Prevention Behaviors and Resilience Among Transgender Women of Color in New York City, 2020–2022
A. Furuya, Y. Ransome I. Kawachi, D. Callander, A. Radix, A. Whalen, C. Herrera, K. Watson, J. Contreras, J. Merriman, K. J. Bhatt, R. Scheinmann, S. Lim, C. Trinh-Shevrin, J. A. Schneider, S. H. Park, and D. T. Duncan

1642 Antitransgender Legislation and Needs of Transgender Floridians, 2018–2024
C. Hummel, K.-P. Truong-Vu, K. Nowotny, A. Mayfaire, B. Ramos, J. McKenzie, C. Copeland, and T. R. Glynn

1652 Discrimination and Sleep Health Among Transgender Women of Color in New York City: Cross-Sectional and Longitudinal Associations From the TURNNT Cohort Study
A. M. Whalen, A. Furuya, J. Contreras, J. A. Schneider, S. Lim, C. Trinh-Shevrin, A. Radix, and D. T. Duncan

1662 Analogous Analogs: Considerations Regarding Off-Label Use of Gonadotropin-Releasing Hormone Analogs Among Transgender Adolescents
S. Murano-Kinney

HEALTH MONITORING

1671 Disaggregating Office of Management and Budget Race/Ethnicity Data to Examine Racial Disparities in Late-Stage HIV Diagnosis, Hawaii, 2010–2022
F. Li, B. K. Gaskov, T. J. McCormick, A. R. Katz, and D. J. Felton

OPEN-THEMED RESEARCH

1681 Inequities in Excess Pandemic Mortality Among Documented and Undocumented Immigrants in California, 2020–2023
A. R. Riley, Y. J. Kim, J. Flores Morales, M.-L. Charpignon, M. A. DeVost, and Y.-H. Chen

1691 Health Hazards of Migration in People Seeking Asylum in New York City, 2023
C. Olivo-Freites, P. Miguez-Arosemena, A. Henao-Martínez, J. A. Suarez, C. Franco-Paredes, D. Edelman, C. Olivo-Freites, J. Marquez, C. Plazola, K. Leschly, J. Leschly, N. Gundacker, and A. M. Mohareb

1700 Impacts of a Healthy Checkout Ordinance on Added Sugars, Sodium, and Other Nutrients at Checkout 1 Year After Implementation: Berkeley, California, 2021–2022
A. E. Reimold, E. C. Wolf, K. J. G. Matas, S. Marinello, L. M. Powell, R. M. Schermbeck, and J. Falbe

1713 Changes in Abortion Access, Travel, and Costs Since the Implementation of State Abortion Bans, 2022–2024
N. F. Berglas, J. T. Barnes, E. Gonzalez, L. Peters, and D. G. Foster

1723 The State of Sexual Education: State Laws and Regulations Mandating Sexual Education in the United States
K. M. Nelson, A. Gray, S. Haiken, and K. Underhill

1734 Self-Managed Medication Abortion: History, Evidence, Models of Care, and Policy Considerations
L. E. Jacobson and C. Gerdts

LAW & ETHICS

1742 Suicide Prevention Training Among Occupational Groups: A Cross-Sectional Study of State-Level Policies as of July 2022
A. E. Massey, A. K. Druyon, S. Roettgering, J. M. Graves, J. Stuber, P. R. Borghesani, A. M. Ratzliff, F. P. Rivara, and A. Rowhani-Rahbar

BACKMATTER

ERRATA

1753 Erratum In: "Collecting Data Is Just the First Step: The Importance of Training Providers for Patient Encounters"

1754 Erratum In: "Association of the COVID-19 Pandemic with Women, Infants, and Children (WIC) Receipt among Pregnant Individuals"

OTHER DEPARTMENTS

1760 Subscription Form

Unprecedented Times Lead to Unprecedented Young Researchers

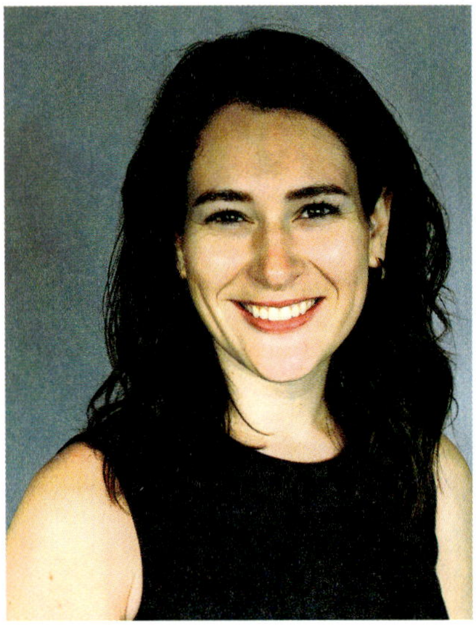

Katherine M. Anderson, MPH
Emory University
Immediate Past Student Editor, *AJPH*

The year 2025 is one of endings for me—I am completing my first grant, my position as *AJPH* student editor, and my doctoral dissertation, the central pursuit of five tumultuous years. Mine is the cohort of investigators entering the public health workforce in these unprecedented times, with the shuttering of career opportunities and longstanding public health infrastructure. But cultural and disciplinary upheaval are not new to us—the newest public health investigators were built within not one, but two consuming public health crises, yielding a group of young researchers unlike any we have seen before.

In the first class of my PhD program, our instructor stood behind a plexiglass booth. In a room built for 40, she faced seven masked-and-distanced students, each of whom had applied to the program before severe acute respiratory syndrome coronavirus 2019 (SARS-CoV-2) existed, yet decided to accept a spot amid its throes. By August 2020, we were exhausted by what the pandemic had already subjected us to, from jobs that pivoted amid COVID-19 to relocating and attempting to create community in a world actively trying to distance. All doctoral students face challenges; the more difficult task was facing them in this context. I wonder still what it would be like to learn with my peers instead of apart from them, and to form community in education and partnership in research, experiences inherent to public health itself. Instead, it was in relative isolation that my cohort and I experienced the stress and demands of an academically rigorous program, coupled with a pandemic raging outside and redefining our work inside. At an (online) interdisciplinary teaching workshop, I remember cautioning a student from another program that COVID-19–centered examples could cause fatigue and emotional disengagement among students, given its daily impact. It was only later that I realized that, compared with the omnipresence I felt, those not in public health might be afforded space from the pandemic, or even temporary escape, through their studies.

As I approach completion of my degree, I recognize that I have only recently been able to emerge from that context and fully participate as a member of the public health community. And years after the pandemic's onset, my peers and I should be embracing that opportunity: the coursework is completed, the exams passed, and we have survived a pandemic-era public health doctoral program, which few alive can say. My cohort is ready to dedicate our resources and abilities to improving the health and well-being of others—just in time to feel like the infrastructure to do so is being torn down around us. Instead of celebrating survival, we must fight for our lives again. And just as we joined our programs with the pandemic, it feels as if we are exiting in consonance with public health itself.

Like many others, I am sad, and I am angry. I have spent almost a decade postcollege working to this point, only to face a crisis of meaning and career imposed by political entities. Like many others, I will also use that frustration and sense of helplessness to find new ways to continue the work of public health. Even as I am still trying to process the hardships and lessons of beginning a PhD in public health during a pandemic, I am making efforts to create space for the new learnings and challenges of ending a PhD in public health during the systematic destruction of public health infrastructure. Whether I want it, I will be a product of these experiences that are, we are continuously reminded, unprecedented. But I take comfort in knowing that, as a member of the newest wave of public health scientists, so are we. AJPH

DOI: https://doi.org/10.2105/AJPH.2025.308211

ORCID iD:
Katherine M. Anderson https://orcid.org/0000-0001-9675-3653

ACKNOWLEDGMENTS

Thank you to Alfredo Morabia for his feedback on an early draft of this article and support throughout the student editorship, to former *AJPH* student editors Steve Fiala and Michelle Livings for their guidance, to Jessica Sales for her mentorship throughout the past five years, and to Kristin Knutzen and Alina Luke for weathering this with me.

From Race and Ethnicity as Proxy Variables to Measuring What It Means: The Next Evolution of Health Equity Research

Joseph Keawe'aimoku Kaholokula, PhD

ABOUT THE AUTHOR

Joseph Keawe'aimoku Kaholokula is a professor and chair of Native Hawaiian Health at the John A. Burns School of Medicine, University of Hawai'i at Mānoa, Honolulu.

See also Li et al., p. 1671.

The aggregation of racial/ethnic data in public health and biomedical research has long obscured the health needs of Asian and Native Hawaiian and Pacific Islander (NHPI) communities. Although the 1997 revisions to Office of Management and Budget (OMB) Directive 15 called for separating these groups, many government agencies and researchers continued to combine them, even up to the present, referring to them as "Asian or Pacific Islander," "Asian," or even "Other." This practice falsely implied uniformity across diverse populations with distinct biological, cultural, and social experiences. As a result, critical health disparities were often masked, sometimes to meet statistical assumptions rather than being empirically informed, which stalled progress toward health equity.

In this issue of *AJPH*, Li et al. (p. 1671) demonstrate the importance of moving from broad, higher-order racial/ethnic categories to more specific, lower-order groupings to uncover health inequities. By disaggregating Asian and NHPI data into distinct Asian and NHPI subgroups, they revealed that only certain subgroups drove the disparities in late-stage HIV diagnosis seen when subsumed under their larger group "Asian and NHPI" compared with Whites. For 2010 through 2014, increased odds were seen among Filipinos, Native Hawaiians, and other Pacific Islanders. From 2015 through 2022, elevated risk remained for Filipinos, Asians with no ethnicity data, and Pacific Islanders other than Native Hawaiians.

IMPROVING THE SPECIFICITY OF RACIAL AND ETHNIC DATA

Li et al.'s study contributes to a growing body of research that goes beyond OMB recommendations by disaggregating Asian and NHPI data into specific subgroups. Similar efforts have been made in studies of COVID-19 risk and mortality,[1] cancer incidence,[2] and cardiovascular disease prevalence.[3] The 2024 revisions to the OMB standards now encourage collecting more granular racial/ethnic data that better reflect individuals' identities. Other scholars have also emphasized the need for culturally respectful and meaningful disaggregation for Asian and NHPI populations.[4,5]

It is important to note that Li et al. separated Native Hawaiians from other Pacific Islander groups but did not further disaggregate smaller subgroups (e.g., Sāmoan or Chuukese), despite collecting race/ethnicity information on 10 distinct NHPI groups, because of small sample sizes (< 10 individuals) and confidentiality concerns. Similarly, for Asians, they collected data for 12 distinct Asian subgroups, but aggregated some of them. Although aggregation is often justified to avoid unreliable risk estimates, broad racial categories can produce misleading and highly inferential results. Nevertheless, their decision to disaggregate at an intermediate level enhanced data granularity beyond their broader, higher-order categories.

Disaggregating racial/ethnic data to the most detailed level can help create effective policies, targeted interventions, and better resource allocation. Li et al.'s work identified Asian and NHPI subgroups at the greatest risk for late-stage HIV diagnosis. Delayed HIV diagnosis can cause severe damage to the immune system, life-threatening infections, premature death, treatment difficulties, psychological distress, and increased transmission risk. Li et al. did suggest that the improvement in late-stage HIV diagnosis in Native Hawaiians over time may be due to the increased attention and resources (e.g., education and access to testing) directed their way. Their findings highlight the need for precise racial/ethnic data to promote health equity.

AJPH October 2025, Vol. 115, No. 10

HANDLING MIXED-RACE/ ETHNICITY DATA

What is not clear in Li et al.'s study is how they treated mixed-race Asians and NHPIs. Following OMB definitions (e.g., "A person having origins in any of the original peoples of Hawaii, Guam, Samoa, or other Pacific Islands"), it is likely that they included both single-race and multirace Asians and NHPIs in their higher-order analysis of racial data. However, how they assigned persons who were Asian + NHPI is not clear in their report. Nevertheless, it highlights an important issue in health equity research: how to fairly classify mixed-race individuals.

According to the 2020 US Census, about 17% of Asians and over half of NHPIs identify with more than one race, yet many may choose their respective Asian or NHPI identity as primary. Unpublished data from the Native Hawaiian Health Research Project show that over 90% of people with Native Hawaiian ancestry prefer this identity despite multiple racial backgrounds. However, a common practice is to separate single-race Asians and NHPIs from their mixed-race counterparts without additional context to guide classification. For example, research that distinguishes between single-race and mixed-race Asians and NHPIs, including combinations like Asian + NHPI or NHPI + White, has found higher rates of cardiovascular disease among mixed-race individuals than their single-race counterparts.[6] Without more detailed information, the causes of these disparities remain unclear, underscoring the need for more nuanced approaches to racial/ethnic categorization.

Recently, researchers have explored improved methods for analyzing multiracial/ethnic data. One study compared two approaches: the additive model, where every race/ethnicity a person selects is counted, and the mutually exclusive model, where individuals are assigned to a single racial/ethnic category.[7] Using 2021 Medicare Consumer Assessment of Healthcare Providers and Systems (CAHPS) survey data and treating all possible race/ethnicity combinations as the gold standard, researchers found that although both models performed similarly in predicting patient experience outcomes, the additive model approach was better at capturing differences related to social determinants of health, such as age, education, and mental health. The additive model avoids assuming that all multiracial individuals share similar experiences or risks.

If we accept that race/ethnicity is a social rather than a biological construct,[8] we must recognize the risk of misclassification when individuals' preferred identities are not captured—for example, by asking, "Which racial/ethnic background most influences who you are?" in the case of multiracial individuals. Without such information, the findings may lack validity because of misclassifications. Even more sophisticated analytical techniques—such as the additive model—which attempt to account for multiracial individuals more inclusively still rely on assumptions other than a person's preferred identity or identities. These limitations underscore that race/ethnicity is a proxy variable—an imperfect stand-in for the complex social, cultural, historical, and structural forces that shape health.

MOVING BEYOND PROXY VARIABLES

There is growing recognition of the need for more nuanced approaches to understanding racial/ethnic disparities. As a social construct, race/ethnicity serves as a proxy for factors that shape health behaviors, risks, and outcomes, such as sociocultural norms and socioeconomic conditions; unequal access to education, quality health care, and other resources; historical and contemporary experiences; exposure to systemic and interpersonal racism; and power dynamics. For example, studies have shown that educational attainment,[9] acculturation-related factors,[10] socioenvironmental conditions,[11] and experiences of racism[12] can help to explain racial/ethnic differences in health risks and outcomes.

To advance health equity, we must move beyond using race/ethnicity as proxies and strive to measure the underlying social, structural, and historical factors they represent. Disaggregating data to more granular subgroups, understanding mixed-race identities, and applying innovative analytical approaches are important and necessary. However, these efforts must be coupled with a greater commitment to understanding and addressing the root causes of disparities, including systemic racism, socioeconomic inequities, and cultural context, and their nuanced effects across distinct racial/ethnic groups. This is the next step in the evolution of health equity research. AJPH

CORRESPONDENCE

Correspondence should be sent to Joseph Keawe'aimoku Kaholokula, PhD, 677 Ala Moana Blvd, Suite 1015, Honolulu, HI 96813 (email: kaholoku@hawaii.edu). Reprints can be ordered at http://www.ajph.org by clicking the "Reprints" link.

PUBLICATION INFORMATION

Full Citation: Kaholokula JK. From race and ethnicity as proxy variables to measuring what it means: the next evolution of health equity research. *Am J Public Health*. 2025;115(10):1551–1553.

Acceptance Date: June 19, 2025.

DOI: https://doi.org/10.2105/AJPH.2025.308232

ACKNOWLEDGMENTS

This work was made possible in part by the National Institute of General Medical Sciences at the National Institutes of Health (grant U54GM138062).

Note. The contents are solely the responsibility of the author and do not necessarily represent the official views of the National Institutes of Health.

CONFLICTS OF INTEREST

The author has no conflicts of interest to declare.

REFERENCES

1. Quint JJ, Van Dyke ME, Maeda H, et al. Disaggregating data to measure racial disparities in COVID-19 outcomes and guide community response—Hawaii, March 1, 2020–February 28, 2021. *MMWR Morb Mortal Wkly Rep.* 2021;70(37):1267–1273. https://doi.org/10.15585/mmwr.mm7037a1
2. Moore KJ, Hubbard AK, Williams LA, Spector LG. Childhood cancer incidence among specific Asian and Pacific Islander populations in the United States. *Int J Cancer.* 2020;147(12):3339–3348. https://doi.org/10.1002/ijc.33153
3. Woodruff RC, Kaholokula JK, Riley L, et al. Cardiovascular disease mortality among Native Hawaiian and Pacific Islander adults aged 35 years or older, 2018 to 2022. *Ann Intern Med.* 2024;177(11):1509–1517. https://doi.org/10.7326/M24-0801
4. Delafield R, Watkins-Victorino L, Quint JJ, et al. No kakou, na kakou—for us, by us: Native Hawaiians and Pacific Islanders informing race data collection standards for Hawai'i. *Hawaii J Health Soc Welf.* 2023;82(10 suppl 1):73–76.
5. Ponce NA, Becker T, Shimkhada R. Breaking barriers with data equity: the essential role of data disaggregation in achieving health equity. *Annu Rev Public Health.* 2025;46(1):21–42. https://doi.org/10.1146/annurev-publhealth-072523-093838
6. Waitzfelder B, Palaniappan L, Varga A, et al. Prevalence of cardiovascular disease among Asian, Pacific Islander and multi-race populations in Hawai'i and California. *BMC Public Health.* 2023;23(1):885. https://doi.org/10.1186/s12889-023-15795-5
7. Martino SC, Dembosky JW, Hambarsoomian K, et al. Comparison of alternative approaches to using race-and-ethnicity data in estimating differences in health care and social determinants of health. *Med Care.* 2025;63(3):241–248. https://doi.org/10.1097/MLR.0000000000002108
8. Lett E, Asabor E, Beltran S, Cannon AM, Arah OA. Conceptualizing, contextualizing, and operationalizing race in quantitative health sciences research. *Ann Fam Med.* 2022;20(2):157–163. https://doi.org/10.1370/afm.2792
9. Goldfarb-Rumyantzev AS, Sandhu GS, Barenbaum A, et al. Education is associated with reduction in racial disparities in kidney transplant outcome. *Clin Transplant.* 2012;26(6):891–899. https://doi.org/10.1111/j.1399-0012.2012.01662.x
10. Divney AA, Echeverria SE, Thorpe LE, Trinh-Shevrin C, Islam NS. Hypertension prevalence jointly influenced by acculturation and gender in US immigrant groups. *Am J Hypertens.* 2019;32(1):104–111. https://doi.org/10.1093/ajh/hpy130
11. Thorpe RJ Jr, Brandon DT, LaVeist TA. Social context as an explanation for race disparities in hypertension: findings from the Exploring Health Disparities in Integrated Communities (EHDIC) Study. *Soc Sci Med.* 2008;67(10):1604–1611. https://doi.org/10.1016/j.socscimed.2008.07.002
12. Beatty Moody DL, Waldstein SR, Leibel DK, et al. Race and other sociodemographic categories are differentially linked to multiple dimensions of interpersonal-level discrimination: implications for intersectional, health research. *PLoS One.* 2021;16(5):e0251174. https://doi.org/10.1371/journal.pone.0251174

Reassessing the Heuristic of the "Healthy Immigrant" in an Era of Turmoil

Jenny S. Guadamuz, PhD, MSPH

ABOUT THE AUTHOR

Jenny S. Guadamuz is with the School of Public Health, University of California, Berkeley.

See also Riley et al., p. 1681.

The COVID-19 pandemic, which stands as one of the most significant public health and economic crises of the past century, drew attention to "essential workers" who could not isolate at home, including at least 10 million immigrants without US citizenship.[1] Early in the pandemic, essential workers, especially Latinos, were found to be at significantly higher risk of dying than other workers.[2] Given that disproportionate numbers of essential workers and Latino adults are noncitizens, immigration status may be an important but underexamined factor of their heightened mortality risk.

In this issue of *AJPH*, Riley et al. (p. 1681) present a novel evaluation of differences in excess mortality across immigration statuses during the COVID-19 pandemic. They leveraged California vital records from 2017 and 2023 and inferred immigration status using indicators for birth country and valid social security numbers. Although overall mortality rose in the postpandemic period compared with prepandemic levels, the excess mortality linked to COVID-19 was much greater among undocumented immigrants. Deaths among undocumented immigrants increased 55%, compared with 22% among documented immigrants and 12% among US-born citizens. This postpandemic mortality increase was most pronounced among undocumented Latino essential workers, who saw a shocking 91% rise in deaths.

These findings challenge the widely held assertion of the "healthy immigrant"—a paradoxical and overly simplistic assertion[3] that immigrants are largely healthier than their US-born counterparts. Instead, Riley et al. illustrate that during times of turmoil, undocumented immigrants are particularly vulnerable to deteriorating health. In this context, this editorial briefly outlines the systemic exclusions that adversely affect the 23 million noncitizens living in the United States, including 11 million undocumented immigrants,[4] as well as recent anti-immigrant policy changes.

Immigrant health trajectories vary widely, depending on immigration status and intersecting axes of oppression related to racial identity, economic status before and after migration, and other socio-structural determinants.[3,5] Immigration status—the extent to which a person has legal rights and protections based on their citizenship and documentation status—influences health via multiple mechanisms of systemic exclusion[5] inflicted by federal and local governments.[5] The stories that emerged during the pandemic illustrate these exclusions in action and begin to elucidate the root causes of the stark inequities observed by Riley et al.

When essential workers needed personal protective equipment and paid time off, noncitizens, especially undocumented immigrants, were less likely to hold jobs that provide access to these resources.[6] Additionally, not only were millions of undocumented immigrants excluded from federal stimulus payments that kept others afloat during the economic crisis,[1] but numerous reports show that undocumented immigrants were unable to obtain testing and vaccinations without providing photo identification or a social security number.[7] Even outside of acute crises, noncitizens are disproportionately employed in physically demanding and often dangerous jobs in agriculture, manufacturing and warehousing, and construction.[1] This means that hazardous jobs are often performed by the most marginalized workers in the United States.

For nearly four decades, the federal government has prohibited the employment of undocumented immigrants.[8] Coupled with inadequate labor protections, state-sanctioned discrimination, increasing law enforcement violence, persistent poverty, language barriers, and ongoing anti-immigrant rhetoric,[3,5] noncitizens live in an environment hostile to their well-being. With workers afraid or unable to speak up or seek legal remedies, they become vulnerable to wage theft, something most common in industries with high numbers of undocumented immigrants (e.g., garment manufacturing and private home services).[9] Similarly, workplace safety violations are prevalent in sectors with substantial informal and contract labor[6]—often the only options for undocumented immigrants without work permits.

Unfortunately, this marginalization extends far beyond laws that facilitate labor exploitations. The exclusion of noncitizens has been embedded in the US immigration system since the introduction of the first immigration law in 1790, which barred non-White immigrants from naturalization—a practice that took more than 150 years to abolish.[8] This racist system continues to negatively affect the health of noncitizens—about 80% of whom are persons of color—by systematically restricting the entry of certain groups into the country (historically non-Europeans), deporting those who are already here (disproportionately Latino immigrants), and denying many their fundamental human rights, including the right to health.[5] Most undocumented immigrants are barred from federally funded health insurance, and even many documented immigrants face exclusions based on their visa, years in the United States, and state of residence.[10]

Alongside the federal exclusions to labor protections and health care discussed here, undocumented immigrants face an increasing threat of deportation. In 2024, about 40% of undocumented immigrants had some form of deportation reprieve because of pending asylum claims, parole, or other temporary authorizations that allowed them to live and work in the country (often because of persecution or unsafe conditions in their home countries).[4] Disturbingly, the Trump administration has threatened to revoke many of these protections, placing millions at renewed risk of deportation—often without due process—as it attempts to expand its deportation authority at the expense of judicial oversight.[11] Although deportation itself destabilizes families, leading to financial instability, mental distress, and long-term health sequelae for the person deported and the family remaining in the United States, it also creates immediate fear and anguish within the broader community.[12] Consequently, many noncitizens, particularly undocumented immigrants, are reluctant to access health care and safety net programs for themselves and their children.[12]

Against this backdrop of federal oppression, several states and localities have made efforts to introduce immigrant-inclusive policies. However, these gains are threatened by federal actions to punish inclusive local governments, including multiple attempts to withhold federal funds from sanctuary cities (which prohibit local police from collaborating with federal immigration enforcement) and investigating state-funded safety net programs for undocumented immigrants for purported but unsubstantiated misappropriations.[13,14] Moreover, when budget shortfalls occur, programs for undocumented immigrants are often among the first to be cut. For instance, Illinois, one of just seven states that expanded Medicaid for some income-eligible undocumented adults using their state coffers, paused enrollment in 2023.[10] Even in California, often praised for its inclusive policies, Governor Newsom called for pausing Medicaid enrollment for undocumented adults amid potential federal cuts to Medicaid and pressure to roll back immigrant-inclusive programs.[13]

We live in an era when noncitizens not only endure long-standing systemic exclusions from health but are also experiencing a dehumanizing erosion of their rights. This erosion is driven by a federal executive branch actively demonizing immigrants, a federal judiciary unable to ensure due process, and state governments hesitant to safeguard the few hard-won protections for undocumented immigrants. Amid these circumstances, the notion of the "healthy immigrant" is not only simplistic but actively harmful. It perpetuates the idea that noncitizens are inherently healthy, endlessly replenishable, and thus disposable. Rather than relying on this reductive heuristic, public health researchers, practitioners, and advocates must acknowledge that the health of undocumented immigrants—and of other increasingly vulnerable noncitizens—is likely to deteriorate in tandem with the erosion of their rights.

Looking forward, immigrant health research must shift toward evaluating the long-term effects of living with precarious and shifting immigration statuses. This includes employing diverse methodological approaches that can capture how immigration status changes over time—both across the life course of an individual and in response to evolving policy contexts—and how those changes affect the health of immigrants and their families via multiple systemic mechanisms of exclusion. AJPH

CORRESPONDENCE

Correspondence should be sent to Jenny S. Guadamuz, MSPH, PhD, University of California, Berkeley, School of Public Health, 2121 Berkeley Way, Berkeley, CA 94720 (e-mail: jennyguadamuz@berkeley.edu). Reprints can be ordered at http://www.ajph.org by clicking the "Reprints" link.

PUBLICATION INFORMATION

Full Citation: Guadamuz JS. Reassessing the heuristic of the "healthy immigrant" in an era of turmoil. *Am J Public Health*. 2025;115(10): 1554–1556.

Acceptance Date: June 11, 2025.

DOI: https://doi.org/10.2105/AJPH.2025.308217

ORCID iD:
Jenny S. Guadamuz https://orcid.org/0000-0002-2312-4140

ACKNOWLEDGMENTS

J. S. Guadamuz is supported, in part, by the Robert Wood Johnson Foundation Health Equity Scholars for Action program.

I thank Maximilian Schmidt for providing thoughtful feedback that strengthened the arguments presented here.

CONFLICTS OF INTEREST

The author has no conflicts of interest to report.

REFERENCES

1. Kerwin D, Nicholson M, Alulema D, Warren R. US foreign-born essential workers by status and state, and the global pandemic. Center for Migration Studies of New York. 2020. Available at: https://cmsny.org/publications/us-essential-workers. Accessed May 25, 2025.
2. Chen YH, Riley AR, Duchowny KA, et al. COVID-19 mortality and excess mortality among working-age residents in California, USA, by occupational sector: a longitudinal cohort analysis of mortality surveillance data. *Lancet Public Health.* 2022; 7(9):e744–e753. https://doi.org/10.1016/S2468-2667(22)00191-8
3. Bacong AM, Menjívar C. Recasting the immigrant health paradox through intersections of legal status and race. *J Immigr Minor Health.* 2021;23(5): 1092–1104. https://doi.org/10.1007/s10903-021-01162-2
4. McCann A, Sun A, Sullivan E. Who are the millions of immigrants Trump wants to deport? *New York Times.* January 18, 2025. Available at: https://www.nytimes.com/interactive/2025/01/17/us/immigrants-trump-deportations.html. Accessed May 27, 2025.
5. Gee GC, Ford CL. Structural racism and health inequities: old issues, new directions. *Du Bois Rev.* 2011;8(1):115–132. https://doi.org/10.1017/S1742058X11000130
6. Valdes M, Ndonwie C, Ivory D, Eder S, Hidalgo S. Death on the night shift at frozen pizza factories in Chicago. *New York Times.* December 21, 2024. Available at: https://www.nytimes.com/2024/12/21/us/immigration-undocumented-workers-jobs.html. Accessed May 27, 2025.
7. Johnson A. For immigrants, IDs prove to be a barrier to a dose of protection. *Washington Post.* April 10, 2021. Available at: https://www.washingtonpost.com/health/2021/04/10/covid-vaccine-immigrants-id. Accessed May 27, 2025.
8. Cohn D. How US immigration laws and rules have changed through history. Pew Research Center. September 30, 2015. Available at: https://www.pewresearch.org/short-reads/2015/09/30/how-u-s-immigration-laws-and-rules-have-changed-through-history. Accessed August 20, 2024.
9. Ferriss S, Yerardi J. Wage theft hits immigrants—hard. Center for Public Integrity. October 14, 2021. Available at: http://publicintegrity.org/inequality-poverty-opportunity/garment-immigrant-workers-wage-theft. Accessed May 27, 2025.
10. KFF. Key facts on health coverage of immigrants. January 15, 2025. Available at: https://www.kff.org/racial-equity-and-health-policy/fact-sheet/key-facts-on-health-coverage-of-immigrants. Accessed February 26, 2025.
11. Feuer A, VanSickle A. Federal courts' emerging bottom line: due process rights for immigrants. *New York Times.* May 17, 2025. Available at: https://www.nytimes.com/2025/05/17/us/politics/courts-immigrants-venezuelans-garcia-trump.html. Accessed May 27, 2025.
12. Pillai A, Pillai D, Artiga S. Potential impacts of mass detention and deportation efforts on the health and well-being of immigrant families. KFF. February 6, 2025. Available at: https://www.kff.org/racial-equity-and-health-policy/issue-brief/potential-impacts-of-mass-detention-and-deportation-efforts-on-the-health-and-well-being-of-immigrant-families. Accessed March 28, 2025.
13. Russell R, Rosenhall L. Republicans push to end immigrant benefits in Democratic states. *New York Times.* May 16, 2025. Available at: https://www.nytimes.com/2025/05/16/us/immigrant-trump-states-california.html. Accessed May 27, 2025.
14. Montague Z. Judge blocks Trump from defunding 16 sanctuary cities: "Here we are again." *New York Times.* April 24, 2025. Available at: https://www.nytimes.com/2025/04/24/us/politics/judge-injuction-sanctuary-city-executive-order.html. Accessed May 27, 2025.

A Case for Welcoming Refugees, Asylees, and Groups of Special Humanitarian Concern to the United States

Colleen Payton, PhD, MPH

ABOUT THE AUTHOR

Colleen Payton is with the School of Nursing and Public Health, Moravian University, Bethlehem, PA.

See also Olivo-Freites et al., p. 1691.

The number of forcibly displaced people across the world has doubled over the past decade—from 59.2 million in 2014 to 122.6 million people in 2024—because of increased persecution, conflict, violence, and human rights violations.[1] This population comprises 68.3 million internally displaced people, 37.9 million refugees, 8 million asylum seekers, and 5.8 million others needing international protection.[1] A refugee is a person who fled their country of origin owing to persecution or fear of persecution because of their race, religion, nationality, membership of a particular social group, or political opinion. An asylum seeker is similar to a refugee, except they are already present or are seeking admission at the border or port of entry. An asylee is a person who was granted asylum.

Refugees and asylum seekers are a diverse population whose backgrounds vary by country of origin, country of transit, and lived experience. Syria, Venezuela, Ukraine, and Afghanistan are among the top countries from which forcibly displaced people originate.[1] The top host countries include Iran, Turkey, Colombia, Germany, and Uganda.[1] The vast majority of refugees (71%) live in low- and middle-income countries, and less than 1% are resettled to third countries such as the United States.[1] High-income countries such as the United States have the capacity to resettle more refugees.

In recent years, refugees who have resettled in the United States have primarily come from the Democratic Republic of the Congo, Afghanistan, and Venezuela, and asylees living in the United States most commonly come from Afghanistan, China, and Venezuela.[2,3] The US president decides on the annual ceiling for refugee admissions in consultation with Congress. Despite the ceiling set to 125 000 from 2022 to 2025, the number of refugees admitted ranged from 25 465 in 2022 to 100 034 in 2024.[2] The number of asylum cases filed in recent years has increased, including a doubling of applications from 2022 to 2023; however, the number of individuals granted asylum ranged from 16 550 in 2021 to 54 350 in 2023.[3]

Forced displacement is a public health and humanitarian issue. Migration experiences in one's country of origin, countries of transit, and host country can influence health. Refugees and asylum seekers are generally healthy. However, hazardous migration conditions, overcrowded environments, limited access to hygiene and sanitation, and food and water insecurity can increase susceptibility to communicable disease and mental health; it can also cause delays in diagnosis and management of noncommunicable disease.[4] Public health leaders have a responsibility to address potential barriers to health, including language and cultural barriers, xenophobia, institutional discrimination, restricted access to health care services, substandard housing, and limited employment and education opportunities.[4]

In this issue of *AJPH*, Olivo-Freites et al. (p. 1691) examined the migration experiences of 1486 asylum seekers in New York City to determine whether migration experiences could predict psychiatric illness. In this population primarily from Venezuela, Ecuador, and Colombia, the authors identified fear of violence (54.9%) and political persecution (21.7%) as the main reasons for displacement. A proportion of asylum seekers experienced extortion (48.3%), physical assault (24.9%), illness (19.4%), kidnapping (4.7%), and sexual assault (1.9%) during the migration journey. Although 17.9% of asylum seekers experienced detention or incarceration during migration, 57.7% experienced detention or incarceration while in the United States, which was associated with psychiatric illnesses.

Previous research among asylum seekers found experiences of violence during migration and fear of returning to their country of origin.[5,6] Previous research demonstrated associations between a history of torture with depression and posttraumatic stress disorder, political violence with lower health-related quality of life,

AJPH October 2025, Vol. 115, No. 10

BOX 1— Example Public Health Initiatives to Create a Welcoming Environment for Refugees and Asylees in the United States Based on the 10 Essential Public Health Services

Core Functions of Public Health[9]	10 Essential Public Health Services[9]	Example Public Health Initiatives to Create a Welcoming Environment for Refugees and Asylees in the United States
Assessment	Assess and monitor population health status, factors that influence health, and community needs and assets	• Identify and monitor the health needs and community assets of refugees and asylees through public health surveillance and quality improvement initiatives at the international, federal, state, and local levels. • Disaggregate data by immigration status, country of origin, country of transit, and language to inform public health follow-up. • Assess vaccination coverage among refugees via the Refugee Immunization Information Systems Exchange Project, which transfers their vaccination records into immunization information systems.
	Investigate, diagnose, and address health problems and hazards affecting the population	• Use the Electronic Disease Notification system, an electronic reporting system to identify health conditions from the overseas and domestic medical examinations that require follow-up for authorized users at health departments and screening clinics.
Policy development	Communicate effectively to inform and educate people about health, factors that influence it and how to improve it	• Educate others about refugee and asylee populations, humanitarian crises, and cultural humility. • Create and promote resources and training for the public health support of refugees and asylees (e.g., Society of Refugee Healthcare Providers, Switchboard, the Migration Health Initiative, the Cultural Orientation Resource Exchange, and Welcoming America). • Provide content in the language preferred by refugees and asylees through language access programs and plans, including interpretation and translation services.
	Strengthen, support, and mobilize communities and partnerships to improve health	• Learn about refugees and asylees by listening to their stories and respecting their culture. • Recognize the identity of each person beyond their immigration status, including how they identify, their needs, and their assets. • Provide affordable housing options to refugees and asylees. • Create supportive school programs to welcome refugees and asylees that meet the needs of learners, including language skills development and information about the education system.[10] • Convene multisector partnerships, e.g., the Philadelphia Refugee Health Collaborative, which includes resettlement agencies, refugee clinics, a health department, community-based organizations, and university collaborators. • Shop at refugee- and asylee-owned businesses. • Donate money or items to organizations that support refugees and asylees (e.g., coat drives for those who arrive in the winter, welcome backpacks for children starting school). • Fundraise with others for collective impact to support refugees and asylees. • Plan community-based events for World Refugee Day on June 20 to honor refugees.
	Create, champion, and implement policies, plans, and laws that affect health	• Ask your government representatives for refugees and asylees to be resettled in your state and have supportive resources. • Introduce new laws that use options for community-based case management services and legal representation rather than immigration detention.[11] • Examine and champion existing laws, including ○ Article 14 of the Universal Declaration of Human Rights (1948), which outlines the right to seek asylum from persecution; ○ The 1951 UN Refugee Convention and its 1967 Protocol, which outlines the definition of a refugee and their rights, including protection from returning to the country where they risk persecution and minimum treatment standards related to housing, work, and education; ○ Title VI of the Civil Rights Act of 1964, which states that language access services are required by programs that receive federal funding; ○ The Refugee Act of 1980, which outlines the procedures for refugee admissions and resettlement to the United States, including the formation of the Office of Refugee Resettlement; and ○ The 1990 Migrant Workers Convention, which is an international treaty that outlines the rights of migrant workers and their families.
	Use legal and regulatory actions designed to improve and protect the public's health	• Follow the technical instructions for panel physicians based on the Centers for Disease Control and Prevention (CDC) regulations evaluating refugees and others required to have an overseas medical examination. • Follow the technical instructions for civil surgeons based on the CDC regulations required to have a medical examination for adjustment of status to permanent resident. • Ensure that employment laws are applied equitably and that refugees are protected from employment discrimination.

Continued

BOX 1— Continued

Core Functions of Public Health[9]	10 Essential Public Health Services[9]	Example Public Health Initiatives to Create a Welcoming Environment for Refugees and Asylees in the United States
Assurance	Ensure an effective system that enables equitable access to the individual services and care needed to be healthy	• Cosponsor a refugee and asylee or family. • Support resettlement agencies, immigration lawyers, medical clinics, community-based organizations, and others that provide services to refugees and asylees (e.g., resettlement support, English as a Second Language classes, community health workers and patient navigators, mental health services, social services, legal advice/representation, community programming, transportation).
	Build and support a diverse and skilled public health workforce	• Use CareRef to complete a domestic medical examination based on CDC Domestic Refugee Screening Guidance. • Use VaxRef to translate immunization records. • Provide your time to support refugees and asylees during the resettlement process (e.g., tutor in English, drive to medical appointments, support a resettlement agency). • Cultivate employees and volunteers who strive for cultural humility. • Employ refugees and asylees in your organizations. • Network and collaborate with others via professional organizations (e.g., Society of Refugee Healthcare Providers, the American Public Health Association).
	Improve and innovate public health functions through ongoing evaluation, research, and continuous quality improvement	• Collaborate on public health surveillance, guidance, clinician training, and newcomer health education (e.g., Minnesota and Colorado Centers of Excellence in Newcomer Health).
	Build and maintain a strong organizational infrastructure for public health	• Ensure equitable access to health insurance, including Refugee Cash Assistance, Refugee Medical Assistance, and the Unaccompanied Refugee Minors Program.

gender-based violence with mental and physical health problems, and sexual violence with sexually transmitted infections, miscarriage, and preterm delivery.[5,6] High-income countries have exacerbated health issues through longer times in detention, restricted health and social services access, deportation threats, and denial of work permission.[5,6] Health is a human right, and the detention of populations of humanitarian concern hinders their physical and mental health both during and after detention.[5] It is essential that government leaders and policymakers seek alternatives to detention.[5]

There are economic, social, and cultural benefits to welcoming refugees and asylees to the United States. Host communities should welcome refugees and asylum seekers because they bring assets at the individual and population levels. Within 15 years, refugees paid $581 billion in taxes and contributed $124 billion more to the US economy than the initial support they received.[7] There were 178 000 refugee entrepreneurs in 2023 who are providing jobs and opportunities in their communities based on their valuable skills and experience.[7] Five-year economic losses in the United States are associated with a 10% reduction in refugees ($1.4 billion loss to the economy and $310 million loss in tax revenue) and a 10% reduction in asylum seekers ($8.9 billion loss to the economy and $1.5 billion loss in tax revenue).[8] Refugees and asylees contribute significantly to the US economy, including by facilitating the diffusion of knowledge and technology. They play a major role in international trade and investment. They also positively affect cultural diversity, community development, and humanitarian values.

Public health professionals can create a welcoming environment for refugees and asylees. Box 1 lists some example initiatives that align with the 10 essential health services—a framework developed by the Centers for Disease Control and Prevention and public health experts and implemented by centers such as the Colorado Center of Excellence in Newcomer Health.[9] Public health professionals can connect refugees and asylees to resettlement agencies, immigration lawyers, medical clinics, and community-based organizations that provide services, such as resettlement support, English as a Second Language classes, support from community health workers and patient navigators, mental health services, legal advice and representation, and community programming. Part of building strengths-based partnerships is recognizing the identity of each person beyond their immigration status, including how they identify, their needs, and their assets.

Public health professionals play a vital role in creating resources and training on the health of refugees and asylees.

Public health professionals can identify and monitor the health needs of refugees and asylees through public health surveillance and quality improvement initiatives. Health registries such as those led by the Centers of Excellence in Newcomer Health focus on refugees and asylees, which is important, as national databases do not disaggregate by immigration status.[12] Public health professionals can examine and champion existing laws, for example, the Refugee Act of 1980. Public health professionals have an important role in monitoring and providing input into laws to ensure health equity for refugees and asylees. This has been increasingly challenging under the xenophobic policies and violent enforcement led by the current federal government, which has restricted new arrivals, increased deportations, and drastically cut funding for resettlement agencies; these policies have led to the separation of families, lack of management of health conditions, and deportations to unsafe third countries.

Refugees and asylees strengthen the United States, and we have a shared responsibility to address global humanitarian concerns. As forced migration increases, future efforts are needed by governments such as the United States to adhere to existing international human rights laws by revising procedures for refugees and asylees at arrival, increasing stay through temporary or permanent residence, and providing resources for integration. There are initiatives that public health professionals can lead to support refugees and asylees in the United States based on the 10 essential public health services. AJPH

CORRESPONDENCE

Correspondence should be sent to Colleen Payton, 1200 Main St, Bethlehem, PA 18018 (e-mail: paytonc@moravian.edu). Reprints can be ordered at https://www.ajph.org by clicking the "Reprints" link.

PUBLICATION INFORMATION

Full Citation: Payton C. A case for welcoming refugees, asylees, and groups of special humanitarian concern to the United States. *Am J Public Health*. 2025;115(10):1557–1560.

Acceptance Date: July 16, 2025.

DOI: https://doi.org/10.2105/AJPH.2025.308253

ORCID iD:
Colleen Payton https://orcid.org/0000-0003-1398-6211

CONFLICTS OF INTEREST

The author has no conflicts of interest to declare.

REFERENCES

1. United Nations High Commissioner for Refugees. Refugee data finder. Available at: https://www.unhcr.org/refugee-statistics. Accessed March 6, 2025.
2. Refugee Processing Center. Admissions & arrivals. June 2025. Available at: https://www.wrapsnet.org/admissions-and-arrivals. Accessed March 6, 2025.
3. Schofield N, Yap A. Annual flow report asylees. October 2024. Available at: https://ohss.dhs.gov/sites/default/files/2024-10/2024_1002_ohss_asylees_fy2023.pdf. Accessed March 6, 2025.
4. World Health Organization. Refugee and migrant health. May 2, 2022. Available at: https://www.who.int/news-room/fact-sheets/detail/refugee-and-migrant-health. Accessed November 5, 2025.
5. Filges T, Bengtsen E, Montgomery E, Kildemoes MW. The impact of detention on the health of asylum seekers: an updated systematic review: a systematic review. *Campbell Syst Rev*. 2024;20(3):e1420. https://doi.org/10.1002/cl2.1420
6. Kalt A, Hossain M, Kiss L, Zimmerman C. Asylum seekers, violence and health: a systematic review of research in high-income host countries. *Am J Public Health*. 2013;103(3):e30–e42. https://doi.org/10.2105/AJPH.2012.301136
7. Church World Service. A closer look: the economic benefits of welcoming refugees. February 26, 2025. Available at: https://cwsglobal.org/blog/a-closer-look-the-economic-benefits-of-welcoming-refugees. Accessed March 6, 2025.
8. Clemens MA. The economic and fiscal effects on the United States from reduced numbers of refugees and asylum seekers. *Oxf Rev Econ Pol*. 2022;38(3):449–486. https://doi.org/10.1093/oxrep/grac012
9. Centers for Disease Control and Prevention. 10 essential public health services. May 16, 2024. Available at: https://www.cdc.gov/public-health-gateway/php/about/index.html. Accessed July 7, 2025.
10. US Department of Education. Chapter 2: Welcoming newcomers to a safe and thriving school environment. 2016. Available at: https://www.ed.gov/sites/ed/files/about/offices/list/oela/newcomers-toolkit/chap2.pdf. Accessed March 6, 2025.
11. American Immigration Lawyers Association. Featured issue: immigration detention and alternatives to detention. March 14, 2025. Available at: https://www.aila.org/library/featured-issue-immigration-detention-and-alternatives-to-detention. Accessed March 6, 2025.
12. Centers for Excellence in Newcomer Health. Colorado Center of Excellence in Newcomer Health. Available at: https://sites.google.com/state.co.us/refugeecoe/home. Accessed July 7, 2025.

Healthy Food at Retail: Supplemental Nutrition Assistance Program Cuts or Food Quality

Jennifer L. Pomeranz, JD, MPH

ABOUT THE AUTHOR

Jennifer L. Pomeranz is with the School of Global Public Health at New York University, New York, NY.

See also Reimold et al., p. 1700.

In their evaluation of the Healthy Checkout Ordinance implemented by Berkeley, California, Reimold et al. (p. 1700) found significant improvements in the healthfulness of food and beverages (collectively food) offered in check-out aisles by most food retailers in the city. Berkeley's Healthy Checkout Ordinance is an example of local government functioning as a laboratory to test new public health policy ideas and highlights the value of local policy implementation.[1]

The authors recommended combining a healthy checkout ordinance with other retail-based policies, such as specific requirements for retailers authorized to accept Supplemental Nutrition Assistance Program (SNAP) benefits. SNAP is a federal program jointly administered by the US Department of Agriculture (USDA) and state governments to provide funding to participants that can be used for all food except "hot foods" and alcohol. There are indeed several legally feasible policy options that could be implemented to improve the food environment through SNAP retailers.[2]

SUPPLEMENTAL NUTRITION ASSISTANCE PROGRAM POLICY

SNAP alleviates food insecurity, which is associated with multiple chronic diseases. Yet, in 2025, members of Congress and the federal administration reported interests in reducing SNAP coverage through policies that would devastate the program—such as cutting SNAP benefits and shifting financial obligations to the states—to those that would drastically reduce benefits or remove food-insecure people from the program—including expanding work requirements[3] and freezing the cost of the Thrifty Food Plan (the basis for SNAP benefits).[4] Although such proposals have been introduced during annual budget discussions, SNAP is historically reauthorized and amended through the Farm Bill, which is scheduled to expire on September 30, 2025. These threats to the program may, therefore, be ongoing.

The Secretaries of Health and Human Services and USDA additionally support amending the definition of food under SNAP pursuant to the president's "Make America Healthy Again" plan. The nonpartisan Congressional Budget Office (CBO) reported that federal lawmakers asked CBO to evaluate how adding nutritional standards to SNAP to "restrict purchases of foods linked to poor health outcomes" might affect the federal budget.[5] There are two primary methods to accomplish this: Congress can revise the federal statutory definition of food, or the USDA can grant waivers to states (or cities) allowing them to implement a revised definition in their jurisdictions. In an example of the first, a bill proposed in Congress, the Healthy SNAP Act of 2025 (HR 479) would remove "soft drinks, candy, ice cream, prepared desserts such as cakes, pies, cookies, or similar products" from the definition of food nationally. For the second, several states have requested waivers from the USDA to restrict SNAP participants from purchasing certain foods like soda and candy with SNAP benefits. As of May 2025, the USDA granted such waivers in Indiana, Iowa, and Nebraska.

FOOD RESTRICTIONS

Restricting specific foods under SNAP is not a new concept. Between 2014 and 2023, one of the most commonly proposed policies relating to sugary beverages at the state, local, and Tribal levels was to request a federal waiver to prohibit the purchase of sugary beverages with SNAP benefits.[6] Indeed, in 2010, New York City requested a two-year demonstration project to remove sugary beverages from SNAP, and in 2013, Senators Tom Harkin (D-IA) and Tom Coburn (R-OK) urged the USDA to engage in demonstration projects in two states to align SNAP benefits with the Dietary Guidelines for Americans. The USDA rejected these proposals at that time, noting the complexity of the issues.

There are substantial differences between sugary beverages and candy and other foods. Sugary beverages are associated with weight gain; obesity; type 2 diabetes; heart, kidney, and liver disease; tooth decay; cavities; and gout. Candy is not.[7] In terms of SNAP purchasing, the USDA does not collect food expenditure data at point-of-sale, so such data are derived from individual studies.[8] In 2016, the USDA estimated that candy purchases made up 2.2% of all SNAP purchases in 2011, while sugary beverages were more than three times this amount (7.1%).[9] Based on 2011 data, it was estimated that the federal government purchased between $1.7 and $2.1 billion annually through SNAP for sugary beverages in grocery stores alone.[10]

For taxation purposes, defining sugary beverages has been straightforward and effective, with multiple US cities enacting sugary beverage taxes. Defining candy has been challenging in practice. Twenty-four state tax laws define candy as not including flour, which results in the exclusion of candies containing flour (e.g., Nestle Crunch, Twizzlers) and noncandy items being taxed as candy (e.g., granola and cereal bars).[11] Furthermore, the SNAP candy exclusion may be a slippery slope. The Healthy SNAP Act proposes removing ice cream and prepared desserts. This elicits questions about why these foods were chosen. Is ice cream for a child's birthday party worse than daily consumption of popular ultra-processed snacks like Doritos or Cheetos?

ADDITIONAL POLICY OPTIONS

Perhaps certain suggested changes to SNAP are not exactly to make America healthy.[12] Indeed, such proposals have been made against a backdrop of proposed cuts to Medicaid, the largest deregulation of environmental protection in US history, severe cuts to federal scientific grant funding, reductions to the federal work force, and discontinuation of other federal programs, including one that delivered fresh produce, meat, and dairy from local farms and ranchers to schools, Tribes, and food banks. If making Americans healthy (and raising revenue or cutting spending) are goals of the federal administration, there are other methods to accomplish them that do not threaten the health of America. For example, taxing sugary beverages is an evidence-based policy that, if accomplished through the federal taxing power, would be a revenue-producing excise tax that raises the base price of the product, thereby applying to all purchases (including those made by SNAP participants).[13]

Another strategy to meet nutrition and fiscal objectives involves incentives and disincentives within SNAP. One study evaluated (1) fruit and vegetable subsidies, (2) fruit and vegetable incentives with sugary beverage restrictions, and (3) a 30% subsidy for fruits and vegetables, nuts, whole grains, fish, and plant-based oils and a 30% disincentive for sugary beverages, junk food, and processed meats.[14] The study found that all modifications would prevent cardiovascular disease events and diabetes, with such health benefits increasing along with the more detailed policies, which were additionally cost-effective, very cost-effective, and cost-saving, respectively.[14] Moreover, SNAP participants have reported support for these types of incentive–disincentive plans.

POLICY IMPLICATIONS

If the federal government were to implement incentives or disincentives, or change the definition of food, it should take a lesson from Berkeley and pilot these policy changes locally. The USDA should grant time-limited waivers—as it has—to allow the agency to study the changes and amend policy accordingly. In this way, the waiver states can serve as laboratories of policy change rather than Congress amending the federal definition of food and using the country as a test site—risking major understudied changes nationally for food-insecure households.

The US Constitution does not require the government to protect or promote Americans' health, as there is no right to health, safety, welfare, or food in the United States. Moreover, the US Supreme Court held that poverty is not a protected category (like race or religion). The United States is thus an outlier among high-income countries in the lack of policy and financial support for many health-related issues (e.g., only Americans go bankrupt because of medical bills). The federal administration has leveraged these gaps to usher in a national experiment at the expense of human and environmental health, safety, welfare, food security, advancements in scientific research, and government oversight, which will have long-term devastating effects on the nation's future. AJPH

CORRESPONDENCE

Correspondence should be sent to Jennifer L. Pomeranz, 708 Broadway 7th Floor, New York, NY 10012 (e-mail: jlp284@nyu.edu). Reprints can be ordered at https://www.ajph.org by clicking the "Reprints" link.

PUBLICATION INFORMATION

Full Citation: Pomeranz JL. Healthy food at retail: Supplemental Nutrition Assistance Program cuts or food quality. *Am J Public Health*. 2025;115(10): 1561–1563.

Acceptance Date: June 18, 2025.

DOI: https://doi.org/10.2105/AJPH.2025.308230

CONFLICTS OF INTEREST

The author has no conflicts of interest to disclose.

REFERENCES

1. Pomeranz JL, Pertschuk M. State preemption: a significant and quiet threat to public health in the United States. *Am J Public Health*. 2017;107(6): 900–902. https://doi.org/10.2105/AJPH.2017.303756
2. Pomeranz JL. Policy opportunities and legal considerations to reform SNAP-authorized food retail environments. *J Public Health Manag Pract*. 2023;29(5):614–621. https://doi.org/10.1097/PHH.0000000000001730
3. Ku L, Brantley E, Pillai D. The effects of SNAP work requirements in reducing participation and benefits from 2013 to 2017. *Am J Public Health*. 2019;109(10):1446–1451. https://doi.org/10.2105/AJPH.2019.305232
4. Bergh K, Hall L. Chair Thompson's plan would cut SNAP benefits and ignore scientific evidence in Thrifty Food Plan updates. Center for Budget and Policy Priorities. April 18, 2024. Available at: https://www.cbpp.org/research/food-assistance/chair-thompsons-plan-would-cut-snap-benefits-and-ignore-scientific. Accessed May 29, 2025.
5. Duchovny N. A call for new research in the area of nutritional standards in SNAP. Congressional Budget Office. May 2, 2025. Available at: https://www.cbo.gov/publication/61290. Accessed May 29, 2025.
6. Davis JN, Goon S, Gouck J, et al. An inventory of proposed and enacted sugar-sweetened beverage policies at the state, local, and Tribal levels in the United States, 2014–2023. *Am J Public Health*. 2024;114(12):1344–1353. https://doi.org/10.2105/AJPH.2024.307855
7. Duyff RL, Birch LL, Byrd-Bredbenner C, et al. Candy consumption patterns, effects on health, and behavioral strategies to promote moderation: summary report of a roundtable discussion. *Adv Nutr*. 2015;6(1):139S–146S. https://doi.org/10.3945/an.114.007302
8. Pomeranz JL. Supplemental Nutrition Assistance Program data: why disclosure is needed. *Am J Public Health*. 2019;109(12):1659–1663. https://doi.org/10.2105/AJPH.2019.305350
9. US Department of Agriculture, Food and Nutrition Service. Foods typically purchased by Supplemental Nutrition Assistance Program (SNAP) households (summary). November 2016. Available at: https://fns-prod.azureedge.us/sites/default/files/ops/SNAPFoodsTypicallyPurchased-Summary.pdf. Accessed May 29, 2025.
10. Andreyeva T, Luedicke J, Henderson KE, Tripp AS. Grocery store beverage choices by participants in federal food assistance and nutrition programs. *Am J Prev Med*. 2012;43(4):411–418. https://doi.org/10.1016/j.amepre.2012.06.015
11. Cole G. Is candy taxed? Here's what to expect this Halloween. October 25, 2024. Available at: https://www.avalara.com/blog/en/north-america/2019/10/state-by-state-guide-to-sales-tax-on-candy-just-in-time-for-halloween.html. Accessed May 29, 2025.
12. Beres D. Maga's era of 'soft eugenics': let the weak get sick, help the clever breed. *The Guardian*. May 4, 2025. Available at: https://www.theguardian.com/us-news/ng-interactive/2025/may/04/maga-soft-eugenics. Accessed May 29, 2025.
13. Pomeranz JL. Implications of the Supplemental Nutrition Assistance Program tax exemption on sugar-sweetened beverage taxes. *Am J Public Health*. 2015;105 (11):2191–2193. https://doi.org/10.2105/AJPH.2015.302850
14. Mozaffarian D, Liu J, Sy S, et al. Cost-effectiveness of financial incentives and disincentives for improving food purchases and health through the US Supplemental Nutrition Assistance Program (SNAP): a microsimulation study. *PLoS Med*. 2018;15(10):e1002661. https://doi.org/10.1371/journal.pmed.1002661

Abortion Bans Do Not End Abortion, but Rather Delay and Complicate Necessary Health Care

Katie Hansen, MD, MPH, and Blair G. Darney, PhD, MPH

ABOUT THE AUTHORS

Both authors are with the Department of Obstetrics and Gynecology, Oregon Health & Science University, Portland.

See also Berglas et al., p. 1713.

On June 24, 2022, the US Supreme Court's *Dobbs v Jackson Women's Health Organization* (*Dobbs*) decision overturned a half century of federal protection for abortion. Since that time, many states have enacted severe abortion restrictions, with immediate and negative impacts on reproductive autonomy and access to health care in the United States. Currently, total abortion bans exist in 13 states, and 28 states ban abortion based on gestational duration.[1] Additional restrictions—many of which were widespread before the *Dobbs* decision—significantly reduce access to abortion, including targeted regulations of abortion providers, mandatory waiting periods, parental consent for minors seeking abortion, and limitations on insurance coverage.

EVIDENCE OF HARM

The substantial harms caused by abortion restrictions were well documented before the *Dobbs* decision. The landmark Turnaway Study, a national longitudinal study conducted from 2008 through 2016 that compared outcomes among women who obtained abortions with those who were denied abortions because they exceeded facility or state gestational duration limits, demonstrated significant negative health and socioeconomic effects of abortion denial on women and their families.[2] Women who could not obtain a desired abortion experienced higher rates of serious medical problems, including chronic pain, hypertension, increased anxiety, and lower self-esteem. They were also more likely to live in poverty and suffer economic hardship. More recent studies focusing on the consequences of state-level bans reveal negative impacts on maternal morbidity and population-level infant mortality and suggest negative impacts on maternal outcomes, although few studies to date have implemented rigorous quasiexperimental methods.[3,4]

TRAVEL, DELAYS, AND FINANCIAL BURDENS

In this issue of *AJPH*, Berglas et al. (p. 1713) present one of the first national studies to directly compare the experiences of individuals seeking abortions both before and after state-level bans. The study documents substantial increases in travel distances, associated financial and logistical burdens, and delays in care. Although most abortion seekers were able to travel to a protected state for care following a ban, they did so at significant personal and financial cost.

Berglas et al. provide empirical evidence confirming that abortion bans cause delays in care in addition to exploring the factors that delay care. Following the implementation of state-level abortion bans, abortion seekers in the study experienced substantial increases in travel times, often exceeding 11 hours, as well as significant reliance on air travel and hotel accommodations for overnight stays. Not surprisingly, the overall amount paid for travel and logistics was significantly greater for those who obtained an abortion after the ban. These logistical hurdles created delays in obtaining care; the proportion of abortions occurring beyond 13 weeks of gestation more than doubled. This finding is consistent with existing state-level data, which have shown an increased proportion of abortions happening in the second trimester following implementation of abortion bans and severe restrictions.

Abortion is safe at any gestational duration, but the risk of complications, time required for care, and costs increase as pregnancy progresses. For example, abortions after 13 weeks can require longer or multiple visits for cervical preparation before the procedure. This additional time needed for more complex care can lead to limited appointment availability and longer wait times for patients. In addition, and as a direct result of bans, there are increasingly limited facilities and providers trained to care for patients at later gestations.[5]

Cost is a key determinant of whether someone who needs an abortion will be able to obtain timely care. The average cost of a first-trimester abortion is $550, which can be a catastrophic health

AJPH October 2025, Vol. 115, No. 10

expense for many.[6] This includes individuals with health insurance, as many states do not allow private health insurance plans to cover abortion care. In addition, the federal Hyde Amendment (enacted annually through appropriations legislation) prohibits the use of federal Medicaid funds for abortion.

Given these widespread insurance restrictions for abortion, it is not surprising that only 4% of abortion seekers in the study by Berglas et al. used insurance to pay for their abortion. Instead, abortion funds—grassroots organizations that provide financial and logistical support to those needing abortion care—provided significant financial support to abortion seekers, substantially lowering out-of-pocket medical costs and likely mitigating travel expenses. However, abortion funds did not completely offset the financial burdens experienced by those forced to travel to another state for care, as the overall travel-related costs increased following a ban. It is also important to note that fewer abortion seekers received support from abortion funds as time progressed following a ban, possibly signaling waning donations to funds. Abortion funds are not an unlimited resource; high caller volume, staff burnout, and decreasing funding availability after the *Dobbs* decision have raised concerns about the ability of abortion funds to support a growing population of people who must travel long distances for care.[7] Abortion funds serve as a critical lifeline for individuals seeking abortion, but more sustainable funding is needed for this essential health service.

ABORTION BANS DO NOT STOP ABORTION

Despite the profound barriers to care created by state-level abortion bans, data suggest that the number of abortions has continued to increase since the *Dobbs* decision, including in states that have implemented bans.[8] Much of this increase has been driven by telehealth medication abortions in combination with shield laws protecting remote clinicians who serve patients in restrictive states.[9] Despite these trends, clinic-based abortion still makes up about 80% of all abortions and, for some—including those at later gestations and those with high medical complexity—may be the safest option. Additionally, procedural abortion is a preferred option for some and ensuring access to all types of abortion is essential for providing person-centered care.[10] Consequently, protecting access to brick-and-mortar abortion facilities remains critical. Although Berglas et al. found that most abortion seekers were able to overcome significant barriers to obtain care out of state, this travel option was not feasible for everyone; between 3% and 11% ended up carrying an unwanted pregnancy to term. Only 1% reported a self-managed abortion, a safe option outside the formal health care system[11] that is common in other countries with restrictive laws and is likely to grow over time in the United States.

Ongoing and future research must continue to expand our understanding of the health and social consequences of abortion bans following the *Dobbs* decision. For example, we have limited data about the experiences of those who seek care outside the formal health care system and those who are uncertain how to or are afraid to access care altogether. Finally, researchers must give enhanced attention to data security for clinical and other qualitative or quantitative data above and beyond normal data stewardship practices and regulations, another consequence of stigma and potential criminalization owing to abortion bans.[12]

Data on the number of abortions after the *Dobbs* decision and Berglas et al. both show that abortion bans do not stop abortion, which is part of a range of normal pregnancy outcomes. They do, however, severely restrict autonomy, exacerbate inequities, and violate human rights. Scientists, advocates, and policymakers need evidence to support political accountability for the effects of bans and ensure the human rights of all individuals capable of pregnancy. AJPH

CORRESPONDENCE

Correspondence should be sent to Blair G. Darney, PhD, MPH, 3181 SW Sam Jackson Park Rd, UHN-50, Oregon Health & Science University, Portland, OR 97239 (e-mail: darneyb@ohsu.edu). Reprints can be ordered at http://www.ajph.org by clicking the "Reprints" link.

PUBLICATION INFORMATION

Full Citation: Hansen K, Darney BG. Abortion bans do not end abortion, but rather delay and complicate necessary health care. *Am J Public Health*. 2025;115(10):1564–1566.

Acceptance Date: June 30, 2025.

DOI: https://doi.org/10.2105/AJPH.2025.308240

ORCID iDs:

Katie Hansen https://orcid.org/0000-0002-1986-6168

Blair G. Darney https://orcid.org/0000-0001-8120-028X

CONTRIBUTORS

B. G. Darney conceptualized the editorial. Both authors made substantial contributions to the design and writing of the work and gave final approval of the version to be published.

CONFLICTS OF INTEREST

B. G. Darney is a member of the board of directors of the Society of Family Planning and a deputy editor at *Contraception*. She has received an honorarium from the American College of Obstetrics and Gynecology for committee work and research funding from Organon, Mexico. K. Hansen has nothing to disclose.

REFERENCES

1. Curhan T, Ephross P. State bans on abortion throughout pregnancy. May 28, 2025. Available at: https://www.guttmacher.org/state-policy/explore/state-policies-abortion-bans. Accessed June 13, 2025.

2. University of California, San Francisco. The Turnaway Study. Available at: https://www.ansirh.org/research/ongoing/turnaway-study. Accessed June 13, 2025.
3. Gemmill A, Franks AM, Anjur-Dietrich S, et al. US abortion bans and infant mortality. *JAMA*. 2025;333(15):1315–1323. https://doi.org/10.1001/jama.2024.28517
4. Society of Family Planning. Post-*Dobbs* research signal. February 20, 2025. Available at: https://societyfp.org/wp-content/uploads/2025/02/Post-Dobbs-Research-Signal_February-20-2025-Final.pdf. Accessed June 16, 2025.
5. Jones RK, Gibson C, Philbin J. The number of brick-and-mortar abortion clinics drops, as US abortion rate rises: new data underscore the need for policies that support providers. June 2024. Available at: https://www.guttmacher.org/report/abortion-clinics-united-states-2020-2024. Accessed June 18, 2025.
6. Harned EB, Fuentes L. Abortion out of reach: the exacerbation of wealth disparities after *Dobbs v Jackson Women's Health Organization*. January 25, 2023. Available at: https://www.guttmacher.org/article/2023/01/abortion-out-reach-exacerbation-wealth-disparities-after-dobbs-v-jackson-womens. Accessed June 14, 2025.
7. White K, Leyser-Whalen O, Whitfield B, et al. Abortion assistance fund staff and volunteers as patient navigators following an abortion ban in Texas. *Perspect Sex Reprod Health*. 2024;56(3):235–243. https://doi.org/10.1363/psrh.12240
8. Society of Family Planning. #WeCount Report: April 2022 through June 2024. October 22, 2024. Available at: https://www.societyfp.org/wp-content/uploads/2024/10/WeCount-Report-8-June-2024-data.pdf. Accessed July 15, 2025.
9. Cohen DS, Donley G, Rebouché R. Abortion shield laws in action. *NEJM Evid*. 2023;2(4):EVIDra2200280. https://doi.org/10.1056/EVIDra2200280
10. Jones RK, Chiu DW, Kohn JE. Characteristics of people obtaining medication vs procedural abortions in clinical settings in the United States: findings from the 2021–2022 Abortion Patient Survey. *Contraception*. 2023;128:110137. https://doi.org/10.1016/j.contraception.2023.110137
11. World Health Organization. WHO guideline on self-care interventions for health and well-being, 2022 revision. June 27, 2022. Available at: https://www.who.int/publications/i/item/9789240052192. Accessed July 15, 2025.
12. Reader R, Schumaker E, Payne D. Abortion researchers' security problem. October 1, 2024. Available at: https://www.politico.com/newsletters/future-pulse/2024/10/01/abortion-researchers-security-problem-00181704. Accessed June 14, 2025.

Mobilizing Public Health to Promote Equitable Access to High-Quality, Life-Enhancing Sex Education in the United States

Eva S. Goldfarb, PhD, and Lisa D. Lieberman, PhD

ABOUT THE AUTHORS

Eva S. Goldfarb and Lisa D. Lieberman are with the Department of Public Health, College for Community Health, Montclair State University, Montclair, NJ.

See also Nelson et al., p. 1723.

Equitable access to high-quality kindergarten through grade 12 (K–12) sex education is vital to the health and well-being of young people and communities. A new study of state mandates and guidelines by Nelson et al. in this issue of *AJPH* (p. 1723) adds new evidence that the United States falls far short of this public health goal. Together with other widely cited analyses, it reveals a factious landscape characterized by a patchwork of policies, divergent objectives, inadequate guidance for local school districts, and a lack of consensus on even basic definitions.[1,2] As a result, students who receive school-based sex education find it lacking,[3,4] and the United States has some of the highest rates of sexually transmitted infections (STIs) and adolescent pregnancies among high-income nations.[5,6]

Unfortunately, a precise accounting of sex education in the United States is elusive. Some analyses identify states as having sex education mandates if they require at least one subject area taught at least one time from grades K–12 (such as a single puberty lesson in grade 5). As noted by Nelson et al., accurate reporting is further impaired by lack of agreement among states on definitions of terms and phrases such as "age appropriate," "consistent with community values," "provided in a factual manner," and even "research based."

Furthermore, despite mandates to teach certain topics, states provide little guidance on how they should be taught. Relegating such decisions to local school districts makes curricular recommendations vulnerable to partisan influence. A state's mandate to teach "healthy relationships," for example, could be met by teaching only violence prevention. Moreover, guidelines that do exist are often contradictory from state to state. For example, Oregon's health education standards insist that teachers discuss "abstinence alongside sexual and reproductive choice in honest, age-appropriate ways that provide space for each student to consider their own personal, familial, and cultural values, health history, and goals while maintaining privacy."[7] Florida law, meanwhile, requires that HIV instruction "Teach abstinence from sexual activity outside marriage as the expected standard for all school-age students, while teaching the benefits of monogamous, heterosexual marriage,"[8] and the Texas Education Code dictates that instruction emphasize "the emotional trauma associated with adolescent sexual activity."[9]

What's more, there is no state-level accountability or enforcement of requirements, further encouraging hyperlocal control and opening the door to political pressure and interference in place of evidence-based programming. Nelson et al. optimistically point out that legislatures can be influenced to improve their state's sex education. The vast majority of pressure on state legislatures of late, however, has resulted in laws antagonistic to evidence-informed, comprehensive, inclusive sex education, such as, forbidding discussion of sexual orientation or gender identity, banning sex education before grade 5, establishing restrictive "opt-in" policies, and requiring crippling oversight by parents and school boards.

Perhaps most challenging are the vast differences in how comprehensive sex education is defined. In fact, sex education programs in the United States typically lack comprehensiveness both in their content and in their delivery. In most states, "comprehensive" refers to narrowly focused behavior change interventions, taught exclusively in middle and high school and focused on preventing pregnancy and STIs. These programs rely primarily on instruction about abstinence, HIV and STIs, and contraception. In some districts, comprehensive sex education also includes

AJPH October 2025, Vol. 115, No. 10

instruction intended to prevent child abuse, sexual assault, and dating and interpersonal violence. The common denominator, however, is danger prevention, meaning that what is called "comprehensive" in the United States is most often limited in scope and characterized by a pathologized view of adolescent sexual expression as something that needs to be carefully controlled and curtailed. When adolescent sexual activity is not treated as a normative part of development, sex education is rendered irrelevant and outdated to students, who consistently report that they want to learn more about emotional aspects of sexual health, navigating relationship dynamics, sexual decision-making, and dealing with breakups and that they want more discussions that acknowledge and address pleasure.[3,4]

The most glaring example of this behavior change model is the abstinence-only approach used in several states. Rebranded as sexual risk avoidance education, these now discredited programs are not based on public health principles but rather rely on fear, stigma, and false or misleading information to prevent any sexual activity outside heterosexual marriage. Not only do they ignore the reality of adolescent sexual experiences—especially sexual- and gender-marginalized adolescent experiences—but they are ineffective in reducing sexual risk.[10] By contrast, programs that include medically accurate information about contraception and safer sex can reduce sexual risks. Even more promising, though, are holistic, positive health-promotion, inclusive approaches based on the broader understanding of sexual health as articulated by the World Health Organization: "a state of physical, emotional, mental and social well-being in relation to sexuality [and] not merely the absence of disease, dysfunction or infirmity."[11] The research shows that such truly comprehensive sex education leads to improved life skills, increased empathy, reduced sexual harassment and homophobic bullying, improved communication, greater acceptance of sexual and gender diversity, and more.[12]

There is a widespread perception that providing sex education in our nation's schools is an inherently controversial proposition, but this is not borne out by the data. In fact, when sex education is clearly explained, the vast majority of parents across the political spectrum support it.[13] Opacity around what is actually being taught across the country, however, creates an opportunity for mis- and disinformation to sow confusion and concern among parents and the public.

Monitoring and reporting on sex education policies and laws across the United States are critical undertakings. These efforts help illuminate where state legislatures are purposefully crafting laws harmful to young people or specifically targeting sexually marginalized youths. Such reporting is far from sufficient, however. There is a need for more research demonstrating the myriad positive outcomes of truly comprehensive, holistic sex education connected to student learning, academic success, safety, and overall well-being. For this to happen, it is crucial for public health advocates to expand beyond the current risk-reduction framework and identify broader comprehensive sex education health-promotion outcomes as public health priorities.

Continued research is necessary to inform best practices for schools and to help ensure that students receive high-quality sex education. Importantly, public health researchers must think beyond peer-reviewed journals. By sharing their expertise through lay publications, including mainstream and social media, researchers can counter dis- and misinformation while building public support for expansive, medically accurate approaches. Furthermore, a more cohesive, coordinated, and assessable approach to sex education can only be established through the development of consistent, universal definitions of comprehensive sex education and terms such as "medical accuracy" and "research based." Policy experts must support and promote adoption of guidelines grounded in public health principles, such as the National Sex Education Standards.[12] These provide minimum requirements for content and learning objectives at each K–12 grade level as well as guidance on teacher preparation.

Professional public health organizations, including the American Public Health Association, should be unified and outspoken in urging states to adequately fund implementation and evaluation of comprehensive sex education and hold school districts accountable for doing so. Although education decisions are the purview of states, the federal government has long shown a penchant for using federal funding streams to influence policies and practices at state and local levels. This makes public health advocacy critical at the national level. One example of such advocacy is urging passage of the Real Education and Access for Healthy Youth Act. Recently reintroduced in Congress, this act would authorize federal grants for comprehensive sex education programs and youth sexual health services that are inclusive of sexual and gender minorities, while ending funding for harmful abstinence-only programs. In short, strong, unified leadership is needed now more than ever to ensure that broad access to high-quality, evidence-based, effective, and comprehensive sex education is treated as essential public health policy. AJPH

CORRESPONDENCE

Correspondence should be sent to Eva S. Goldfarb, PhD, Department of Public Health, Montclair State University, UN 4175, 1 Normal Ave, Montclair, NJ 07043 (e-mail goldfarbe@montclair.edu). Reprints can be ordered at https://www.ajph.org by clicking the "Reprints" link.

PUBLICATION INFORMATION

Full Citation: Goldfarb ES, Lieberman LD. Mobilizing public health to promote equitable access to high-quality, life-enhancing sex education in the United States. *Am J Public Health*. 2025;115(10): 1567–1569.

Acceptance Date: July 18, 2025.

DOI: https://doi.org/10.2105/AJPH.2025.308255

ORCID iD:
Eva S. Goldfarb https://orcid.org/0000-0002-9794-5777

CONTRIBUTORS

The authors contributed equally to the conceptualization, writing, and revising of this work.

CONFLICTS OF INTEREST

The authors have no conflicts of interest to report.

REFERENCES

1. Sexuality Information and Education Council of the United States. State profiles. Available at: https://siecus.org/siecus-state-profiles. Accessed June 13, 2025.
2. Guttmacher Institute. State laws and policies: sex education and HIV education. July 23, 2025. Available at: https://www.guttmacher.org/state-policy/explore/sex-and-hiv-education. Accessed July 31, 2025.
3. Goldfarb E, Lieberman L, Bible J. High school sex education in the context of state mandates and policies in New Jersey: a qualitative retrospective study of student experiences. *Sex Res Soc Policy*. 2023;20(1):141–152. https://doi.org/10.1007/s13178-022-00739-2
4. Corcoran JL, Davies SL, Knight CC, Lanzi RG, Li P, Ladores SI. Adolescents' perceptions of sexual health education programs: an integrative review. *J Adolesc*. 2020;84:96–112. https://doi.org/10.1016/j.adolescence.2020.07.014
5. Crowley JS, Geller AB, Vermund SH, eds. *Sexually Transmitted Infections: Adopting a Sexual Health Paradigm*. Washington, DC: National Academies Press; 2021.
6. World Population Review. Teenage pregnancy rates by country. Available at: https://worldpopulationreview.com/country-rankings/teenage-pregnancy-rates-by-country. Accessed July 17, 2025.
7. Oregon Department of Education. Oregon health standards. 2023. Available at: https://www.oregon.gov/ode/educator-resources/standards/health/Documents/Health%20Standards%20Adopted%2010.19.23.pdf. Accessed June 13, 2025.
8. FindLaw. Florida Statutes Title XLVIII K-20 Education Code § 1003.46 Health education; instruction in acquired immune deficiency syndrome. January 1, 2023. Available at: https://codes.findlaw.com/fl/title-xlviii-k20-education-code/fl-st-sect-1003-46. Accessed June 26, 2025.
9. FindLaw. Texas Education Code – EDUC § 28.004 Local School Health Advisory Council and Health Education Instruction. January 1, 2024. Available at: https://codes.findlaw.com/tx/education-code/educ-sect-28-004. Accessed June 20, 2025.
10. Santelli JS, Bell DL, Trent M, et al. School-based sex education in the US at a crossroads: taking the right path. *J Adolesc Health*. 2021;69(6): 886–890. https://doi.org/10.1016/j.jadohealth.2021.09.007
11. World Health Organization. Sexual and reproductive health and research (SRH). Available at: https://www.who.int/teams/sexual-and-reproductive-health-and-research/key-areas-of-work/sexual-health/defining-sexual-health. Accessed June 23, 2025.
12. Goldfarb E, Lieberman L. Three decades of research: the case for the National Sex Education Standards, K–12. *J Adolesc Health*. 2021;68(1): 13–27. https://doi.org/10.1016/j.jadohealth.2020.07.036
13. Szucs LE, Harper CR, Andrzejewski J, Barrios LC, Robin L, Hunt P. Overwhelming support for sexual health education in US schools: a meta-analysis of 23 surveys conducted between 2000 and 2016. *J Adolesc Health*. 2022;70(4):598–606. https://doi.org/10.1016/j.jadohealth.2021.05.016

MAHA's Hallucinations

Amy A. Eyler, PhD, Jenine K. Harris, PhD, and Kimberly J. Johnson, PhD

ABOUT THE AUTHORS

Amy A. Eyler, Jennie K. Harris, and Kimberly J. Johnson were with Brown School's Master of Public Health Program, Washington University in St. Louis at the time of this study.

Since his confirmation in February, US Health and Human Services Secretary Robert F. Kennedy Jr. has spearheaded the Make America Healthy Again (MAHA) Commission. In May, the White House released the commission's report on the roots of childhood chronic disease.[1]

This is a worthy subject. But if a student turned this report in as an assignment for any of our classes, they would not get a passing grade. In fact, the student would likely be referred to the academic integrity committee for improper use of artificial intelligence (AI).

We teach in the Brown School's Master of Public Health Program. Our courses (biostatistics, epidemiology, and research methods) require students to write reports incorporating scientific evidence from peer-reviewed literature. We instill in our students the importance of understanding existing evidence and correctly citing the studies that provide this evidence.

In many ways, technology has made research easier. There are software programs that instantly format research articles, including the citations. There are very effective literature search programs to identify relevant scientific studies. AI can be helpful in generating outlines and improve writing.

But, we warn our students, AI also has major pitfalls. One of the hallmarks of AI misuse is the inclusion of made-up references that look like they could be real. These AI "hallucinations" are well known and well documented. While testing AI's capabilities and ethical use, we have all observed them firsthand. And as recent media coverage has documented, such hallucinations riddle the MAHA report.[2]

Federal reports can have huge long-term positive public health consequences. For example, the 1964 Surgeon General's report on smoking started the nation down a successful decades-long path that greatly reduced smoking, preventing disease and death for millions of Americans. We applaud the idea of a report that could do the same for the health of American children.

Many issues presented in the MAHA report, including pervasive poor diet and lack of physical activity, deserve increased policy and research attention. Too many US children and adults are overweight or obese. Too many have diabetes and other preventable chronic diseases. And although it receives far too little attention compared with treatment, prevention is a core tenant of public health. A tremendous amount of data to guide prevention priorities already exists.

Some of these data are presented in the MAHA report. But they are undermined by two egregious flaws. First are the AI hallucinated citations for research that does not exist. Second, the authors frequently cite evidence for their policy preferences while ignoring evidence that conflicts or adds important context. For example, the report flags increased autism rates but ignores how this coincides with improved diagnostic tools and changes in how autism is defined.

At a minimum, the authors of the MAHA report should be held to the same standards of scientific integrity that we require from public health students.

If the intention of this report is to support devoting taxpayer dollars to the most effective ways of improving child health, it must be based on a thorough review of the highest quality scientific evidence. It also must grapple with the risks and benefits of different approaches. Lacking that foundation, we risk spending US taxpayer resources on new programs and policies that are ineffective. We also risk redoing science that has already been done and reinstating approaches we already know do not work.

This will not make children in the United States healthier. Indeed, it may pull critical resources away from other areas that do help improve children's health. So let's not waste this opportunity to do for children's health what we did for smoking. Let's actually try to "Make America Healthier." AJPH

CORRESPONDENCE

Correspondence should be sent to Amy A. Eyler, PhD, Brown School, Washington University in St. Louis, One Brookings Dr, CB 1196, St. Louis, MO 63130 (e-mail: aeyler@wustl.edu). Reprints can be ordered at http://www.ajph.org by clicking the "Reprints" link.

PUBLICATION INFORMATION

Full Citation: Eyler AA, Harris JK, Johnson KJ. MAHA's hallucinations. *Am J Public Health*. 2025; 115(10):1570–1571.

Acceptance Date: July 16, 2025.

DOI: https://doi.org/10.2105/AJPH.2025.308252

ORCID iDs:
Amy A. Eyler https://orcid.org/0000-0001-8417-1656

Jenine K. Harris https://orcid.org/0000-0002-3576-5906

CONTRIBUTORS

A. A. Eyler originated the idea for and finalized the editorial. J. K. Harris and K. J. Johnson helped revise the editorial for important intellectual content. All authors wrote the editorial and approved the final version.

ACKNOWLEDGMENTS

The authors would like to thank the past and present master of public health students for their willingness to learn that good science benefits public health.

CONFLICTS OF INTEREST

The authors have no conflicts of interest to disclose.

REFERENCES

1. Make America Healthy Again Commission. Make our children healthy again: assessment. February 13, 2025. Available at: https://www.whitehouse.gov/wp-content/uploads/2025/05/MAHA-Report-The-White-House.pdf. Accessed July 16, 2025.
2. Kennard E, Manto M. The MAHA report cites studies that don't exist. May 29, 2025. Available at: https://www.notus.org/health-science/make-america-healthy-again-report-citation-errors. Accessed July 16, 2025.

Can War Help in Better Understanding of Burnout?

Jakub Owoc, PhD, Małgorzata Mańczak, PhD, Robert Olszewski, MD, PhD, Oksana Shevchuk, MD, PhD, Stepan Zaporozhan, MD, PhD, and Mykhaylo Korda, MD, PhD

ABOUT THE AUTHORS

Jakub Owoc, Małgorzata Mańczak and Robert Olszewski are with the National Institute of Geriatrics, Rheumatology and Rehabilitation, Warsaw, Poland. Oksana Shevchuk, Stepan Zaporozhan and Mykhaylo Korda are with the Ivan Horbachevsky Ternopil National Medical University, Ternopil, Ukraine.

Burnout among medical staff has been one of the most extensively studied phenomena in health care over recent decades. The concept gained significant attention shortly after Herbert Freudenberger, a German-born American psychologist, first referred it to medical staff in 1974. Since then, a myriad of studies—continuing to emerge each year—has demonstrated that burnout affects nearly every aspect of health care. Its effects are evident at the organizational level (e.g., reduced quality of care, compromised patient safety and satisfaction, increased absenteeism, and higher staff turnover), the individual level (e.g., depression, diminished well-being, and disruptions to work–life balance), and the financial level.[1] Burnout prevalence has remained alarmingly high for years, and the COVID-19 pandemic, which pushed medical staff to their limits, has exacerbated it further. A methodologically consistent longitudinal study of American physicians reported burnout levels of 45.5% in 2011, 54.4% in 2014, 43.9% in 2017, 38.2% in 2020, and a staggering 62.8% in 2021, following the initial waves of COVID-19.[2]

Freudenberger's original concept of burnout described its emergence among physicians working after hours in a free clinic for people living with substance use disorder. Christina Maslach later expanded on this by identifying burnout in lawyers working with impoverished clients. In both cases, burnout was rooted in the emotional toll of assisting individuals in crisis, where the act of caregiving itself exacted a significant personal cost.

In 2019, the National Academy of Sciences published a comprehensive report that identified three levels of systemic factors contributing to burnout: the external environment (e.g., the health care industry, regulations, and standards), health care organizations (e.g., leadership and management practices), and frontline care delivery (e.g., work conditions, technology, and relationships with patients).[3] This model illustrates how systemic factors interact with individual variables to initiate and perpetuate burnout. Notably, in this framework, patients have become just one of many contributing factors, marking a significant evolution from the original concept, which primarily centered on emotionally demanding interactions with individuals in need.

As early as 1989, Freudenberger expressed concern that the term burnout had, astonishingly quickly, become a buzzword used to describe a wide array of personal and societal issues. He cautioned that its overuse risked rendering the term meaningless.[4] In the same article, Freudenberger's vision for the future of burnout research sounds disturbingly familiar even today: the need for models that identify interactions between personal and organizational variables, validated norms and instruments to measure burnout, and prevention strategies as the foundation for future work. Despite decades of research, burnout remains fraught with inconsistencies and ongoing debates.

Even the Maslach Burnout Inventory—the most widely used and long-standing tool for assessing burnout in health care—faces criticism. Objections include its one-sided wording (predominantly positive or negative statements within domains), which may lead to acquiescence bias,[5] and its failure to account for factors outside the work environment that could yield similar outcomes.[6] Rotenstein et al. identified at least 142 unique definitions for burnout or its subscales, reporting prevalence rates among medical staff ranging from 0% to 80.5%.[7] Additionally, although modern conceptualizations of burnout tend to emphasize systemic roots, the Maslach Burnout Inventory's focus remains largely on attitudes toward people rather than on broader organizational or structural factors. This raises an important question: is the burnout of today the same phenomenon that Freudenberger described half a century ago?

Have we truly gained a deeper understanding of burnout over the decades? Does the term burnout continue to

AJPH October 2025, Vol. 115, No. 10

TABLE 1— Factors Associated With Burnout Among a Convenience Sample of 926 Medical Staff Members: Ukraine, 2023

	OR (95% CI)	
Variable	**Univariable**	**Multivariable**
Sex (men)	2.26 (1.66, 3.06)	1.14 (0.68, 1.91)
Profession (physician)	2.54 (1.91, 3.38)	2.97 (1.85, 4.74)
Dealing with war victims (very often + often)	1.58 (1.19, 2.10)	1.25 (0.85, 1.83)
Region (ref. Lviv)		
Ternopil	0.56 (0.37, 0.86)	1.33 (0.60, 2.93)
Zhytomir	0.54 (0.34, 0.85)	1.36 (0.57, 3.23)
Vinnytsia	0.70 (0.43, 1.15)	1.48 (0.63, 3.52)
Other	1.91 (0.58, 6.36)	1.99 (0.29, 13.83)
Age	0.98 (0.97, 0.99)	0.98 (0.96, 0.99)
Fatigue	1.57 (1.45, 1.70)	1.36 (1.24, 1.50)
WHO-5 Well-Being Index	0.96 (0.96, 0.97)	0.96 (0.95, 0.97)

Note. CI = confidence interval; OR = odds ratio. The WHO-5 Well-Being Index is a continuous measure from 0 to 100. Fatigue is measured on a continuous scale from 1 (minimum fatigue) to 10 (maximum fatigue).

suggest a personal failing, or has it evolved to represent the inevitable toll on professionals navigating increasingly complex and demanding health care systems? Although research has undoubtedly advanced since Freudenberger's pioneering work, the fundamental questions he posed remain unresolved, challenging us to continue refining our understanding of this pervasive issue.

We investigated burnout in a cross-sectional study conducted in February 2023 in war-torn Ukraine. The study utilized a convenience sample of 926 medical staff members, comprising physicians (386; 43%) and nurses (520; 57%) working in six Ukrainian hospitals. The war in Ukraine, which began in February 2022, has plunged this large European, democratic, and independent nation into a full-scale conventional military conflict following an invasion by an external aggressor. This conflict has resulted in hundreds of thousands of casualties and represents the first such situation in Europe since World War II.

The objective of the study was to assess the level of burnout and associated factors among medical staff operating under these unprecedented conditions of warfare. We aimed to explore how work-related factors, including assisting wounded civilians and soldiers defending the nation's independence, were associated with the staff's burnout levels, well-being, and fatigue.

Research on burnout during wartime is scarce and has previously focused only on internal conflicts in Syria[8] and Libya[9]—countries with significantly lower scores on the Human Freedom Index and not classified as liberal democracies. Our results revealed that physicians were more likely to experience burnout than nurses, with 169 physicians (44%) and 122 nurses (23%) reporting burnout. However, overall burnout levels among participants, particularly nurses, were relatively low compared not only to Western countries and studies from Syria and Libya, but also to prewar Ukrainian data.[10] Although staff members who frequently or often assisted war victims appeared to face a higher risk of burnout, multivariable analysis indicated that this factor was not statistically significant (Table 1). Detailed methodology and results are provided in the Appendix (available as a supplement to the online version of this article at http://www.ajph.org).

The results, along with the design of the study and the methodological obstacles discussed in the online Appendix, limit the ability to draw firm conclusions but raise intriguing questions about the unexpectedly low levels of burnout observed. Could the staff's deeper sense of purpose, brought about by the wartime circumstances, play a role? Some studies suggest that a sense of meaning at work is a significant predictor of burnout levels.[11] Dean et al. describe burnout as a form of moral injury, stemming from the distress of knowing the care a patient needs but being unable to provide it because of systemic constraints.[12] If the frequency of assisting war victims was not associated with burnout, can one speculate that war circumstances reduce some of the organizational and systemic "noise" inherent in modern health care under routine conditions? By focusing efforts on helping as many patients as possible, may these conditions paradoxically mitigate burnout?

The current wartime conditions in Ukraine, although tragic, present a unique opportunity to conduct a comprehensive randomized study on physician burnout. Such a study could address long-standing questions and deepen our understanding of burnout in health care. Despite extensive research on this phenomenon over recent decades—demonstrating its widespread impact on both personal well-being and organizational efficiency—its full conceptualization remains elusive. The National Academy of Sciences' model identifies systemic factors as central to burnout, marking a significant evolution from Freudenberger's original concept. It is now evident that simply working in health care and assisting patients constitute a major risk factor for burnout. What was once thought to arise primarily from the caregiver's personal experience has increasingly been recognized as a burden imposed by systemic deficiencies within health care organizations. If unexpected and extraordinary circumstances, such as war, provide an enhanced sense of purpose that mitigates burnout, this could offer critical insights for its prevention and management in the future. AJPH

CORRESPONDENCE

Correspondence should be sent to Jakub Owoc, Narodowy Instytut Geriatrii, Reumatologii i Rehabilitacji, ul. Spartańska 1, 02-637 Warsaw, Poland (e-mail: Jakub.owoc@spartanska.pl). Reprints can be ordered at http://www.ajph.org by clicking the "Reprints" link.

PUBLICATION INFORMATION

Full Citation: Owoc J, Mańczak M, Olszewski R, Shevchuk O, Zaporozhan S, Korda M. Can war help in better understanding of burnout? *Am J Public Health*. 2025;115(10):1572–1574.

Acceptance Date: April 25, 2025.

DOI: https://doi.org/10.2105/AJPH.2025.308181

ORCID iDs:

Jakub Owoc https://orcid.org/0000-0001-6513-4040

Małgorzata Mańczak https://orcid.org/0000-0002-0736-0389

Robert Olszewski https://orcid.org/0000-0002-4210-5279

Oksana Shevchuk https://orcid.org/0000-0003-2473-6381

Stepan Zaporozhan https://orcid.org/0000-0002-4038-2010

Mykhaylo Korda https://orcid.org/0000-0003-0676-336X

CONTRIBUTORS

All authors approved the final version to be published. J. Owoc designed the study and wrote the article. O. Shevchuk, S. Zaporozhan, and M. Korda chose partner hospitals and managed all aspects of data collection and management. J. Owoc, M. Mańczak, and R. Olszewski analyzed and interpreted all data. M. Mańczak conducted statistical analyses.

ACKNOWLEDGMENTS

This project was funded by the affiliated institutions and their statutory funds.

We thank all the involved hospitals and their efforts in conducting this study: Ternopil Regional Hospital, Ternopil Psychoneurological Hospital, Ternopil Municipal Hospital No 3, Zhytomyr Regional Hospital, Vinnytsia Regional Hospital, and Lviv Military Hospital.

CONFLICTS OF INTEREST

The authors have no conflicts of interest to disclose.

HUMAN PARTICIPANT PROTECTION

This study was approved by the Bioethics Committee of Ivan Horbachevsky Ternopil National Medical University.

REFERENCES

1. Shanafelt TD, Dyrbye LN, West CP, Sinsky CA. Potential impact of burnout on the US physician workforce. *Mayo Clin Proc*. 2016;91(11):1667–1668. https://doi.org/10.1016/j.mayocp.2016.08.016
2. Shanafelt TD, West CP, Dyrbye LN, et al. Changes in burnout and satisfaction with work-life integration in physicians during the first 2 years of the COVID-19 pandemic. *Mayo Clin Proc*. 2022; 97(12):2248–2258. https://doi.org/10.1016/j.mayocp.2022.09.002
3. National Academies of Sciences, National Academy of Medicine, and Committee on Systems Approaches to Improve Patient Care by Supporting Clinician Well-Being. 2019. *Taking Action Against Clinician Burnout: A Systems Approach to Professional Well-Being*. Washington, DC: National Academies Press; 2019. https://doi.org/10.17226/25521
4. Freudenberger H. An overview of burnout: past, present and future concerns. *Loss Grief Care*. 1989;3:1–2. Available at: https://www.tandfonline.com/doi/pdf/10.1300/J132v03n01_01. Accessed February 16, 2024.
5. Demerouti E, Bakker AB, De Jonge J, Janssen PP, Schaufeli WB. Burnout and engagement at work as a function of demands and control. *Scand J Work Environ Health*. 2001;27(4):279–286. https://doi.org/10.5271/sjweh.615
6. Bianchi R, Schonfeld IS, Laurent E. Burnout–depression overlap: a review. *Clin Psychol Rev*. 2015;36:28–41. https://doi.org/10.1016/j.cpr.2015.01.004
7. Rotenstein LS, Torre M, Ramos MA, Rosales RC, Guille C, Sen S, Mata DA. Prevalence of burnout among physicians: a systematic review. *JAMA*. 2018;320(11):1131–1150. https://doi.org/10.1001/jama.2018.12777
8. Alhaffar BA, Abbas G, Alhaffar AA. The prevalence of burnout syndrome among resident physicians in Syria. *J Occup Med Toxicol*. 2019;14:31–38. https://doi.org/10.1186/s12995-019-0250-0
9. Elhadi M, Msherghi A, Elgzairi M, et al. Burnout syndrome among hospital healthcare workers during the COVID-19 pandemic and civil war: a cross-sectional study. *Front Psychiatry*. 2020;11: 579563. https://doi.org/10.3389/fpsyt.2020.579563
10. Botiakova VV. Prevalence of burnout syndrome among medical professionals in Ukraine from 2018 to 2022. *Art of Medicine*. 2023:92–100. http://dx.doi.org/10.21802/artm.2023.1.25.92
11. Ben-Itzhak S, Dvash J, Maor M, Rosenberg N, Halpern P. Sense of meaning as a predictor of burnout in emergency physicians in Israel: a national survey. *Clin Exp Emerg Med*. 2015;2(4): 217–225. https://doi.org/10.15441/ceem.15.074
12. Dean W, Talbot S, Dean A. Reframing clinician distress: moral injury not burnout. *Fed Pract*. 2019;36(9):400–402. https://pmc.ncbi.nlm.nih.gov/articles/PMC6752815

The Changing Landscape of Maternal Health Care in the United States: A Call to Action

Pamela Xaverius, PhD, MEd, CPH, S. Marie Harvey, DrPH, MPH, Michele Kiely, DrPH, and Pam Factor-Litvak, PhD

ABOUT THE AUTHORS

Pamela Xaverius is with the Parkinson School of Health Sciences and Public Health, Loyola University Chicago, Chicago, IL. S. Marie Harvey is with the College of Health, Oregon State University, Corvallis, OR. Michele Kiely is with the CUNY Graduate School of Public Health & Health Policy, New York, NY. Pam Factor-Litvak is with the Mailman School of Public Health, Columbia University, New York, NY.

Maternal mortality is a persistent problem in the United States, and most of it is preventable.[1] Maternal mortality rates (MMR: deaths per 100 000 live births within 42 days after birth) expose sharp disparities, with rates for non-Hispanic Black and Indigenous women significantly higher than for non-Hispanic White and Hispanic women.[2] Pregnancy-related mortality expands the MMR to 365 days after birth, exposing even higher rates of mortality for Black and Indigenous women.[3] Although the MMR decreased in 2023 for non-Hispanic White women, statistics remain unchanged and disturbing for other racial/ethnic groups.[2] Indeed, the United States ranks last in a comparison of MMR among developed countries, with Black and Indigenous women having rates over 10 times higher compared with countries such as Germany, Japan, and the Netherlands.[4]

In this article, we contend that now, more than ever, policy changes at all levels of the government and the private sector are critical to reducing maternal deaths. We focus on diminished access to reproductive health services and the critical role of the maternity care workforce in addressing this maternal health crisis. We describe structural and geographic barriers to accessing maternity care, underscoring the harmful effects of these obstacles that exacerbate health inequities and diminish overall population health. We provide evidence that the overturning of *Roe v Wade* has affected the availability of all forms of reproductive health care, including the provision of maternity care. We issue a call to action for advancing public health efforts to ensure equitable access to reproductive health care; increasing federal, state, and private sector funding for workforce development and training; and prioritizing the voices of historically marginalized groups.

BARRIERS TO MATERNITY CARE ACCESS

The United States faces a maternal health crisis that is shaped by a complex interplay of structural, geographic, and policy-related barriers. These barriers are not experienced equally across populations and regions, leading to stark disparities in access, quality, and outcomes of care.

Structural Barriers

The provision of maternal care during pregnancy, the immediate postpartum period, and intrapartum in the United States is woefully inadequate. Compared with other developed countries such as Sweden, Austria, Norway, Germany, and the United Kingdom, the United States has the lowest number of maternity care providers (16 per 100 000 deliveries).[5] Although most developed countries provide postpartum home visits as a universal benefit, the United States offers only sporadic and fragmented home visiting programs that are not available to all. The option for states to extend Medicaid postpartum coverage to 12 months became permanent in 2023. However, if the current administration cuts Medicaid, these extensions will likely be rescinded.[6] Additionally, the United States is the only high-income country that does not guarantee paid parental leave and universal health care, leaving families to face economic hardship, stress, and poor maternal health.[3]

Geographic Barriers

Where you live matters. More than one third of all counties in the United States have neither birthing facilities nor maternity care providers.[7] A recent study found that between 2010 and 2022, 500 hospitals closed their maternity wards, which resulted in 52% of rural hospitals no longer having delivery services.[8] Furthermore, the types of services provided in rural areas are less comprehensive than those offered in urban areas.[9] Individuals in rural areas also face higher out-of-pocket costs for reproductive health services because of travel expenses. These challenges are exacerbated by state-level policies that can create additional barriers to accessing reproductive health services, such as medication abortion restrictions, targeted regulation of abortion providers, parental consent laws, insurance coverage restrictions, and waiting periods.[10] This lack of access results in higher rates of inadequate prenatal care, higher risk of preterm births, and greater risk of maternal death.[11]

Overturning of *Roe v Wade*

On June 24, 2022, access to abortion suffered a severe setback when the US Supreme Court overturned *Roe v Wade* with the *Dobbs v Jackson Women's Health Organization* decision. As of January 22, 2025, 19 states have protections in place for abortion services whereas 32 have restrictions.[12] In addition to state-level restrictions, the election of Donald Trump as president of the United States has introduced further national restrictions. These national limits include reinstating the global gag rule that prevents organizations from even discussing abortion as an option, fortifying the Hyde Amendment (prohibiting the use of federal funds for abortions), and even pardoning several antiabortion activists convicted of blocking access to abortion clinics. The newest expansion of the gag rule also affects funding for HIV/AIDS, malaria, tuberculosis, nutrition, maternal health, and health systems. The devastating consequences of the gag rule are widespread, particularly for women, young people, lesbian, gay, bisexual, transgender, queer, and intersex (LGBTQI) people, poor people, religious minorities, and people living in rural areas. Further, these harmful policies will decrease access to services and increase unwanted pregnancies, abortion rates, maternal and child mortality rates, and HIV rates.[13]

Abortion bans and restrictions discourage many doctors, including those who specialize in maternal–fetal medicine and high-risk pregnancies, from choosing residency programs in affected states.[14] In 2023, obstetrician-gynecologist (OB-GYN) residency applications declined more sharply in states with bans (10.5%) than in those without bans (5.2%). Many surveys indicate that a majority of medical students and physicians prefer states without abortion limits, influencing residency application decisions.[15] Because many doctors choose to train where they intend to practice, the location of training programs is an essential determinant of care availability. A recent analysis found that fewer applicants are pursuing emergency medicine residencies in states with bans, emphasizing how *Dobbs* continues to have a broad impact on health care access nationwide.[16] With these reductions in health care providers in states with abortion bans and restrictions, fewer practices are available to provide other reproductive services, including cancer and sexually transmitted infection screenings, regular exams, and contraception provisions, weakening opportunities for maternal health and wellness.

HEALTH EQUITY AND DISPARITIES

Racial disparities in maternal and infant health have persisted in the United States for decades despite advances in medical care. The impact of the COVID-19 pandemic and the overturning of *Roe v Wade* have exacerbated the disparities.[17] Indeed, the COVID-19 pandemic was associated with a doubling of maternal mortality among Indigenous women, higher than for any other racial/ethnic group, with larger increases in non-Medicaid expansion states.[18] Barriers include lack of health insurance coverage, social and economic factors (e.g., income, education), limited availability of providers, and racism and historical trauma.[5,6,19,20] Women experiencing intersectional discrimination based on race, ethnicity, immigration status, and gender identity likely experience more than one of these barriers.[7,21] Notably, the lack of access to evidence-based approaches to maternity care before, during, and after pregnancy disproportionately affects low-income women and those from marginalized racial and ethnic groups.[22] The current administration's dismantling of diversity, equity, and inclusion activities, which are designed to reach these marginalized groups, will likely reduce the educational preparation of people of color entering health care education programs and exacerbate poor health outcomes.

CALL TO ACTION

We champion and call for compelling policies to address structural barriers to maternity care access. Women's health and the health of children, families, and communities require nothing less than a renewed commitment within our public health discipline to address these challenges with steadfast courage, tenacity, and resilience. Prioritizing efforts to ensure affordable, available, and accessible maternity care will contribute to closing the gap in reproductive health disparities in our country, of which MMR is only the tip of the iceberg.

Ensuring a robust workforce is critical. We are losing skilled and compassionate maternal health professionals, especially in states with abortion restrictions. Incentive programs such as those that provide student loan forgiveness to providers who practice in rural communities are necessary to entice a new generation of practitioners to these geographic areas. We encourage states to implement policies and programs that support maternal health care providers and services, including lactation services, postpartum coverage, midwives and doulas, perinatal community health workers, presumptive eligibility, home visiting, perinatal quality collaboratives, and maternal mortality review committees.[23]

Even in states without abortion restrictions, ensuring a robust maternal health–focused workforce is crucial. We join the call for federal and state funding for workforce development and training to ensure a competent workforce. National and local groups are advocating for increased funding for workforce development and training of OB-GYNs, midwives, doulas, and community health workers. Lobbying groups affiliated with specialty organizations, such as the American College of Obstetrics and Gynecology, the American College of Nurse-Midwives, and the Childbirth and Postpartum Professional Association (representing doulas, childbirth educators, and lactation experts), are providing leadership for these activities. Leading public health organizations (e.g., the American Public Health Association), academic institutions, key advocacy groups, and funding foundations, such as the Kaiser Family Foundation, Guttmacher Institute, and the Commonwealth Fund, are also contributing to these efforts. Such providers will require special training in providing services to women considering the emerging legal challenges.

Strong skills in research and policy development are needed to provide evidence that will increase access to care and translate into community-based programs designed to decrease maternal morbidity and mortality. In support of a strong workforce, state and local health departments must continue to collect data and compile statistics on racial and ethnic disparities in the United States and to reinstate funding for research databases and surveillance systems such as the Pregnancy Risk Assessment Monitoring System (PRAMS), which was previously funded by the Centers for Disease Control and Prevention.[24] Data are essential to provide guidance for the most efficient use of limited resources. More than ever, data-driven policies are vital to addressing women's reproductive health and changing health priorities at the federal level.

To address persistent health disparities among low-income women and those from marginalized racial and ethnic groups, we must center the voices of those most affected by poor maternal health and diminished access to maternity care. Amplifying the perspectives of Black, Indigenous, and other marginalized groups in maternal health research and policies ensures that solutions reflect their needs. We call for a culturally humble, culturally aligned, and respectful maternal care workforce that is trained to address issues of implicit bias and create a sense of belonging for historically marginalized groups. When individuals feel valued and included, their voices and experiences contribute to shaping federal and state policies and programs that drive meaningful changes and increase access to maternal care.

Finally, political will for policy and advocacy for women's reproductive health on the federal, state, and local levels is essential for advancing equitable access to reproductive health. Political will is needed to advocate for increased education, more targeted workforce development in the maternity care field, increased access to high-quality care, continuity of care, and specialized programs at all levels. For example, community-driven programs and increased access to midwifery and doula services can provide much-needed support. The Michigan Momnibus legislation is one example of a state-led effort to improve racial equity in maternal health care by supporting community-driven programs and ensuring accountability for health care providers.[25] Unfortunately, such programs are targeted for defunding under the current administration.

Public health efforts are now more critically important than ever. We strongly advocate and call for compelling policies, increased health surveillance, strong community-based practices, public health education, and health equity. The authors of this article are women who are beyond their childbearing years. We remember the signing of *Roe v Wade* in 1973 and have raised daughters who now have far fewer rights than we had. We are not, however, discouraged; we stand united in support of and defense of bold efforts that will lead to transformative changes and ensure the health and well-being of all women. AJPH

CORRESPONDENCE

Correspondence should be sent to Pamela Xaverius, PhD, MEd, CPH, Associate Dean for Research and Scholarship, Professor, Public Health Sciences, Parkinson School of Health Sciences and Public Health, Loyola University Chicago, Health Sciences Campus, 2160 S. First Ave, Maywood, IL 60153 (e-mail: pxaverius@luc.edu). Reprints can be ordered at https://www.ajph.org by clicking the "Reprints" link.

PUBLICATION INFORMATION

Full Citation: Xaverius P, Harvey SM, Kiely M, Factor-Litvak P. The changing landscape of maternal health care in the United States: a call to action. *Am J Public Health*. 2025;115(10):1575–1578.

Acceptance Date: June 22, 2025.

DOI: https://doi.org/10.2105/AJPH.2025.308236

ORCID iD:

Pamela Xaverius https://orcid.org/0000-0001-8824-2933

CONTRIBUTORS

All authors contributed equally to designing this article, drafting and revising the intellectual content, and providing final approval of the published version.

ACKNOWLEDGMENTS

We acknowledge a fifth contributor to this article who asked to be removed from authorship in an abundance of caution regarding the current political environment for institutions of higher education in their state.

CONFLICTS OF INTEREST

There are no potential or actual conflicts of interest regarding this work.

REFERENCES

1. Thoma ME, Declercq ER. Changes in pregnancy-related mortality associated with the coronavirus disease 2019 (COVID-19) pandemic in the United States. *Obstet Gynecol*. 2023;141(5):911–917. https://doi.org/10.1097/AOG.0000000000005182
2. Hoyert DL. Maternal mortality rates in the United States, 2023. *NCHS Health E-Stats*. 2025. https://doi.org/10.15620/cdc/174577
3. Centers for Disease Control and Prevention. Maternal mortality. Available at: https://www.cdc.gov/womens-health/features/maternal-mortality.html. Accessed May 5, 2025.
4. Munira Z, Gunja M, Tikkanen R, Seervai S, Collins SR. Insights into the US maternal mortality crisis: an international comparison. Commonwealth Fund. June 2024. https://doi.org/10.26099/cthn-st75
5. Tikkanen R, Gunja MZ, FitzGerald M, Zephyrin L. Maternal mortality and maternity care in the United States compared to 10 other developed countries. Commonwealth Fund. November 2020. https://doi.org/10.26099/411v-9255
6. Kaiser Family Foundation. Medicaid postpartum coverage extension tracker. January 17, 2025. Available at: https://www.kff.org/medicaid/issue-brief/medicaid-postpartum-coverage-extension-tracker/#note-0-44. Accessed May 5, 2025.
7. Tanne JH. Nearly six million women in the US live in maternity care deserts. *BMJ*. 2023;382:1919. https://doi.org/10.1136/bmj.p1919
8. Kozhimannil KB, Interrante JD, Carroll C, et al. Obstetric care access at rural and urban hospitals in the United States. *JAMA*. 2025;333(2):166–169. https://doi.org/10.1001/jama.2024.23010
9. Adler A, Biggs MA, Kaller S, Schroeder R, Ralph L. Changes in the frequency and type of barriers to reproductive health care between 2017 and 2021. *JAMA Netw Open*. 2023;6(4):e237461. https://doi.org/10.1001/jamanetworkopen.2023.7461
10. Center for Reproductive Rights. Systemic racism and reproductive injustice in the United States: a report for the UN Committee on the Elimination of Racial Discrimination. 2022. Available at: https://reproductiverights.org/wp-content/uploads/2022/08/2022-CERD-Report_Systemic-Racism-and-Reproductive-Injustice.pdf. Accessed May 3, 2025.
11. Kozhimannil K, Hung P, Henning-Smith C, Casey MM, Prasad S. Association between loss of hospital-based obstetric services and birth outcomes in rural counties in the United States. *JAMA*. 2018;319(12):1239–1247. https://doi.org/10.1001/jama.2018.1830
12. Guttmacher Institute. Interactive map: US abortion policies and access after Roe. 2025. Available at: https://states.guttmacher.org/policies/?gad_source=1&gad_campaignid=22269387563&gbraid=0AAAAAD-Q3trrh_IhfFPMX0kwLZHYVq5Je. Accessed May 3, 2025.
13. MSI Reproductive Choices. The impact of the Global Gag Rule on reproductive health services worldwide. January 2021. Available at: https://www.msichoices.org. Accessed May 5, 2025.
14. Becker's Hospital Review. The states where physicians can be sentenced to prison for abortions. 2025. Available at: https://www.beckershospitalreview.com/legal-regulatory-issues/the-states-where-physicians-can-be-sentenced-to-prison-for-abortions. Accessed May 5, 2025.
15. Orgera K, Grover A. States with abortion bans see continued decrease in US MD senior residency applicants. Association of American Medical Colleges. 2024. https://doi.org/10.15766/rai_dnhob2ma
16. American Association of Medical Colleges. Emergency doctors grapple with abortion bans. 2024. Available at: https://www.aamc.org/news/emergency-doctors-grapple-abortion-bans. Accessed May 3, 2025.
17. Hill L, Rao A, Artiga S, Ranji U. Racial disparities in maternal and infant health: the current status and efforts to address them. Kaiser Family Foundation. 2024. Available at: https://www.kff.org/racial-equity-and-health-policy/issue-brief/racial-disparities-in-maternal-and-infant-health-current-status-and-efforts-to-address-them. Accessed May 3, 2025.
18. Rowley DL, Anyanwu K, Crosby A, Phillips KS, Hutchins S. Pregnancy-related mortality disparities during the COVID-19 pandemic. *Am J Public Health*. 2024;114(S9):S723–S730. https://doi.org/10.2105/AJPH.2024.307814
19. Sutton MY, Anachebe NF, Lee R, Skanes H. Racial and ethnic disparities in reproductive health services and outcomes. *Obstet Gynecol*. 2021;137(2):225–233. https://doi.org/10.1097/AOG.0000000000004224
20. López JD, Sriprasert I, Wilson ML. Inequities and disparities in reproductive health: reproductive epidemiology. *Front Reprod Health*. 2024;6:1419178. https://doi.org/10.3389/frph.2024.1419178
21. Guttmacher Institute. Any restrictions on reproductive health care harm reproductive autonomy: evidence from four states. 2023. Available at: https://www.guttmacher.org/report/any-restrictions-reproductive-health-care-harm-reproductive-autonomy-evidence-four-states. Accessed May 3, 2025.
22. Njoku A, Evans M, Nimo-Sefah L, Bailey J. Listen to the whispers before they become screams: addressing black maternal morbidity and mortality in the United States. *Healthcare (Basel)*. 2023;11(3):438. https://doi.org/10.3390/healthcare11030438
23. Johnson R, Eldridge GN, Khanal P, Zephyrin LC. State policy trends to improve perinatal health outcomes. To the Point [blog], Commonwealth Fund. November 20, 2023. Available at: https://doi.org/10.26099/2w1h-h609. Accessed May 3, 2025.
24. Handler A, Johnson K, Rankin K, Velonis A, James A, Kotelchuck M. Shuttering the Pregnancy Risk Assessment Monitoring System (PRAMS): a dangerous attack on US mothers and infants. *Am J Public Health*. 2025;115(6):848–850. https://doi.org/10.2105/AJPH.2025.308107
25. Planet Detroit. Maternal health "momnibus" bills pass Michigan Senate. October 22, 2024. Available at: https://planetdetroit.org/2024/10/michigan-senate-committee-maternal-health-reform. Accessed May 3, 2025.

Public Health Education and Training in Sex, Gender, and Transgender Health: A Course to Advance Health at a US School of Public Health

Sari L. Reisner, ScD, MA, and Kieren P. Todd, PhD, MPH

We describe the development and evaluation of "Women, Gender, and Health 230: The Health of Transgender and Gender Diverse People," a course at Harvard T. H. Chan School of Public Health that aims to equip future leaders in public health with conceptual frameworks and research methods to address sex- and gender-based population health inequities. We explain the pedagogy, course rationale, design, and implementation of the course for faculty, designers of educational curricula, and public health institutions to integrate transgender, nonbinary, and gender diverse population health. (*Am J Public Health*. 2025;115(10):1579–1583. https://doi.org/10.2105/AJPH.2025.308222)

AJPH October 2025, Vol. 115, No. 10

"Women, Gender, and Health 230: The Health of Transgender and Gender Diverse People" (WGH 230) was developed to address the gap in curricula on sex and gender health in schools and programs of public health. We explain the pedagogy, rationale, design, and implementation of the course.

INTERVENTION AND IMPLEMENTATION

Our goal was for the course to serve as a way for faculty, educational curricula designers, and public health institutions to integrate transgender, nonbinary, and gender diverse (TGD) population health into their offerings while simultaneously helping students to enhance skills and competencies necessary to address sex- and gender-based health inequities.

For course objectives, we wanted students to be able to (1) describe terminology, history, and inequities pertaining to TGD populations and health; (2) identify and critically discuss concepts, theories, and frameworks guiding a multidisciplinary understanding of TGD public health; (3) identify best practices, gaps, and opportunities in research methodologies for TGD health, including study design, sampling, community engagement, and measurement of gender identity and sex; and (4) critically evaluate interventions that address TGD population health in different countries and contexts.

The goal of WGH 230 was to introduce students to TGD population health, an emerging multidisciplinary field focused on the health of TGD people (see Figure 1 for logic model).[1] The course draws from three primary sensitizing frameworks: health equity,[2] gender analysis,[3] and intersectionality.[4] Students acquired foundational knowledge to understand TGD population health, including terminology, history of TGD health and medicine, composition and experiences of TGD communities, and current controversies and scientific debates. Students in WGH 230 also learned the theories and frameworks that explain morbidity and mortality in TGD physical and mental health and the determinants of TGD health inequities. This included an emphasis on how intersectional stigma and oppression, such as cissexism and racism, contribute to adverse health outcomes. In addition, students learned best practices in research methodologies, such as measurement of gender identity and community-engaged research methods. Students discussed issues on health care access for TGD people and learned about models of TGD care,

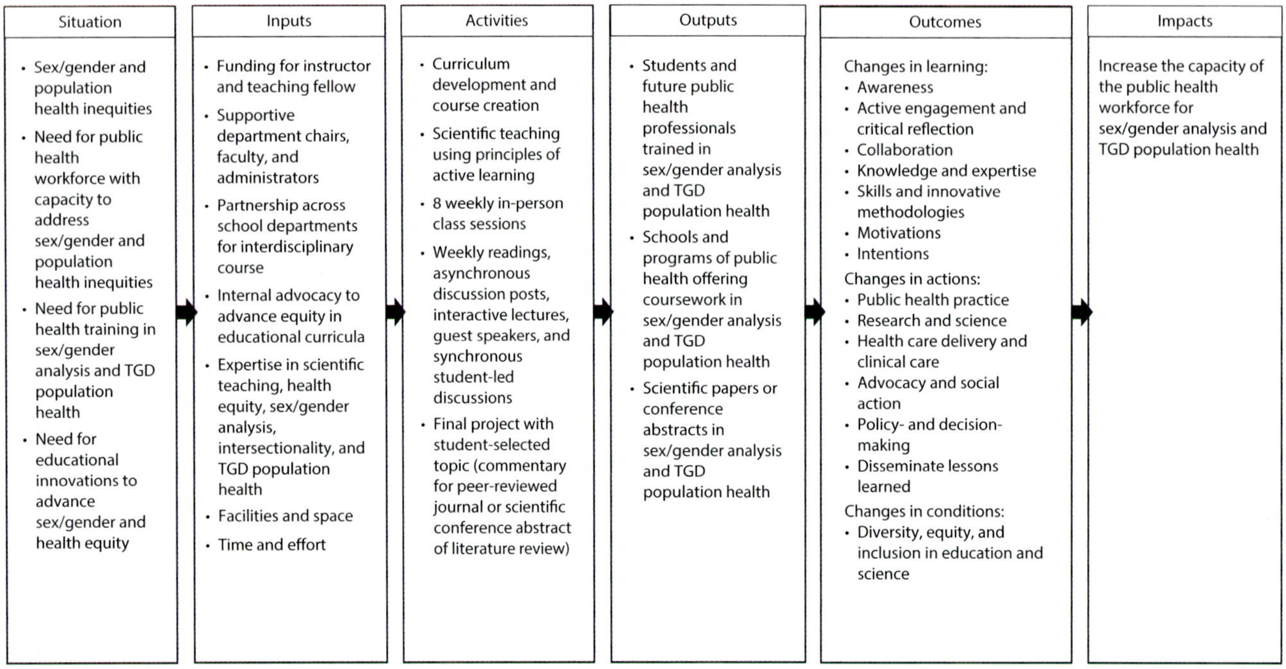

FIGURE 1— Logic Model for "Women, Gender, and Health 230: The Health of Transgender and Gender Diverse People"

Note. TGD = transgender, nonbinary, and gender diverse. The course, developed by a student group and instructors in the Women, Gender, and Health Interdepartmental Concentration based in the Department of Epidemiology at the Harvard T. H. Chan School of Public Health (Boston, Massachusetts), was first offered in 2022.

evidence-based health interventions, and considerations for policy, advocacy, and human rights. The course provided readings and discussions on multiple aspects that influence the lives, health, and well-being of TGD populations (e.g., sociocultural, structural, political, legal). We aimed for the course to take an intersectional approach, highlighting that gender modality is but one dimension of social position and underscoring the importance of considering how multiple intersecting forms of power and privilege fuel health inequities along race, ethnicity, classism, ableism, and other forms of oppression.

PLACE, TIME, AND PERSONS

WGH 230 has been offered as part of the Women, Gender, and Health Interdepartmental Concentration based in the Department of Epidemiology at the Harvard T. H. Chan School of Public Health in Boston, Massachusetts, in academic years 2022 and 2023, and had 16 and 17 students, respectively. WGH 230 is a graduate-level elective course consisting of three-hour sessions with 15-minute breaks during an eight-week period (Box 1).

To develop the course, the instructor held a semester-long independent study in 2020, working with six students. Students mapped TGD health courses and content offered by accredited US schools and programs of public health. Students systematically searched the most recent course catalogs. Where no information was available, students e-mailed school administrators, registrars, or professors directly with relevant research interests using a standardized e-mail template. Of the 67 Council on Education for Public Health–accredited schools and programs at that time,[5] information from 50 schools and programs was collected (74.6% response rate). Among the 50 schools and programs, four (8.0%) had a course solely dedicated to TGD health, and two reported having TGD health courses under development. Students met weekly to reflect on and discuss the process and findings. This activity helped students to gain research experience and demonstrated the gap that the current course would fill at Harvard and in public health education more broadly.

PURPOSE

WGH 230 emerged from multiple student requests for more curricular

BOX 1— Weekly Content, Final Project Type, and Examples of Student-Selected Projects for "Women, Gender, and Health 230: The Health of Transgender and Gender Diverse People"

Week and Session Title or Final Project Type	Session Content or Student Example
Session title	
Week 1: Transgender public health, gender affirmation, terminology, and lived experiences	Content • Overview of terminology related to sex and gender • Exploration of transgender social and health inequities • Opportunities for transgender health • Mini-lecture: discussion group facilitation skills
Week 2: Key concepts, theories, and frameworks	Content • Defining theory, theory types, and conceptual frameworks • Importance of theories, frameworks, and models and selection thereof • Case study: masculine identity development for transmasculine individuals
Week 3: Intersectionality, identity, and fluidity	Content • Origins of Black feminism and intersectionality theories • Methodological challenges of empirical intersectionality research • Case study: participatory action research in Ecuador
Week 4: Methodologies for health research with TGD populations	Content • Data needs and research priorities • Measures, sampling, and study designs
Week 5: Physical health research and interventions	Content • National LGBTQIA+ Education Health Center lectures and videos
Week 6: Mental health research, interventions, and systems	Content • Mental health burden in TGD populations • Conceptual models and applications • Interventions and participatory population perspective for transgender health equity
Week 7: Health care systems, delivery, services, and utilization; policy, law, and advocacy	Content • Development of patient-reported outcome measures in gender-affirming surgeries • Anti- and protective legislation for TGD health in the United States • Geographic implications for health equity
Week 8: Intersex populations	Content • Intersex advocacy • Intersex terminology and concepts • Intersex young people
Final project type	
Option 1: commentary formatted for submission to the peer-reviewed journal *Transgender Health*	Student example • Gaps in measures of structural cisgenderism and recommendations for future measurement and research • Criminal justice data sources and ways to increase reporting of violent crimes by sex and gender and for transgender and nonbinary people • Stigma reduction for TGD patients having a gender dysphoria diagnosis in their medical record by using Z codes for billing in the *Diagnostic and Statistical Manual of Mental Disorders* rather than a diagnosis of gender dysphoria • Inequitable Medicaid block grant structures in Puerto Rico that affect low-income TGD residents
Option 2: Literature review with abstract and poster for submission to the American Public Health Association annual meeting	Student example • Scoping review of studies on the intersection of neurodiversity and gender diversity • Systematic review of studies on food insecurity in TGD populations • Narrative review of interventional research on suicidality and mental health • Scoping review of genetic counseling in TGD people

Note. LGBTQIA+ = lesbian, gay, bisexual, transgender, queer/questioning, intersex, asexual+; TGD = transgender, nonbinary, and gender diverse. The course, developed by a student group and instructors in the Women, Gender, and Health Interdepartmental Concentration based in the Department of Epidemiology at the Harvard T. H. Chan School of Public Health (Boston, Massachusetts), was first offered in 2022.

content and training in sex- and gender-based research methods and TGD health research. Sex, gender, and their intersection shape the distribution, causes, and conditions that produce and sustain population health inequities.[1] Historically, sex and gender have been conflated in public health; however, they are distinct constructs.[1,3,6,7] Sex refers to biology, including chromosomes, reproductive anatomy, and hormones; gender describes the sociocultural dimensions mapped onto biology and includes gender identity, expression, and roles.[8]

Although sex and gender have been traditionally conceptualized as binary, both are increasingly understood to be on a continuum.[8]

The practice of treating sex and gender as interchangeable and binary has obfuscated research in the population health of individuals who are transgender, nonbinary, or hold other diverse gender identities that do not correspond to the sex assigned to them at birth.[1] During the past decade, public health and epidemiology have documented a range of physical, mental, and social health inequities by gender modality—with TGD populations disproportionately affected compared with cisgender populations.[1,9] TGD health research also provides a springboard for analyses of ways that interlocking systems of oppression—such as cissexism, racism, and classism—drive poor health outcomes among people who are at the intersection of multiple marginalized social locations (e.g., for people who are transgender, Latine, and living in poverty).[10]

EVALUATION AND ADVERSE EFFECTS

The average course ratings were 4.9 and 5.0 (of 5.0), respectively. Students were enthusiastic about the course and appreciated the emphasis on applications beyond TGD health. On formal evaluations, students noted the following: (1) student-led discussions allowed for effective peer learning environments to share experiences and learn from each other, (2) lectures were interactive and accessible to students, and (3) students felt empowered to consider their own experiences with research and programming to better center experiences on TGD population health. Because the course was an elective, students self-selected to enroll in WGH 230 and may have been more comfortable with or interested in the topic area than those who did not enroll.

One challenge is that the course draws master's and doctoral students with varying levels of exposure to TGD health. The master's and doctoral students are from diverse backgrounds, including clinicians-in-training, researchers, practitioners, and policymakers. Finding the "sweet spot," where students are challenged no matter what their familiarity was with TGD population health, was leveraged by the teaching team through creation of colearning opportunities such as cofacilitating group discussions.

New opportunities to engage on TGD population health topics and with sex and gender research were facilitated through the students' final projects. The flexibility for students to choose their topic and format opened new areas for exploration based on their interests (Box 1); students submitted projects to peer-reviewed journals or to scientific meetings or used projects to inform their dissertation prospectus or for community advocacy efforts.

The evaluation highlights the potential of this course to enhance training in sex and gender research methods within public health schools and programs. As the course is offered to graduate students at Harvard, we suggest it be replicated in other institutions. Comparing course evaluations across institutions could help gather valuable insights for public health education.

SUSTAINABILITY

The small class size allowed students to become familiar with others in the class, build trust, and test new ideas in a safe and respectful space; small class size enhanced collaborative learning opportunities and ensured accountability across sensitive topics. Group presentations and conversations facilitated peer learning, including allowing students to critically think about their roles and responsibilities as future public health researchers and practitioners pertaining to sex and gender. The focus on applied learning, by engaging students in TGD population health challenges, was intentionally designed so that students would grapple with core issues in which no simple answer in public health yet exists. The success of the course and positive student feedback have resulted in an institutional commitment to offer the course annually. The course has continued amid multiple changes, including the founding instructor moving institutions in January 2024 and the US Presidential Executive Order targeting "gender ideology" in January 2025.

PUBLIC HEALTH SIGNIFICANCE

Sex and gender are determinants of population health,[1,3] and global calls have been made to address sex and gender in public health, including policies by funders that require reporting on sex and gender to ensure scientific rigor and reproducibility.[11–14] Formal integration of sex- and gender-based medicine into medical and allied health professional education has also been proposed.[15] However, a need continues for public health training in sex and gender research methods, gender analysis, and TGD population health. Having this training requires innovations in public health education, such as WGH 230. Furthermore, given the intersectional nature of health inequities along other axes besides sex and gender (e.g., race, ethnicity, socioeconomic status, sexual orientation, immigration),[1,9] students need to be sensitized to the issues, concerns, and needs of specific populations and where these needs intersect. Key to achieving health equity is educating and equipping future public health leaders with the skills and competencies to advance the science and praxis of using an intersectional lens for sex and gender analysis. AJPH

ABOUT THE AUTHORS

Sari L. Reisner is affiliated with the Department of Epidemiology, University of Michigan School of Public Health, Ann Arbor, MI, and Department of Epidemiology, Harvard T. H. Chan School of Public Health, Boston, MA. Kieran P. Todd is affiliated with the Department of Social and Behavioral Sciences, Harvard T. H. Chan School of Public Health.

CORRESPONDENCE

Correspondence should be sent to Sari L. Reisner, ScD, MA, 1415 Washington Heights, SPH-2649A, Ann Arbor, MI 48109 (e-mail: sreisner@umich.edu). Reprints can be ordered at https://ajph.org by clicking the "Reprints" link.

PUBLICATION INFORMATION

Full Citation: Reisner SL, Todd KP. Public health education and training in sex, gender, and transgender health: a course to advance health at a US school of public health. *Am J Public Health.* 2025;115(10):1579–1583.

Acceptance Date: June 16, 2025.

DOI: https://doi.org/10.2105/AJPH.2025.308222

ORCID iD:
Sari L. Reisner https://orcid.org/0000-0001-7868-4746

CONTRIBUTORS

S. L. Reisner conceptualized, drafted, and revised the article. K. P. Todd critically reviewed and edited the article. Both authors take full responsibility for the content.

ACKNOWLEDGMENTS

The authors acknowledge the graduate students and trainees in the 2020 independent study course at Harvard T. H. Chan School of Public Health for their assistance in developing the course through researching course offerings at accredited schools and programs of public health. We thank Nancy Krieger, PhD, professor of social epidemiology, American Cancer Society clinical research professor, Department of Social and Behavioral Sciences, and chair of the Women, Gender, and Health Concentration at Harvard T. H. Chan School of Public Health, for advocating and supporting the development of this course and for comments to and review of the syllabus. We also thank the Women, Gender, and Health faculty and working group for their review of the course syllabus.

CONFLICTS OF INTEREST

The authors report no conflicts of interest.

HUMAN PARTICIPANT PROTECTION

This article reports on a course evaluation and does not involve human participants.

REFERENCES

1. Reisner SL, Poteat T, Keatley J, et al. Global health burden and needs of transgender populations: a review. *Lancet.* 2016;388(10042):412–436. https://doi.org/10.1016/S0140-6736(16)00684-X
2. Peterson A, Charles V, Yeung D, Coyle K. The Health Equity Framework: a science- and justice-based model for public health researchers and practitioners. *Health Promot Pract.* 2021;22(6):741–746. https://doi.org/10.1177/1524839920950730
3. Krieger N. Genders, sexes, and health: what are the connections—and why does it matter? *Int J Epidemiol.* 2003;32(4):652–657. https://doi.org/10.1093/ije/dyg156
4. Bowleg L. The problem with the phrase women and minorities: intersectionality—an important theoretical framework for public health. *Am J Public Health.* 2012;102(7):1267–1273. https://doi.org/10.2105/AJPH.2012.300750
5. Council on Education for Public Health. List of accredited schools and programs. Available at: https://ceph.org/about/org-info/who-we-accredit/accredited/#programs. Accessed May 10, 2024.
6. Clayton JA, Tannenbaum C. Reporting sex, gender, or both in clinical research? *JAMA.* 2016;316(18):1863–1864. https://doi.org/10.1001/jama.2016.16405
7. Rich-Edwards JW, Kaiser UB, Chen GL, Manson JE, Goldstein JM. Sex and gender differences research design for basic, clinical, and population studies: essentials for investigators. *Endocr Rev.* 2018;39(4):424–439. https://doi.org/10.1210/er.2017-00246
8. Bauer GR. Sex and gender multidimensionality in epidemiologic research. *Am J Epidemiol.* 2023;192(1):122–132. https://doi.org/10.1093/aje/kwac173
9. Scheim AI, Rich AJ, Zubizarreta D, et al. Health status of transgender people globally: a systematic review of research on disease burden and correlates. *PLoS One.* 2024;19(3):e0299373. https://doi.org/10.1371/journal.pone.0299373
10. Restar AJ, Sherwood J, Edeza A, Collins C, Operario D. Expanding gender-based health equity framework for transgender populations. *Transgend Health.* 2021;6(1):1–4. https://doi.org/10.1089/trgh.2020.0026
11. Arnegard ME, Whitten LA, Hunter C, Clayton JA. Sex as a biological variable: a 5-year progress report and call to action. *J Womens Health (Larchmt).* 2020;29(6):858–864. https://doi.org/10.1089/jwh.2019.8247
12. Heidari S, Babor TF, De Castro P, Tort S, Curno M. Sex and gender equity in research: rationale for the SAGER guidelines and recommended use. *Res Integr Peer Rev.* 2016;1:2. https://doi.org/10.1186/s41073-016-0007-6
13. Hunt L, Nielsen MW, Schiebinger L. A framework for sex, gender, and diversity analysis in research. *Science.* 2022;377(6614):1492–1495. https://doi.org/10.1126/science.abp9775
14. White J, Tannenbaum C, Klinge I, Schiebinger L, Clayton J. The integration of sex and gender considerations into biomedical research: lessons from international funding agencies. *J Clin Endocrinol Metab.* 2021;106(10):3034–3048. https://doi.org/10.1210/clinem/dgab434
15. Khamisy-Farah R, Bragazzi NL. How to integrate sex and gender medicine into medical and allied health profession undergraduate, graduate, and post-graduate education: insights from a rapid systematic literature review and a thematic meta-synthesis. *J Pers Med.* 2022;12(4):612. https://doi.org/10.3390/jpm12040612

Implementation of Doxy-PEP in a Diverse Sexual Health Program in Northern Manhattan: The Doxy-Care Study

Simian Huang, MPH, Caroline Carnevale, DNP, MPH, Natalie Neu, MD, MPH, Joshua Klein, BS, Daniela Quigee, MPH, Edward Perez, FNP-C, Lauren Burrell, FNP-C, Kathrine Meyers, DrPH, MSc, MPP, Jacob McLean, MD, Magdalena E. Sobieszczyk, MD, MPH, Delivette Castor, PhD, and Jason Zucker, MD

This prospective cohort study evaluated the real-world effectiveness of doxycycline postexposure prophylaxis use in reducing bacterial sexually transmitted infections (STIs) within a diverse urban sexual health program. Propensity-matched analyses showed significant STI reductions, particularly in rectal *Chlamydia trachomatis* infections, among early adopters. Uptake was disproportionately higher in non-Hispanic White individuals and those more engaged in care. Findings emphasize the need for targeted outreach to improve care engagement and equitable access to this STI prevention strategy. (*Am J Public Health*. 2025;115(10):1584–1588. https://doi.org/10.2105/AJPH.2025.308209)

AJPH October 2025, Vol. 115, No. 10

One promising strategy to reduce the burden of bacterial sexually transmitted infections (STIs) is doxycycline postexposure prophylaxis (doxy-PEP).

INTERVENTION AND IMPLEMENTATION

Doxy-PEP involves taking a 200-milligram dose of doxycycline within 72 hours after sexual activity to reduce the risk of acquiring bacterial STIs such as syphilis, chlamydia, or gonorrhea.[1] The Centers for Disease Control and Prevention (CDC) recommends that providers discuss doxy-PEP with gay, bisexual, and other men who have sex with men (gbMSM), as well as transgender women who have been diagnosed with a bacterial STI in the past 12 months.[1] The adoption of new sexual health preventive measures is influenced by both patient and provider factors, which can lead to disparities even among clients within the same practice.[2,3] Similar to HIV preexposure prophylaxis (PrEP), doxy-PEP uptake may be inequitable, delaying access for those most vulnerable, such as Black and Latinx/Hispanic gbMSM.[4]

PLACE, TIME, AND PERSONS

The study was conducted at the Comprehensive Health Program (CHP), which provides status-neutral care within the New York–Presbyterian Hospital Columbia University Irving Medical Center (NYP/CUIMC). The CHP, located in Northern Manhattan, serves racial and ethnically diverse communities with high STI rates, including Washington Heights, Harlem, and the South Bronx. This longitudinal observational study using real-world data included patients who received care at CHP sites between April 26, 2023, and February 26, 2024.

Formal doxy-PEP guidance from the New York State AIDS Institute was first released on September 25, 2023; before the release of guidelines, prescriptions were primarily made on the basis of patient requests.[5] Between July and December 2023, an average of 12 patients initiated doxy-PEP per month. This number tripled to 46 per month between January and June 2024 (Figure A, available as a supplement to the online version of this article at https://ajph.org). To estimate real-world doxy-PEP effectiveness, we assembled an Early Adopter of Doxy-PEP (EADP) cohort and, using electronic health records, selected non-EADP comparators through propensity-score matching.

The EADP cohort in this analysis consisted of the first 100 individuals who initiated doxy-PEP at the CHP. EADP participants were aged 18 years or older, assigned male sex at birth, identified as either a gbMSM or a transgender woman who had sex with men and had not received doxycycline in the 14 days before inclusion.

The non-EADP cohort consisted of patients who sought care at the CHP during the same observation period but had not initiated doxy-PEP. These participants had been screened for or diagnosed with gonorrhea, chlamydia, or early syphilis in the previous 12 months. We developed a propensity score of doxy-PEP exposure using the following variables: (1) initiation time of doxy-PEP (exposure assignment), (2) five-year age band, (3) racial/ethnic identity, (4) duration of observation before, and (5) duration of observation after the date of matching to the doxy-PEP start date.[6]

PURPOSE

Randomized trials of doxy-PEP in gbMSM and transgender women demonstrated significant reductions in chlamydia and syphilis, contributing to early adoption in the sexual health community, even before national guidelines were released in June 2024.[7–11] Early real-world data on doxy-PEP have shown promise, but comprehensive assessments across diverse, often marginalized populations with limited health care access remain lacking.[8,12,13] To address these gaps, our study aimed to characterize early adopters of doxy-PEP, describe factors related to inequitable access, and evaluate its impact on STI rates among early adopters compared with propensity-matched comparators (unexposed).

EVALUATION AND ADVERSE EFFECTS

In this prospective cohort study of early adopters, individuals receiving doxy-PEP showed significant reductions in overall STI and chlamydia incidence and modest reductions in gonorrhea at specific anatomical sites. When compared with the non-EADP propensity score–matched cohort, prescribing doxy-PEP did not reach statistical significance in reducing overall STI or gonorrhea incidence but was effective in reducing rectal chlamydia incidence. Non-Hispanic White individuals and those more engaged in care were more likely to use doxy-PEP than their propensity score–matched comparators. During the study period, overall STI incidence in the comparator group remained stable, but chlamydia incidence decreased, further highlighting the effectiveness of doxy-PEP in this subgroup.

Early Adopters

The 100-person EADP cohort had a median age of 36 years (interquartile range [IQR] = 32.0–39.2). The cohort was predominantly composed of minoritized individuals; 41% self-identified as Hispanic, 12% as Black/African American, and 30% as White. Approximately 21% of participants were uninsured, and 49% had Medicaid. People with HIV comprised 12% of the sample, and all were on antiretroviral therapy. Among participants without HIV, all were on PrEP, with 97% using daily oral PrEP (Table A, available as a supplement to the online version of this article at https://ajph.org).

Matched Cohort of Non–Early Adopters

Propensity matching yielded 355 comparators in the non-EADP cohort, resulting in 97 matched EADP participants at a 3.7:1 ratio. The median age was similar between the non-EADP and EADP cohorts (35 years; IQR = 31–39). The cohorts were also well-matched on exposure assignment time, with a median difference of 7 days (IQR = 3–9) between the doxy-PEP start date and matched visit date. However, racial/ethnic composition differed significantly ($P = .012$), with a higher proportion of non-Hispanic White participants in the EADP cohort (31% vs 18%) and a lower proportion of unknown race/ethnicity (4.1% vs 12%). Despite these differences, the non-EADP matched set still included 60% minoritized individuals, with 46% identifying as Hispanic and 14% as Black. EADP participants also had a higher median number of visits before initiating doxy-PEP (3 vs 2; $P < .001$) and a statistically significant difference in postinitiation visits despite the same median value ($P = .043$; Table B, available as a supplement to the online version of this article at https://ajph.org).

Comparison of Demographic Characteristics

The median age in the nonuser cohort was 33 years (IQR = 28–39), compared with 36 years (IQR = 32–39) in the doxy-PEP cohort ($P = .008$; Table D, available as a supplement to the online version of this article at https://ajph.org). A higher proportion of the nonuser cohort was younger than

AJPH October 2025, Vol. 115, No. 10

25 years (16.5% vs 1.0%), while fewer were aged 36 to 40 years (16% vs 32%). A smaller proportion identified as White (17% vs 30%; *P* = .001), while a higher percentage identified as Hispanic (48% vs 41%) or Black/African American (19% vs 12%; Table D, available as a supplement to the online version of this article at https://ajph.org).

Early Adopters Effectiveness (Within-Person)

The positivity rate for any new STI decreased from 14% (96 cases) in the 9 months before doxy-PEP prescription to 7.9% (34 cases) in the 9 months after (incidence rate ratio [IRR] = 0.56; 95% confidence interval [CI] = 0.37, 0.81; Table 1). The most notable decrease was observed for chlamydia positivity at any anatomical site, which decreased from 12% (40 cases) to 2.8% (6 cases; IRR = 0.24; 95% CI = 0.09, 0.51). Rectal chlamydia decreased from 10% (33 cases) to 2.5% (5 cases; IRR = 0.24; 95% CI = 0.08, 0.55), and pharyngeal chlamydia decreased from 1.2% (4 cases) before doxy-PEP to 0% after initiation. Gonorrhea positivity did not show a meaningful decrease at any anatomical site. In the unmatched (unexposed) sample, gonorrhea and chlamydia trends varied by bacterial agent and clinical site (Figure 1).

Primary Outcome, Effectiveness

Reduction in overall STI incidence in the EADP cohort compared with the non-EADP cohort (IRR = 0.69; 95% CI = 0.41, 1.15) did not reach statistical significance. Gonorrhea incidence did not decrease overall (IRR = 0.95; 95% CI = 0.49, 1.82) or at specific anatomical sites (rectal and pharyngeal). Conversely, overall chlamydia incidence rates decreased significantly (IRR = 0.30; 95% CI = 0.10, 0.75), as did rectal chlamydia rates (IRR = 0.23; 95% CI = 0.07, 0.63; Table 1).

SUSTAINABILITY

In this diverse urban care setting, we applied rigorous methodology to improve causal inference using readily available, lower-cost data sources and demonstrated doxy-PEP effectiveness for overall STIs and chlamydia in real-world settings. The findings align with observations from clinical trials and the few real-world studies conducted to date.[7–11] The rapid uptake of doxy-PEP in this study highlights its acceptability among populations at risk for STIs and mirrors trends observed in other health care settings.[12] This underscores doxy-PEP's potential as a preventive intervention for individuals at risk for bacterial STIs. Implementation studies in rural and other geographically distinct settings with different health care access and utilization patterns are needed. Equitable implementation, including universal education and targeted outreach, is essential for maximizing doxy-PEP's public health impact.

TABLE 1— Reduction in Bacterial Sexually Transmitted Infections (STIs) in the 9 Months Before the Intervention and 9 Months After the Intervention: Northern Manhattan, NY, 2022–2024

	Early Adopters of Doxy-PEP Cohort (n = 100)			Early Doxy-PEP Adopters (n = 97) vs Comparator (n = 355)[a]	
STI	Positivity Before Doxy-PEP, No. (%)	Positivity After Doxy-PEP, No. (%)	RR (95% CI)	Unadjusted RR (95% CI)	Adjusted RR (95% CI)
All STIs	96 (14.2)	34 (7.9)	0.56 (0.37, 0.81)	0.66 (0.40, 1.09)	0.69 (0.41, 1.15)
Gonorrhea overall	56 (16.6)	28 (13.0)	0.78 (0.49, 1.22)	0.88 (0.46, 1.69)	0.95 (0.49, 1.82)
Chlamydia overall	40 (11.9)	6 (2.8)	0.24 (0.09, 0.51)	0.30 (0.10, 0.74)	0.30 (0.10, 0.75)
Gonorrhea site					
Urine	14 (4.2)	4 (1.9)	0.45 (0.13, 1.25)	0.62 (0.12, 3.06)	0.64 (0.12, 3.20)
Rectal	41 (13.0)	19 (9.4)	0.72 (0.41, 1.22)	0.84 (0.38, 1.86)	0.89 (0.39, 1.98)
Pharyngeal	25 (7.6)	14 (6.7)	0.87 (0.44, 1.65)	0.85 (0.32, 2.16)	0.91 (0.34, 2.34)
Chlamydia site					
Urine	7 (2.1)	1 (0.5)	0.23 (0.01, 1.26)	0.72 (0.03, 6.17)	0.79 (0.04, 6.80)
Rectal	33 (10.4)	5 (2.5)	0.24 (0.08, 0.55)	0.23 (0.07, 0.62)	0.23 (0.07, 0.63)
Pharyngeal	4 (1.2)	0 (0.0)	NA	NA	NA

Note. CI = confidence interval; doxy-PEP = doxycycline postexposure prophylaxis; NA = not applicable; RR = cumulative risk ratio.
[a]Early doxy-PEP users were propensity score–matched 1:4 to comparators (unexposed).

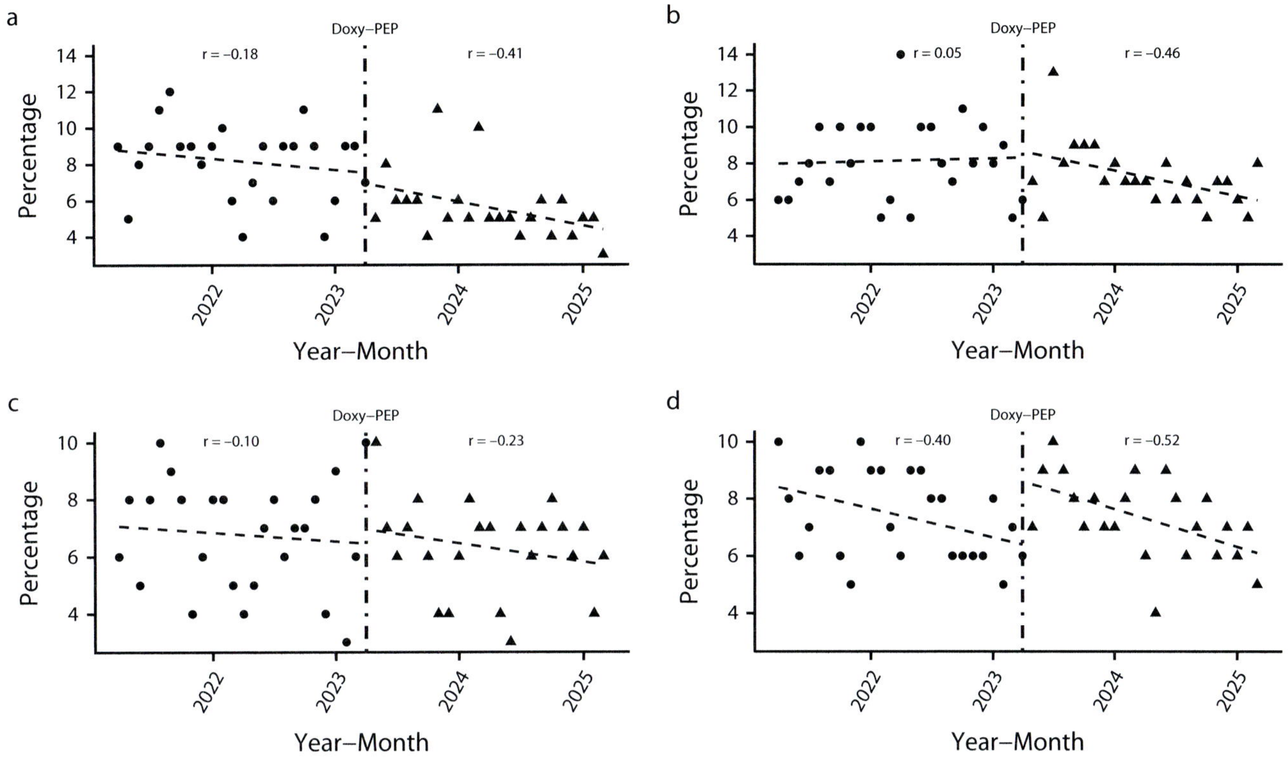

FIGURE 1— **Prevalence Before and After the Implementation of Doxycycline Postexposure Prophylaxis (Doxy-PEP) of (a) Chlamydia Positivity at the Comprehensive Health Program Sexual Health Clinic, (b) Gonorrhea Positivity at the Comprehensive Health Program Sexual Health Clinic, (c) Chlamydia Positivity at the HIV Program, and (d) Gonorrhea Positivity at the HIV Program: Northern Manhattan, NY, 2022–2024**

PUBLIC HEALTH SIGNIFICANCE

This study underscores the critical role of STI prevention strategies in public health. The real-world effectiveness of doxy-PEP in reducing STIs was more pronounced for chlamydia than for gonorrhea. The concordance of these findings with clinical trials and other real-world effectiveness studies reinforces the inclusion of doxy-PEP in the prevention armamentarium to address the STI epidemic. Doxy-PEP uptake was rapid, yet even in this diverse urban setting, disparities in early adoption favored White individuals with greater health care engagement, mirroring patterns seen with HIV PrEP. Targeted outreach efforts must prioritize populations with the highest STI burden, including younger individuals and racially and ethnically minoritized populations. Comprehensive service models can mitigate inequities in access and uptake, maximizing doxy-PEP's public health benefit.

Equitable implementation strategies—including universal education, provider training, and integration into routine sexual health and primary care—are critical to ensuring broad doxy-PEP uptake and reducing STI incidence. AJPH

ABOUT THE AUTHORS

Simian Huang, Joshua Klein, Daniela Quigee, Kathrine Meyers, Jacob McLean, Magdalena E. Sobieszczyk, Delivette Castor, and Jason Zucker are with the Division of Infectious Diseases, Department of Medicine, Columbia University Vagelos College of Physicians and Surgeons, New York, NY. Natalie Neu is with the Division of Infectious Diseases, Department of Pediatrics, Columbia University Vagelos College of Physicians and Surgeons. Caroline Carnevale, Edward Perez, and Lauren Burrell are with New York–Presbyterian Hospital, New York, NY.

CORRESPONDENCE

Correspondence should be sent to Jason Zucker, 630 W 168th St, Presbyterian Hospital PH-876A, New York, NY 10032 (e-mail: jz2700@cumc.columbia.edu). Reprints can be ordered at https://ajph.org by clicking the "Reprints" link.

PUBLICATION INFORMATION

Full Citation: Huang S, Carnevale C, Neu N, et al. Implementation of doxy-PEP in a diverse sexual health program in Northern Manhattan: the doxy-care study. *Am J Public Health*. 2025; 115(10):1584–1588.

Acceptance Date: May 25, 2025.

DOI: https://doi.org/10.2105/AJPH.2025.308209

ORCID iDs:

Simian Huang https://orcid.org/0000-0001-5536-1231

Caroline Carnevale https://orcid.org/0000-0002-7701-3569

Natalie Neu https://orcid.org/0000-0001-5462-2938

Joshua Klein https://orcid.org/0009-0002-3039-8016

Edward Perez https://orcid.org/0009-0002-3080-7641

Kathrine Meyers https://orcid.org/0000-0002-8573-1958

Jacob McLean https://orcid.org/0000-0002-4961-3487

Delivette Castor https://orcid.org/0000-0002-0988-9489

Jason Zucker https://orcid.org/0000-0001-6987-6412

CONTRIBUTORS

S. Huang, C. Carnevale, N. Neu, and J. Klein contributed equally to this work and are co–first authors. D. Castor and J. Zucker contributed equally to this work and are co–senior authors. S. Huang, C. Carnevale, N. Neu, J. Klein, D. Quigee, K. Meyers, J. McLean, M. E. Sobieszczyk, D. Castor, and J. Zucker made substantial contributions to the conceptualization or design of the work, or the acquisition, analysis, or interpretation of data for the work. All authors were involved in drafting the article or revising it critically for important intellectual content and approved the final version for publication. S. Huang, C. Carnevale, N. Neu, J. Klein, D. Castor, and J. Zucker accept full accountability for all aspects of the work, ensuring accuracy and integrity.

ACKNOWLEDGMENTS

Research reported in this publication was supported by the National Institute of Allergy and Infectious Diseases of the National Institutes of Health under award K23AI150378, R56AI182347.

Note. The content is solely the responsibility of the authors and does not necessarily represent the official views of the National Institutes of Health.

CONFLICTS OF INTEREST

J. Zucker receives salary support from the Centers for Disease Control and Prevention and has received honoraria for sexual health education from academic medical centers, the New York State Clinical Education Initiative, AIDS Education and Training Centers, the International Antiviral Society–USA, the Infectious Diseases Society of America, and the American Medical Association.

HUMAN PARTICIPANT PROTECTION

This study was approved by the Columbia University institutional review board with a waiver of informed consent.

REFERENCES

1. Bachmann LH, Barbee LA, Chan P, et al. CDC clinical guidelines on the use of doxycycline postexposure prophylaxis for bacterial sexually transmitted infection prevention, United States, 2024. *MMWR Recomm Rep.* 2024;73(2):1–8. https://doi.org/10.15585/mmwr.rr7302a1
2. Carter G, Tavares T. PrEP prescription in Indiana 2017–2022: implications for clinical practice. *Res Nurs Health.* 2024;47(1):49–59. https://doi.org/10.1002/nur.22354
3. Pleuhs B, Quinn KG, Walsh JL, Petroll AE, John SA. Health care provider barriers to HIV pre-exposure prophylaxis in the United States: a systematic review. *AIDS Patient Care STDS.* 2020;34(3):111–123. https://doi.org/10.1089/apc.2019.0189
4. Kamitani E, Johnson WD, Wichser ME, Adegbite AH, Mullins MM, Sipe TA. Growth in proportion and disparities of HIV PrEP use among key populations identified in the United States national goals: systematic review and meta-analysis of published surveys. *J Acquir Immune Defic Syndr.* 2020;84(4):379–386. https://doi.org/10.1097/QAI.0000000000002345
5. New York City Department of Health and Mental Hygiene, Bureau of Hepatitis, HIV, and Sexually Transmitted Infections. Sexually transmitted infections surveillance report, 2023. December 2024. Available at: https://www.nyc.gov/assets/doh/downloads/pdf/std/sti-2023-report.pdf. Accessed February 15, 2025.
6. Brookhart MA, Wyss R, Layton JB, Stürmer T. Propensity score methods for confounding control in nonexperimental research. *Circ Cardiovasc Qual Outcomes.* 2013;6(5):604–611. https://doi.org/10.1161/CIRCOUTCOMES.113.000359
7. Chan PA, Malyuta Y, Parent H, et al. Early adopters of doxycycline as post-exposure prophylaxis to prevent bacterial sexually transmitted infections in a real-world clinical setting. *Sex Transm Infect.* 2024;100(6):339–342. https://doi.org/10.1136/sextrans-2024-056152
8. Sankaran M, Glidden DV, Kohn RP, et al. Doxycycline postexposure prophylaxis and sexually transmitted infection trends. *JAMA Intern Med.* 2025;185(3):266–272. https://doi.org/10.1001/jamainternmed.2024.7178
9. Molina J-M, Charreau I, Chidiac C, ANRS IPERGAY Study Group, et al. Post-exposure prophylaxis with doxycycline to prevent sexually transmitted infections in men who have sex with men: an open-label randomised substudy of the ANRS IPERGAY trial. *Lancet Infect Dis.* 2018;18(3):308–317. https://doi.org/10.1016/S1473-3099(17)30725-9
10. Molina JM, Bercot B, Assoumou B, et al. Doxycycline prophylaxis and meningococcal group B vaccine to prevent bacterial sexually transmitted infections in France (ANRS 174 DOXYVAC): a multicentre, open-label, randomised trial with a 2×2 factorial design. *Lancet Infect Dis.* 2024;24(10):1093–1104. https://doi.org/10.1016/S1473-3099(24)00236-6
11. Stewart J, Oware K, Donnell D, et al. Doxycycline prophylaxis to prevent sexually transmitted infections in women. *N Engl J Med.* 2023;389(25):2331–2340. https://doi.org/10.1056/NEJMoa2304007
12. Traeger MW, Leyden WA, Volk JE, et al. Doxycycline postexposure prophylaxis and bacterial sexually transmitted infections among individuals using HIV preexposure prophylaxis. *JAMA Intern Med.* 2025;185(3):273–281. https://doi.org/10.1001/jamainternmed.2024.7186
13. Ogunbajo A, Henry C, Barney A, Anderson T, Brown J, Hickson D. Predictors of receiving a doxycycline postexposure prophylaxis (doxy-PEP) prescription for the prevention of bacterial sexually transmitted infections (STIs) in a community-based clinic: a case-control study. *Sex Transm Infect.* 2025;101(1):68–69. https://doi.org/10.1136/sextrans-2024-056291

Ending the HIV Epidemic: Development and Evaluation of CyberGIS-HIV, a Web-Based Prediction Application

Man-pui Sally Chan, PhD, Bita Fayaz-Farkhad, PhD, Su Yeon Han, PhD, Jinwoo Park, PhD, Shaowen Wang, PhD, and Dolores Albarracin, PhD

Officials from US state and county health departments perceive the need to adopt new methods for making epidemiological decisions about HIV. Hence, a web-based prediction modeling application, CyberGIS-HIV, was developed and systematically compared with currently used approaches (e.g., community consultation) in a sample of 42 state and federal public health officials as well as senior and junior modelers. Overall, CyberGIS-HIV had more favorable public health and modeling ratings than other approaches currently used by the participants. (*Am J Public Health*. 2025;115(10):1589–1593. https://doi.org/10.2105/AJPH.2025.308194)

AJPH October 2025, Vol. 115, No. 10

We developed a web-based Geographic Information System (GIS) application—CyberGIS-HIV—based on Sass and colleagues'[1] two-part model using nine data sources,[2] including the National Center for HIV, Viral Hepatitis, STD, and Tuberculosis Prevention of the Centers for Disease Control and Prevention (CDC). The CyberGIS-HIV application, backed by the CyberGISX platform,[3,4] adopts an open science framework that allows users to download source codes from GitHub.

INTERVENTION AND IMPLEMENTATION

The main features of CyberGIS-HIV include analyzing and visualizing spatiotemporal HIV rates and displaying results based on user-defined scenarios. Users can visually compare the spatial differences by displaying two maps of HIV rates from different years (e.g., 2020 and 2026) for a particular county. For example, two maps can be displayed side by side: the 2020 HIV rates on the left and the 2026 HIV rates on the right (Figure 1). The application also automatically shows line graphs to illustrate temporal changes in HIV rates and each key predictor from 2020 to 2026. In addition, CyberGIS-HIV offers lasso or zoom features that enable users to select one or more counties to visualize spatiotemporal and temporal patterns of HIV rates in those circumscribed areas. Four training videos were created[2]: logging in to CyberGISX, running CyberGIS-HIV, plotting spatial patterns, and exploring temporal patterns.

An HIV prediction application should meet several goals. We defined our goals according to the guidelines of the World Health Organization,[5] national health agencies,[6] and the Johns Hopkins Bloomberg School of Public Health.[7] From a public health perspective, a new HIV prevention method should offer population benefit by providing information that improves prevention planning. It should also support the identification of vulnerable regions and be useful at a large scale (e.g., by all relevant health department personnel). Moreover, models should offer automation and efficiency and be statistically sound, with precise statistical estimates. Thus, we conducted a study in which users evaluated CyberGIS-HIV versus the method they were currently using to forecast HIV patterns and make service provision decisions.

PLACE, TIME, AND PERSONS

The evaluation leveraged a within-participants design to obtain 360-degree feedback on CyberGIS-HIV.[8,9] We preregistered the study at https://osf.io/nr4hw. Participants used their system-generated credentials to log into CyberGIS-HIV and self-paced through the training. Next, they

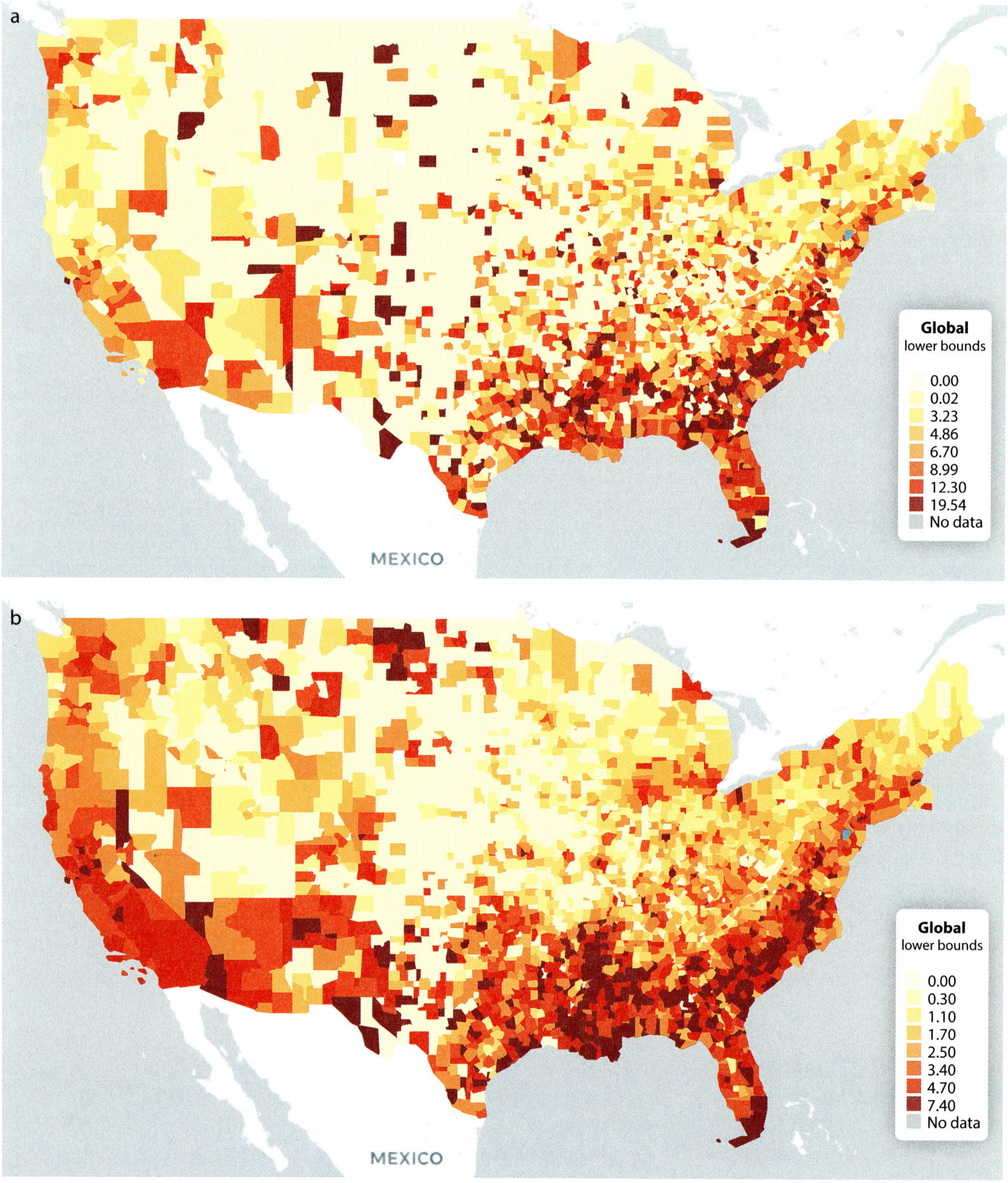

FIGURE 1— HIV Rates Across US Counties: (a) 2020 Actual Data and (b) 2026 Predicted Data

Source. CyberGIS-HIV Web User Interface.
Note. Other plots are provided in Figure B, available as a supplement to the online version of this article at http://www.ajph.org.

completed 12 evaluation items (six for their current approach and six for CyberGIS-HIV) using a 10-point scale and provided open-ended comments about the new method. Each participant received $200 for taking part in the study.

Public health personnel, senior modelers, and junior modelers (i.e., junior researchers with modeling expertise) were recruited at a ratio of 5:1:4. We used a snowball sampling method to recruit health departments and other agencies. We contacted researchers through their online profiles and via coordinators of public health programs (details are provided in the appendix, available as a supplement to the online version of this article at http://www.ajph.org). Forty-two participants completed the study (22 public health personnel, five senior modelers, and 16 junior modelers), constituting an approximately 70% completion rate and a 38% response rate.

We used a weighted-decision matrix with six items rated on a scale from 1 (does not describe the approach) to 10 (truly describes the approach). Three items measured public health goals: (1) population benefit, (2) constituency perspectives, and (3) administrative feasibility. Another three measured modeling goals: (1) automation and efficiency, (2) statistical soundness, and (3) satisfactory level of uncertainty (see the appendix). For each item, respondents were asked about the approach they were currently using and the CyberGIS-HIV application. The raw scores for each rating were summed after multiplying each item by its weight (public health at 0.3, 0.5, and 0.2 and modeling at 0.33, 0.33, and 0.33; see the appendix). These indexes were then compared across the CyberGIS-HIV application and the approach respondents were using at the time.

PURPOSE

The prevalence and incidence of HIV infections in the United States remain troubling and inequitable despite the availability of successful biomedical interventions.[10] Difficulties achieving critical health milestones (e.g., the National HIV/AIDS Strategy[11]) can be attributed in part to delayed surveillance data reporting within regions, lags in preexposure prophylaxis use or HIV status awareness, and limited access to Federally Qualified Health Centers. Some of these problems might have been avoided if public health officials had been able to forecast them. Integrating a predictive model of HIV epidemiology into a cyber-based GIS framework[12,13] enables public health officials and researchers to make more accurate predictions about future HIV trends. It also allows them to assess the impact of changes in intervention strategies. Thus, the public health system needs methods to make service decisions by predicting HIV epidemiology within and across areas,[14,15] considering social determinants of health, and contemplating different prediction scenarios.

To date, however, existing methods involve spreadsheets and, occasionally, heat maps of regional epidemiology in addition to informal knowledge of the area in question and insights from community partners. As noted, we collected field data on the perceived need for statistical prediction tools, developed a web-based GIS application, and evaluated the application among public health personnel and modelers.

EVALUATION AND ADVERSE EFFECTS

Table 1 reports descriptive statistics by evaluation item and approach. Examples of current approaches included relying on data from America's HIV Epidemic Analysis Dashboard, AIDSVu, the Enhanced HIV/AIDS Reporting System, and CDC's HIV reports. Thirty-seven percent of the approaches currently used by respondents involved displaying surveillance data without any predictive modeling. These applications provided data mainly at the state level and included no predictive results.

On our 1 to 10 weighted scale, CyberGIS-HIV mean scores ranged from 7.91 to 8.54, whereas scores on currently used approaches ranged from 3.06 to 5.92. Thus, across dimensions, CyberGIS-HIV was rated more favorably than the approach respondents were using at the time, and the findings were similar for different user populations (Table 1). In addition, considering each rating individually, CyberGIS-HIV received more positive ratings than the approach currently used for all six evaluation items (Figure A, available as a supplement to the online version of this article at http://www.ajph.org).

Many respondents also provided comments about the application. These comments were classified as pertaining to functionality, visualization, or statistics. Table A (available as a supplement to the online version of this article at http://www.ajph.org) indicates whether the comments had been addressed in a new system. Most comments suggested making minor layout changes and adding details to CyberGIS-HIV, and these suggestions have been implemented. Moreover, CyberGIS-HIV was developed on the Python Jupyter

TABLE 1— Evaluation Item Responses From 42 State and Federal Public Health Study Respondents: CyberGIS-HIV Web User Interface and Other Approaches, 2020

	CyberGIS-HIV Item Score, Mean (SD)	Current Approach Item Score, Mean (SD)	Difference Between Means (95% CI)
Public health items			
Public health personnel	7.91 (1.63)	4.03 (2.98)	3.88 (2.62, 5.15)
Senior modelers	8.23 (0.96)	5.05 (3.11)	3.18 (−0.62, 6.97)
Junior modelers	8.53 (0.75)	5.92 (2.93)	2.61 (0.89, 4.34)
Overall	8.18 (1.31)	4.85 (3.03)	3.33 (2.41, 4.25)
Modeling items			
Public health personnel	7.92 (1.68)	3.06 (2.66)	4.86 (3.58, 6.15)
Senior modelers	8.00 (0.47)	4.08 (2.54)	3.92 (−0.29, 8.12)
Junior modelers	8.54 (0.89)	5.44 (2.91)	3.10 (1.65, 4.55)
Overall	8.17 (1.36)	4.06 (2.91)	4.11 (3.21, 5.00)

Note. CI = confidence interval. Public health items measured population benefit, constituency perspectives, and administrative feasibility, whereas modeling items measured automation and efficiency, statistical soundness, and satisfactory level of uncertainty.

Notebook user interface. The interface requires users to enter codes or commands and obtain results. A few comments requested a more straightforward user interface without any coding and with side-by-side scenario comparisons, which we are developing for CyberGIS-HIV 2.0. There were two comments about user-friendliness, which can be fully addressed only with a major update of the CyberGISX system in the future.

This study has several limitations. First, the cross-sectional nature of the evaluation, even with a within-participants design, may have influenced the findings. In addition, the visualization of national county maps does not consider population sizes or densities, which could affect data interpretation if users do not consider the other provided charts and figures. Furthermore, the proposed tool cannot provide predictions over shorter time periods (e.g., monthly or quarterly intervals) because of limitations in the input data. The use of the Python Jupyter Notebook interface, rather than a "what you see is what you get" interface, might also affect usability. Finally, participants' ratings were subjective and might not correspond to real-world service design and implementation. The relationship between the evaluation ratings and real-world implementation has not yet been explored and is an empirical question for future research.

SUSTAINABILITY

CyberGIS-HIV allows for the analysis and visualization of spatiotemporal HIV rates based on user-defined scenarios in real time. The administrative feasibility item raw scores were higher for CyberGIS-HIV (mean = 7.94, SD = 1.77) than for the current approach respondents were using (mean = 4.64, SD = 3.25), $t(41) = 6.10$, 95% confidence interval [CI] = 2.21, 4.39, suggesting that CyberGIS-HIV is easier to use and scale up than most approaches. However, 30% of our participants did not complete the study and stopped at the video tutorial stage. Future studies can investigate these difficulties and ways to overcome them.

PUBLIC HEALTH SIGNIFICANCE

Here we have reported fieldwork about public health prediction tools, specifically comparing CyberGIS-HIV with the approach our study respondents were currently using. CyberGIS-HIV outperformed currently used approaches on public health and modeling criteria and among public health personnel, senior modelers, and junior modelers. These findings underscore the potential for CyberGIS-HIV to significantly improve HIV epidemiology decision-making after refinement of the system's interface.

To maximize its impact, CyberGIS-HIV should be disseminated at public health conferences, journals, and Centers for AIDS Research to ensure that it remains accessible to researchers and public health officials at no cost. It is crucial to regularly update the associated data and codes to maintain their relevance and accuracy. Public health agencies and nongovernmental organizations should take advantage of these data in their decision-making processes and publish their results.

Finally, modeling researchers are encouraged to enhance prediction algorithms and integrate them with other implementation data to improve forecasting capabilities within a dynamic social context. AJPH

ABOUT THE AUTHORS

Man-pui Sally Chan and Bita Fayaz-Farkhad are with the Annenberg School for Communication and the Annenberg Public Policy Center, University of Pennsylvania, Philadelphia. Su Yeon Han is with the Department of Geography and Environmental Studies, Texas State University, San Marcos. Jinwoo Park is with the Department of Geography and the Department of Climate-Social Science Convergence, Kyung Hee University, Seoul, Republic of Korea. Shaowen Wang is with the Department of Geography and Geographic Information Science, University of Illinois at Urbana-Champaign. Dolores Albarracin is with the Annenberg School for Communication, the Annenberg Public Policy Center, the Department of Psychology, the Department of Family and Community Health, and Wharton Health Care Management, University of Pennsylvania, Philadelphia.

CORRESPONDENCE

Correspondence should be sent to Man-pui Sally Chan, PhD, Annenberg School for Communication, University of Pennsylvania, 3620 Walnut St, Philadelphia, PA 19104 (e-mail: sallycmp@upenn.edu). Reprints can be ordered at https://www.ajph.org by clicking the "Reprints" link.

PUBLICATION INFORMATION

Full Citation: Chan MS, Fayaz-Farkhad B, Han SY, Park J, Wang S, Albarracin D. Ending the HIV epidemic: development and evaluation of CyberGIS-HIV, a web-based prediction application. *Am J Public Health*. 2025;115(10):1589–1593.

Acceptance Date: May 7, 2025.

DOI: https://doi.org/10.2105/AJPH.2025.308194

ORCID iDs:

Man-pui Sally Chan https://orcid.org/0000-0003-2984-0487

Bita Fayaz-Farkhad https://orcid.org/0000-0002-2669-9986

Su Yeon Han https://orcid.org/0000-0002-3906-4533

Jinwoo Park https://orcid.org/0000-0002-6774-216X

CONTRIBUTORS

M. S. Chan and D. Albarracin originated and developed the study's concept and hypothesis and contributed to the conclusions and preparation of the article. M. S. Chan and B. Fayaz-Farkhad contributed to interpretation of the results. B. Fayaz-Farkhad administered the study and conducted the analysis. S. Y. Han and J. Park designed the user interfaces, developed the training videos, programmed the codes, and implemented the system. S. Wang developed the idea of CyberGIS-HIV and gave feedback on the features.

ACKNOWLEDGMENTS

This research was supported by the National Institute on Drug Abuse (award DP1 DA048570), the National Institute of Mental Health (awards R01MH114847 and R01MH132415), and the National Institute of Allergy and Infectious Diseases (award R01AI147487).

We thank Alexander Christopher Michels for providing technical support for the CyberGIS-HIV and Shiyu (Zoe) Zhang for recruiting the participants and preparing the data set.

Note. The content is solely the responsibility of the authors and does not necessarily represent the official views of the National Institutes of Health.

CONFLICTS OF INTEREST

The authors have no conflicts of interest to report.

HUMAN PARTICIPANT PROTECTION

This study was approved by the institutional review board of the University of Pennsylvania. Participants provided informed consent.

REFERENCES

1. Sass D, Farkhad BF, Li B, Sally Chan MP, Albarracín D. Are spatial models advantageous for predicting county-level HIV epidemiology across the United States? *Spat Spatiotemporal Epidemiol.* 2021;38:100436. https://doi.org/10.1016/J.SSTE.2021.100436
2. CyberGIS Center. CyberGIS-HIV 1.0 documentation. Available at: https://cybergis.github.io/CyberGIS_HIV_document/build/index.html. Accessed August 21, 2024.
3. Wang S, Goodchild MF. CyberGIS for transforming geospatial discovery and innovation. In: Wang S, Goodchild MF, eds. *CyberGIS for Geospatial Discovery and Innovation.* New York, NY: Springer; 2019:3–10.
4. Padmanabhan A, Wang S, Cao G, et al. FluMapper: a cyberGIS application for interactive analysis of massive location-based social media. *Concurrency and Computation Pract Exp.* 2014;26(13):2253–2265. https://doi.org/10.1002/cpe.3287
5. World Health Organization. Standards for quality HIV care: a tool for quality assessment, improvement, and accreditation. Available at: https://iris.who.int/bitstream/handle/10665/43093/9241592559.pdf?sequence=1&isAllowed=y. Accessed August 21, 2024.
6. US Department of Health and Human Services. Decision matrix. Available at: https://digital.ahrq.gov/health-it-tools-and-resources/evaluation-resources/workflow-assessment-health-it-toolkit/all-workflow-tools/decision-matrix. Accessed August 21, 2024.
7. Weiner J. Health policy analysis checklist: for the development, selection, and assessment of program policies within health care organizations. Available at: https://studylib.net/doc/8369349/health-policy-analysis-checklist—johns-hopkins-bloomber...%20https://studylib.net/doc/8369349/health-policy-analysis-checklist—johns-hopkins-bloomber. Accessed August 21, 2024.
8. Bracken DW, Rose DS, Church AH. The evolution and devolution of 360° feedback. *Ind Organ Psychol.* 2016;9(4):761–794. https://doi.org/10.1017/iop.2016.93
9. Chandler N, Henderson G, Park B, Byerley J, Brown WD, Steiner MJ. Use of a 360-degree evaluation in the outpatient setting: the usefulness of nurse, faculty, patient/family, and resident self-evaluation. *J Grad Med Educ.* 2010;2(3):430–434. https://doi.org/10.4300/JGME-D-10-00013.1
10. Centers for Disease Control and Prevention. Social determinants of health among adults with diagnosed HIV infection, 2019. Available at: http://www.cdc.gov/hiv/library/reports/hiv-surveillance.html. Accessed June 27, 2024.
11. US Department of Health and Human Services. National HIV/AIDS Strategy: what you need to know. Available at: https://files.hiv.gov/s3fs-public/NHAS-2022-2025-2Pager.pdf. Accessed March 6, 2025.
12. Liu Y, Padmanabhan A, Wang S. CyberGIS Gateway for enabling data-rich geospatial research and education. Available at: https://ieeexplore.ieee.org/document/6702694. Accessed March 6, 2025.
13. Wang S. A CyberGIS framework for the synthesis of cyberinfrastructure, GIS, and spatial analysis. *Ann Assoc Am Geogr.* 2010;100(3):535–557. https://doi.org/10.1080/00045601003791243
14. Sanchez T, Zlotorzynska M, Sineath C, Kahle E, Sullivan P. The annual American Men's Internet Survey of behaviors of men who have sex with men in the United States: 2014 key indicators report. *JMIR Public Health Surveill.* 2016;2(1):e23. https://doi.org/10.2196/publichealth.5476
15. Jeffries WL, Greene KM, Paz-Bailey G, et al. Determinants of HIV incidence disparities among young and older men who have sex with men in the United States. *AIDS Behav.* 2018;22(7):2199–2213. https://doi.org/10.1007/s10461-018-2088-3

Transgender Public Health Today

B. Ethan Coston, PhD

ABOUT THE AUTHOR

B. Ethan Coston is an associate professor of Gender, Sexuality and Women's Studies, Virginia Commonwealth University, Richmond, and is the founding director of the Sexual Health Exploration Project, Richmond, VA.

See also LGBTQ+ Transgender Health, pp. 1598–1670.

Within the past decade in the United States, an increasing amount of legislation has been proposed, passed, and enacted that aims to undermine transgender people's health and well-being, severely restricting their ability to participate in social, economic, and civil life. This includes making it a felony to provide best practice gender-affirming care to youths. It also involves restricting youths from participating in sports, banning the discussion of LGBTQ+ (lesbian, gay, bisexual, transgender, queer, questioning, asexual, intersex, and other nonheterosexual, noncisgender) people and history in schools, censoring LGBTQ+ content on public-facing governmental websites, and paving the way for the reinstatement of conversion therapy practices for youths. Although the total number of bills is ever changing, the antitrans legislation tracker reported that 948 state- and national-level bills were introduced or carried over into 2025 (as of July 10, 2025), including 114 passed and signed into law.[1–7] This has had far-reaching and devastating consequences.

The Trevor Project's 2024 National Survey on LGBTQ+ Youth Mental Health found that almost half of all transgender and nonbinary young people seriously considered attempting suicide in the past year, with 90% saying that their mental health was negatively affected by recent sociopolitical events.[8] The 2022 US Trans Survey report also indicated that 50% of transgender people were either forced to or seriously considered relocating to a different state because of legislative changes and gender-affirming care bans; and 25% avoided necessary health care owing to fear (half of the people who did seek out care reported experiencing discrimination from their health care providers).[9]

The past year has brought additional challenges and setbacks, both in the United States and globally. This includes the recent Supreme Court decision in *United States v Skrmetti* (No. 23-477), which essentially allows current bans on gender-affirming care for youths to stand. In their opinions, the majority justices referred to gender-affirming care for youths being "risky," questioning the scientific evidence on the matter.[10]

However, in the face of this sociopolitical violence, there has also been significant and powerful resistance. This includes, but is certainly not limited to, a number of prominent professional organizations affirming transgender people's right to exist, receive comprehensive care, and be treated with dignity. These organizations include the American Academy of Child and

HISTORY CORNER

17 YEARS AGO

Sexual and Gender Minority Health: What We Know and What Needs to Be Done

Transgender health in general has not been a focus of specialized clinical care because of an even greater lack of data and resources than with gay and lesbian health. Transgender individuals have had to struggle to have their clinical issues taken seriously and to find appropriate resources for care. Guidelines for the care of transgender people are available online but are not yet widely disseminated or taught. Transgender people also face financial barriers to care, given that transitional therapies with either medication or surgery are expensive and rarely covered by insurers in the United States. . . . Culturally appropriate programs need to be developed and refined to improve disparities in smoking, alcohol use, mental health, healthy weight, cancer prevention activities, and sexually transmitted infections. Federal agencies and public health organizations must disseminate the best practices of successful programs.

From *AJPH*, June 2008, pp. 992, 994

AJPH October 2025, Vol. 115, No. 10

Adolescent Psychiatry—which opposes all efforts to restrict youths' access to care[11]—and the Society for Adolescent Health and Medicine—which called on "community members, health professionals, institutional leaders, and policymakers to support and protect transgender and nonbinary adolescents and young adults, their families, and the clinicians who serve them."[12] In addition to clear support for youths, other organizations have affirmed their commitment to the transgender community more broadly. For example, the American Psychiatric Association approved a landmark policy that takes aim at the spread of misleading, unfounded, and stigmatizing narratives about transgender people and care,[13] and the American Medical Association noted in its 2021 letter to the National Governors Association that they oppose "the dangerous intrusion of government into the practice of medicine and the criminalization of health care decision-making."[14]

Given the increasing need to provide comprehensive, evidence-based insights into transgender health and well-being, *AJPH* invited the submission of articles in several critical areas related to the state of transgender public health and health equity today; this special section is the result of those efforts. In what follows, 55 coauthors across eight articles explore a number of pressing public health issues.

To start, Babbs et al. (p. 1605) discuss the lack of gender identity and gender modality in federal surveys and nationally representative data sources, which has led researchers to use administrative claims data to make generalizations. They note the utility and pitfalls of researchers' attempts to identify and classify transgender people through such data and provide a five-step roadmap for conducting rigorous and ethical claims-based research on transgender and gender-diverse populations—including ethical considerations, inclusion and exclusion criteria, and analytical issues. Shifting to applied research, Minalga and Feuer (p. 1621) report on and test the HIV Research Scorecard for transgender (TGD) Inclusivity, which consists of "14 yes-or-no indicators spanning four domains of clinical trials: study design, study implementation, study reporting, and language." Using the scorecard in a cross-sectional review of HIV clinical trials, they find that only two studies (of 41 eligible) receive an A grade. They provide actionable advice for researchers and advocates to use in designing and implementing clinical trials in the future.

In looking at gender-affirming health care itself, Stetten et al. (p. 1598) describe their cross-national research with health care providers, examining those providers' current practices during a moment when the legality of such care is often tenuous. They find that gender-affirming care providers—in continued alignment with the informed consent model—follow clinical standards for the provision of care, mitigating risks and maximizing benefits, for their transgender patients. On the patient side of the equation, Murano-Kinney (p. 1662) explores how gonadotropin-releasing hormone analog prescription and use among adolescents is complicated by gender modality. Although these medications have been used on-label for three decades to pause early onset puberty among cisgender girls, it is considered "off-label"—a categorization that gives bad faith actors the ability to call such use experimental and dangerous—for use to pause incongruent pubertal development in transgender youths. Murano-Kinney's

HISTORY CORNER

24 YEARS AGO

Enhancing Transgender Health Care

Individuals both within and allied to the transgender community believe that the standards of care imposed by the Harry Benjamin International Gender Dysphoria Association are regarded as authoritative by providers but as restrictive by many clients. In addition, these guidelines have given rise to small groups of "experts" within specific areas whose services are sought by all transgender persons wishing to medically change their gender; those living in isolated areas may not have ready access to such "experts" and may have to find other ways to go about their transition. Current constraints on access to medical care related to gender changes may place people at risk by forcing them to seek unsafe methods of making these changes (e.g., using hormones bought off the street, sharing needles while injecting hormones). The constraints for transgender youths are even greater; often, such youths are denied the ability to change their social gender in any way within institutional settings, which may force them back into situations that can place them at great risk. There is some support for allowing transgender youths to begin the process of changing their gender; many do so without trouble.

From *AJPH*, June 2001, p. 870

AJPH October 2025, Vol. 115, No. 10

extensive and thoroughly supported documentation of gonadotropin-releasing hormone analogs shows that their use in gender-affirming pediatric care is—as editorialist Rory O'Brien notes—an "evidence-based, safe, efficacious standard of care."

A number of contributions explore how the current sociopolitical landscape is affecting transgender people themselves. Lampe and Sumerau (p. 1616) investigate how older adults are managing their mental health. They reveal the importance of framing transgender identities, bodies, and experiences as life-affirming as well as the role chosen families have in providing invaluable emotional, logistical, and financial support. They affirm the need for more "governmental and private sector efforts to facilitate more structured social opportunities (e.g., support groups, online communities, book clubs) for trans older adults."

Whalen et al. (p. 1652) report findings from the Trying to Understand Relationships, Networks and Neighborhoods Among Trans Women of Color (TURNNT) Cohort Study. They find that transgender women of color do not receive an adequate amount of sleep, that their sleep is often of poor quality, and that those who face discrimination are particularly susceptible to these issues. They conclude that it is imperative that effective sleep interventions be adapted to transgender people's experiences and that "combating provider-based discrimination and increasing affordable and sustainable access to gender-affirming care" is "an active priority for public health." Furuya et al. (p. 1631) also use data from the TURNNT Cohort Study and examine the importance of community connectedness in HIV prevention and care outcomes among transgender women of color. Specifically, in looking at increases in condom use and sexually transmitted infection testing, they conclude that "connectedness can be thought of as a manifestation of resilience—a construct that enables marginalized individuals to practice healthy behavior and maintain good health statuses even despite encountering interlocking systems of oppression on a daily basis."

Finally, Hummel et al. (p. 1642) examine the health impacts of antitrans legislation in Florida, finding that an increasing number of transgender people sought services from organizations each year, with 92% requesting help with legally changing their names or updating their identification documents and 50% requesting health care services or referrals. Importantly, they discover that "antitransgender legislation prompts transgender people to seek support, resources, and protection from advocacy groups, which are an important source of resistance" for those in the community.

Rounding out this special section is an editorial by Martha O. de la Paz and Harry Barbee (p. 1611) that marshals evidence that access to gender-affirming care is integral to the HIV care continuum, specifically noting through a thorough review of the literature that offering preexposure prophylaxis in a gender-affirming context improves engagement, normalizing HIV testing in routine gender-affirming care increases testing uptake, and integrating HIV treatment into gender-affirming care provision increases retention. de la Paz and Barbee end their article by highlighting what is necessary to achieve HIV health equity for transgender and gender-diverse people today, writing, "public health professionals, policymakers, and advocates have a responsibility to ensure that TGD people enjoy access to the care they need to thrive."

As the American Public Health Association affirmed in 2016,[15] the Public Health Code of Ethics demands that all public health practitioners and policymakers value the protection of human dignity, including the development of scientific knowledge that will improve and ensure public health for all. Nearly a decade later, the evidence is clear: bias, stigma, discrimination, and erasure in housing, health care, the workplace, educational systems, and public accommodations have contributed to the rise in distress, isolation, feelings of hopelessness, and suicidality among transgender youths and adults.[15]

Ultimately, we hope that this special section adds to the growing chorus of support for transgender people, communities, and health. It highlights the dire consequences of antitrans rhetoric and policy. It also underscores the work that lies ahead for public health practitioners and policymakers to create inclusive health services, sustain multilevel health interventions, and enact multisector nondiscrimination policies. As the context of transgender public health is ever changing, *AJPH* will continue to publish in this area in the future and welcomes future submissions in this and related areas anytime. AJPH

CORRESPONDENCE

Correspondence should be sent to B. Ethan Coston, 919 W. Franklin St, Richmond, VA 23284 (e-mail: bmcoston@vcu.edu). Reprints can be ordered at https://www.ajph.org by clicking the "Reprints" link.

PUBLICATION INFORMATION

Full Citation: Coston BE. Transgender public health today. *Am J Public Health*. 2025;115(10): 1594–1597.

Acceptance Date: July 15, 2025.

DOI: https://doi.org/10.2105/AJPH.2025.308251

ORCID iD:
B. Ethan Coston https://orcid.org/0000-0002-6511-4362

ACKNOWLEDGMENTS

I would like to thank every transgender person who came before me for their vibrancy, beauty, and rebellious spirit. To all those who come after, I hope you know you are seen, you are loved, and you are worthy of a thriving life. May we all be the sugar in the cement and not the cog in the wheel.

CONFLICTS OF INTEREST

The author has no conflicts of interest to disclose.

REFERENCES

1. Dawson L, Kates J. Policy tracker: youth access to gender affirming care and state policy restrictions. June 18, 2025. Available at: https://www.kff.org/other/dashboard/gender-affirming-care-policy-tracker. Accessed July 25, 2025.
2. Movement Advancement Project. Bans on transgender people using bathrooms and facilities according to their gender identity. July 25, 2025. Available at: https://www.lgbtmap.org/equality-maps/nondiscrimination/bathroom_bans. Accessed July 25, 2025.
3. Yamat R. What to know about the US Supreme Court's ruling on public school lessons using LGBTQ books. June 28, 2025. Available at: https://apnews.com/article/supreme-court-ruling-lgbtq-books-e91c0e7bb4359a05adf7b1079709e76b. Accessed July 25, 2025.
4. Reed E. The painful history of forced outing and anti-LGBTQ+ school policies. October 11, 2023. Available at: https://lalgbtcenter.org/vanguard/the-painful-history-of-forced-outing-and-anti-lgbtq-school-policies. Accessed July 25, 2025.
5. Jingnan H. Here are all the ways people are disappearing from government websites. March 19, 2025. Available at: https://www.npr.org/2025/03/19/nx-s1-5317567/federal-websites-lgbtq-diversity-erased. Accessed July 25, 2025.
6. Movement Advancement Project. Conversion "therapy" laws. July 25, 2025. Available at: https://www.lgbtmap.org/equality-maps/conversion_therapy. Accessed July 25, 2025.
7. Trans Legislation Tracker. 2025 Anti-trans bills tracker. 2025. Available at: https://translegislation.com. Accessed July 25, 2025.
8. Trevor Project. 2024 US national survey on the mental health of LGBTQ+ young people. 2024. Available at: https://www.thetrevorproject.org/survey-2024. Accessed July 25, 2025.
9. US Trans Survey. 2025. Available at: https://ustranssurvey.org. Accessed July 25, 2025.
10. Ring T. 5 Takeaways from the Supreme Court ruling on gender-affirming care. June 19, 2025. Available at: https://www.advocate.com/news/5-takeaways-skrmetti-ruling. Accessed July 10, 2025.
11. AACAP statement responding to efforts to ban evidence-based care for transgender and gender diverse youth. *American Academy of Child and Adolescent Psychiatry.* November 8, 2019. Available at: https://www.aacap.org/AACAP/Latest_News/AACAP_Statement_Responding_to_Efforts-to_ban_Evidence-Based_Care_for_Transgender_and_Gender_Diverse.aspx. Accessed July 25, 2025.
12. Society for Adolescent Health and Medicine. SAHM supports protecting access to gender-affirming clinical care for transgender and nonbinary AYA. August 15, 2023. Available at: https://adolescenthealth.org/press_release/sahm-supports-protecting-access-to-gender-affirming-clinical-care-for-transgender-and-nonbinary-aya. Accessed July 25, 2025.
13. American Psychological Association. APA adopts groundbreaking policy supporting transgender, gender diverse, nonbinary individuals. February 28, 2024. Available at: https://www.apa.org/news/press/releases/2024/02/policy-supporting-transgender-nonbinary. Accessed July 25, 2025.
14. American Medical Association. AMA reinforces opposition to restrictions on transgender medical care. June 15, 2021. Available at: https://www.ama-assn.org/press-center/ama-press-releases/ama-reinforces-opposition-restrictions-transgender-medical-care. Accessed July 25, 2025.
15. American Public Health Association. Promoting transgender and gender minority health through inclusive policies and practices. October 31, 2016. Available at: https://www.apha.org/policy-and-advocacy/public-health-policy-briefs/policy-database/2017/01/26/promoting-transgender-and-gender-minority-health-through-inclusive-policies-and-practices. Accessed July 25, 2025.

Understanding Provider Treatment Approaches for the Provision of Gender-Affirming Hormones in the Current US Political Climate

Nichole E. Stetten, PhD, MPH, CPH, Patrick J. A. Kelly, MPH, Theresa I. Shireman, PhD, Em Balkan, MSW, Gray Babbs, MPH, Ash B. Alpert, MD, MFA, Hill L. Wolfe, PhD, MPA, David J. Meyers, PhD, MPH, and Jaclyn M. W. Hughto, PhD, MPH

See also LGBTQ+ Transgender Health, pp. 1594–1670.

Transgender people's access to gender-affirming hormone therapy (GAHT) is under attack in the United States. In 2024, we interviewed US providers about how they prescribe GAHT. In accordance with informed consent models, providers reported that they reviewed patients' medical history, social supports, and comorbidities; prescribed GAHT formulations that aligned with patients' goals; monitored health regularly; and maintained open communication with patients. The GAHT prescribers followed clinical standards to mitigate risks and maximize benefits, following similar standards of care for cisgender patients. (*Am J Public Health*. 2025;115(10):1598–1601. https://doi.org/10.2105/AJPH.2025.308143)

AJPH October 2025, Vol. 115, No. 10

Gender-affirming hormone therapy (GAHT) is often the first and sometimes only medical intervention used by transgender and gender diverse (TGD) people.[1]

STUDY OBJECTIVE

We sought to identify the practices that US-based health care providers use when (1) assessing TGD patients' readiness to begin GAHT, (2) initiating patients on GAHT, and (3) managing the long-term use of GAHT among TGD patients.

RESEARCH QUESTIONS

Research questions included the following: (1) How do providers assess and manage health risks and maximize health benefits when prescribing GAHT? (2) How do TGD patients' characteristics—such as age, sex assigned at birth, health comorbidities, and gender affirmation goals—affect how providers prescribe GAHT?

PARTICIPANTS, SAMPLE, GEOGRAPHIC LOCATION, SETTING, AND YEAR OF STUDY

Between March and April 2024, we interviewed 10 GAHT providers (specialty: primary care [n = 7]; endocrinology [n = 3]) from across the United States (West [n = 1]; Southwest [n = 2]; Midwest [n = 2]; Southeast [n = 1]; Northeast [n = 4]). Providers were recruited from the World Professional Association for Transgender Health (WPATH) provider directory. Semistructured interviews averaged 30 minutes (range = 30–45 minutes).

METHODS

Informed by the literature and clinical care guidelines, we developed an interview guide that focused on how providers determined patients' capacity to consent to GAHT and patients' comorbidities, gender affirmation goals, and insurance coverage; providers' processes for developing GAHT treatment plans; and whether providers received formal or informal training in GAHT prescribing. Using the national WPATH provider directory, we compiled an initial list of 66 primary care providers and endocrinologists stratified by geographic region. Providers were eligible if they were 18 years of age or older, prescribed GAHT in the United States, spoke English, and were able to provide informed consent. Of the 66 providers contacted, 11 agreed to be interviewed, and 10 were eligible, consented to, and completed an interview over Zoom. Interviews were conducted until data saturation was reached. All participants were compensated $25 for their time.

Interviews were recorded, transcribed, de-identified, and analyzed (by N. E. S. and P. J. A. K.) using a 5-step rapid qualitative analysis approach that triangulates and iteratively analyzes data to form an initial understanding of a phenomenon.[2–8] Steps 1, 4, and 5 of rapid qualitative analysis employ the constant comparison method,[9] whereby researchers systematically compare summaries across analysts to ensure reliability in summary generation.

The social positions of the authorship team, including our gender identities, race/ethnicity (all authors identify as White), and life experiences as clinicians, scientists, and patients, influenced the interview guide and how we interpreted the data in known and unknown ways. To mitigate potential biases and ensure that we are ethical stewards of our data, we held regular meetings with the interviewer, analysts, and the larger study team to collectively interpret findings and prevent analysts' viewpoints from being presented as results. We also thoughtfully wrote up our findings in ways that would reduce the misinterpretation and politicization of our findings by external actors. Finally, we supported one another by acknowledging the impact that legislative efforts to restrict access to care for TGD people has on us, professionally and personally.

KEY FINDINGS

We interviewed providers from across the United States with a range of experience providing gender-affirming care to TGD people. Results are categorized according to three primary themes: (1) assessing treatment goals and readiness, (2) addressing and optimizing mental health, and (3) navigating physical health risks to maximize benefits. Exemplar quotes for each theme are shown in Table A (available as a supplement to the online version of this article at http://www.ajph.org).

Theme 1: Assessing Treatment Goals

Providers emphasized the importance of using a patient-centered approach to assess patients' treatment goals and provide accurate information on the expected outcomes, including risks and benefits, prior to initiating GAHT. Understanding patients' goals allowed providers to convey the potential outcomes of different GAHT formulations and the likely persistence of physical changes. To ensure patient readiness to initiate treatment, some providers also reported discussing expected outcomes with patients across several appointments to allow time for the patients to consider their options and ask further questions before starting GAHT.

Theme 2: Addressing and Optimizing Mental Health

Providers underscored the importance of prioritizing patient safety by addressing any serious mental health concerns, including suicidality, prior to initiating GAHT. Providers reported sharing data with their patients on the mental health benefits of GAHT, including reductions in gender dysphoria. Providers also reported ensuring that patients were aware that they may experience brief, temporary periods of worsened mental health following hormone initiation, such as depression or mood disorder exacerbation, as they adjust to GAHT levels. Accordingly, providers emphasized evaluating whether a patient had access to adequate mental health care and social support services prior to initiating GAHT. Some participants practiced at institutions where mental health services are co-located with their clinical services, making it easier to refer patients to mental health care when necessary.

Theme 3: Navigating Physical Health Risks

Providers took care to ensure that comorbid physical conditions were identified and managed to maximize GAHT benefits. Clinicians stated that reviewing a patient's medical history is crucial to understanding whether the patient has or is at risk for developing comorbid conditions that may place them at greater risk of experiencing GAHT complications. If patients had physical comorbidities, clinicians ensured these were optimally managed prior to GAHT initiation or would adjust treatment plans accordingly. For example, for patients with high-risk comorbidities such as clotting disorders and cardiovascular disease, clinicians started with lower doses or topical formulations of GAHT because these methods afford greater dose control and confer fewer side effects than standard doses, injections, or pills. Providers also distinguished health risks by GAHT type (i.e., testosterone, estrogens, antiandrogens). Notably, all providers acknowledged that smoking tobacco is associated with the development and worsening of comorbidities that could exacerbate the risk of adverse events related to hormone use and thus ensured that they conveyed this information to patients and provided support to reduce or cease tobacco use. Providers also reported routinely monitoring for pulmonary and metabolic conditions, pregnancy, thromboembolism, weight, liver enzymes, lipid profile, bone health, diabetes, and hormone-sensitive cancers and tumors, among other conditions.

Multiple providers explained that older age is associated with a greater prevalence of comorbidities that could exacerbate the risk of adverse events related to hormone use, including thrombosis and malignancies. As such, providers adopted a life-course model wherein they adapted patients' starting dose and speed of titration based on the risks of side effects for their age. Accordingly, providers monitored older patients more regularly for complications.

EVALUATION, TRANSFERABILITY, AND ADVERSE EFFECTS

In this study, we found that providers consider a host of factors when creating patients' new and ongoing GAHT treatment plans. Providers described asking patients about their treatment goals to tailor GAHT regimens and manage their expectations of outcomes. Further, providers highlighted the importance of mental health supports for patients, including facilitating access to mental health care if needed. Finally, providers described how they helped patients to manage existing comorbidities, and tailored treatment plans according to specific patient attributes, such as age.

This study recruited providers affiliated with WPATH, so findings may not transfer to all GAHT care providers in the United States, as all providers in this study followed WPATH's current evidence-based practices and standards of care. Nonetheless, we ensured geographic variability in the sample and ultimately reached qualitative data saturation.[10] Given that the political climate has continued to evolve since these data were collected in 2024, ongoing research exploring the provision of GAHT care across US regions could help to identify emerging trends.

SCALABILITY

This study highlights several avenues for future research. First, additional research should explore patients' experiences communicating with providers about their needs and preferences for obtaining GAHT and managing their related care. Future work should also examine the heterogeneity of health care providers' experiences based on the political climate of the state in which they provide care, particularly as new state and federal policies and policy responses emerge. Finally, our research focused on providers' conversations about GAHT use with TGD people. Additional research could explore similarities and differences in patient–provider communication about hormone therapies (e.g., hormonal birth control, postmenopausal hormone replacement therapy) for cisgender patients.

PUBLIC HEALTH SIGNIFICANCE

TGD populations face unique barriers to receiving GAHT because of cisnormativity, rampant misinformation, and recent legislative efforts to restrict GAHT access.[11–13] These barriers occur even though GAHT is a medically necessary and effective treatment for TGD people seeking medical gender affirmation. To that end, GAHT reduces gender dysphoria and is associated with improved mental health and quality of life for TGD people.[1,14,15] Although the risks of exogenous hormones in TGD and cisgender people are similar and are overwhelmingly outweighed by the benefits, legislative actions to block hormone utilization have focused exclusively on the use of GAHT by TGD people. Findings from our cross-national sample of GAHT providers illustrate that these providers know how to safely prescribe GAHT to mitigate risks, maximize benefits, and ensure patient safety. These findings should be taken into consideration in legislative and legal proceedings to preserve access to these medically necessary medications for TGD people. AJPH

ABOUT THE AUTHORS

Nichole E. Stetten, Theresa I. Shireman, and David J. Meyers are with the Center for Gerontology & Healthcare Research, Brown University School of Public Health, Providence, RI. Patrick J. A. Kelly and Jaclyn M. W. Hughto are with the Department of Behavioral and Social Sciences, Brown University School of Public Health. Em Balkan and Gray Babbs are with the Department of Health Services, Brown University School of Public Health. Ash B. Alpert is with the Yale Cancer Center, Yale School of Medicine, Yale University, New Haven, CT. Hill L. Wolfe is with the Yale School of Medicine, Yale University, New Haven.

CORRESPONDENCE

Correspondence should be sent to Nichole Stetten, 155 S. Main St, Providence RI 02903 (e-mail: nichole_stetten@brown.edu). Reprints can be ordered at https://www.ajph.org by clicking the "Reprints" link.

PUBLICATION INFORMATION

Full Citation: Stetten NE, Kelly PJA, Shireman TI, et al. Understanding provider treatment approaches for the provision of gender-affirming hormones in the current US political climate. *Am J Public Health*. 2025;115(10):1598–1601.

Acceptance Date: March 31, 2025.

DOI: https://doi.org/10.2105/AJPH.2025.308143

ORCID iDs:

Nichole E. Stetten https://orcid.org/0000-0001-7993-9851

Patrick J. A. Kelly https://orcid.org/0000-0003-1462-1150

Theresa I. Shireman https://orcid.org/0000-0001-6846-8783

Em Balkan https://orcid.org/0009-0001-0333-9312

Gray Babbs https://orcid.org/0000-0003-4060-571X

Hill L. Wolfe https://orcid.org/0000-0001-8834-1560

Jaclyn M. W. Hughto https://orcid.org/0000-0003-4722-8179

CONTRIBUTORS

N. E. Stetten and J. M. W. Hughto designed the study. All authors reviewed study design and interview questions. N. E. Stetten recruited participants and conducted interviews. N. E. Stetten and P. J. A. Kelly analyzed the data and wrote the Methods and Results sections of the manuscript. All authors contributed to writing the other sections of the manuscript, reviewing, and providing edits.

ACKNOWLEDGMENTS

This work was supported in part by grant R01AG073440-01A1 from the National Institute on Aging and the Brown University Center for Gerontology & Healthcare Research.

CONFLICTS OF INTEREST

The authors have no conflicts of interest to declare.

HUMAN PARTICIPANT PROTECTION

The institutional review board at Brown University reviewed the study and deemed it exempt.

REFERENCES

1. Coleman E, Radix AE, Bouman WP, et al. Standards of care for the health of transgender and gender diverse people, version 8. *Int J Transgend Health*. 2022;23(suppl 1):S1–S259. https://doi.org/10.1080/26895269.2022.2100644
2. Hamilton AB. Qualitative methods in rapid turn-around health services research. Presented at: VA HSR&D Cyberseminar Spotlight on Women's Health; 2013. VA Women's Health Network Research Network. Available at: https://www.betterevaluation.org/tools-resources/qualitative-methods-rapid-turn-around-health-services-research. Accessed December 6, 2024.
3. Hamilton AB, Finley EP. Qualitative methods in implementation research: an introduction. *Psychiatry Res*. 2019;280:112516. https://doi.org/10.1016/j.psychres.2019.112516
4. Vindrola-Padros C, Johnson GA. Rapid techniques in qualitative research: a critical review of the literature. *Qual Health Res*. 2020;30(10):1596–1604. https://doi.org/10.1177/1049732320921835
5. Beebe J. *Rapid Assessment Process: An Introduction*. Walnut Creek, CA: AltaMira Press; 2001.
6. Beebe J. *Rapid Qualitative Inquiry*. 2nd ed. Lanham, MD: Rowman & Littlefield; 2014.
7. Gale RC, Justina W, Erhardt T, et al. Comparison of rapid vs in-depth qualitative analytic methods from a process evaluation of academic detailing in the Veterans Health Administration. *Implement Sci*. 2019;14(1):11–12. https://doi.org/10.1186/s13012-019-0853-y
8. Taylor B, Henshall C, Kenyon S, et al. Can rapid approaches to qualitative analysis deliver timely, valid findings to clinical leaders? A mixed methods study comparing rapid and thematic analysis. *BMJ Open*. 2018;8(10):e019993. https://doi.org/10.1136/bmjopen-2017-019993
9. Glaser BG, Strauss AL. *The Discovery of Grounded Theory: Strategies for Qualitative Research*. Chicago, IL: Aldine De Gruyter; 1967.
10. Hennink M, Kaiser BN. Sample sizes for saturation in qualitative research: a systematic review of empirical tests. *Soc Sci Med*. 2022;292:114523. https://doi.org/10.1016/j.socscimed.2021.114523
11. Dutton HJ, Breder K, Ma C. Exploring the relationship between gender-affirming care delivery and health outcomes in transgender and gender-diverse adults: an integrative review. *Transgender Health*. 2024; Epub ahead of print. https://doi.org/10.1089/trgh.2023.0087
12. Schall TE, Moses JD. Gender-affirming care for cisgender people. *Hastings Cent Rep*. 2023;53(3):15–24. https://doi.org/10.1002/hast.1486
13. Lampe NM. Accounting for cisnormativity: understanding transgender and non-binary young people's strategies to resist and reduce inequality in healthcare. *Soc Curr*. 2024;11(1):3–21. https://doi.org/10.1177/23294965231179432
14. White Hughto J, Reisner S. A systematic review of the effects of hormone therapy on psychological functioning and quality of life in transgender individuals. *Transgend Health*. 2016;1(1):21–31. https://doi.org/10.1089/trgh.2016.0005
15. Hughto JM, Gunn HA, Rood BA, Pantalone DW. Social and medical gender affirmation experiences are inversely associated with mental health problems in a US non-probability sample of transgender adults. *Arch Sex Behav*. 2020;49(7):2635–2647. https://doi.org/10.1007/s10508-020-01655-5

Public Health's Defense of Pediatric Gender-Affirming Care

Rory P. O'Brien, PhD

ABOUT THE AUTHOR

Rory P. O'Brien is with the University of Michigan School of Social Work, Ann Arbor.

See also LGBTQ+ Transgender Health, pp. 1594–1670.

In this issue of the *American Journal of Public Health*, Murano-Kinney (p. 1662) details how pediatric use of gonadotropin-releasing hormone analogs (GnRHAs, commonly referred to as "puberty blockers") for gender dysphoria is safe, effective, reversible, and supported by decades of medical research. Despite being an evidence-based standard of care for pediatric gender dysphoria, GnRHAs are primarily approved for precocious puberty and are prescribed off-label for gender dysphoria. Given that off-label pediatric prescription is commonplace and a prescription's off-label status does not indicate a lack of evidence, safety, or efficacy, Murano-Kinney presents a strong argument that supplemental indication of GnRHAs to treat pediatric gender dysphoria by the US Food and Drug Administration could help counter mischaracterizations of pediatric gender-affirming care (PGAC) as "experimental." This article adds to a growing call for the field of public health to defend transgender, nonbinary, and gender-diverse (hereafter, "trans") youths by addressing misinformation and expanding access.

PGAC refers to a range of services, including social transition supports, mental health care, use of GnRHAs to delay the onset of secondary sex characteristics, and, in later adolescence and early adulthood, hormone replacement therapy. Youths may desire only some or all of these interventions, and youths who receive PGAC exhibit reductions in depression and suicide attempt.[1,2] However, the current PGAC medico-legal landscape induces extreme regional variation in PGAC access. An estimated 300 100 trans children aged 12 to 17 years live across the United States,[3] including in states with PGAC shield laws, no PGAC protections, and PGAC bans. State bans on PGAC threaten patients with litigation for accessing care out of state, parents with child protective service investigations, and providers with criminal charges, fines, and license revocation.[4]

Under the Trump administration, the landscape of PGAC—and public health generally—shifts rapidly week by week. Public health professionals are tasked in this great historical moment of uncertainty to defend access to care where it is threatened and to expand it wherever possible. Under Executive Order 14187, "Protecting Children From Chemical and Surgical Mutilation," the Trump administration proclaims that "medical professionals are maiming and sterilizing a growing number of impressionable children . . . through a series of irreversible medical interventions."[5] The order dictated that "it is the policy of the United States that it will not fund, sponsor, promote, assist, or support the so-called 'transition' of a child from one sex to another."[5] Although currently subject to court injunction, this order carries widespread implications for trans children, their parents, providers, clinics and hospitals, and researchers. As the nation's highest office peddles in misinformation and mischaracterizes PGAC as abuse with irreversible consequences, the defense of public health must necessarily avoid such biased reasoning, anecdotes, and improvisation.[6] Public health policy, researchers, and trans communities must work together to defend and expand access to care. Murano-Kinney's article corrects disinformation and outlines one strategy—albeit now a long-term strategy given today's federal context—to expand access where it is still permitted in the United States. These are important components of a public health defense of PGAC. A strong public health defense should include maintaining and expanding access to care, supporting legislation to shield patients and providers, combatting misinformation, and—because of threats against patients and providers—bolstering security.[7] In this editorial, I discuss current threats and barriers to accessing PGAC and ways to defend it.

In addition to variation in state law, PGAC access depends on parental support, access to health insurance that does not discriminate by denying coverage, proximity to the limited number of PGAC-trained providers, and long waitlists for care.[3,8,9] Echoing Murano-Kinney's argument that off-label prescription is used to argue for PGAC bans, off-label prescription is also used to deny insurance claims.[10] These barriers help explain why PGAC remains widely inaccessible for youths who need timely access to this

AJPH October 2025, Vol. 115, No. 10

preventative form of health care. Timely access to GnRHAs is a key method of prevention of violence and mental distress for trans children, so long waitlists for PGAC can present serious and preventable risks to children's safety and mental health. States where PGAC remains legal are already receiving medical refugees from states with PGAC bans,[8] and they must be ready to receive and connect them with medical, social service, financial, educational, and community supports.

As noted by Murano-Kinney and Kim et al.,[7] misinformation and disinformation, such as in the *Cass Review*, have fueled PGAC bans. Executive Order 14187 instructed that the secretary of health and human services, Robert F. Kennedy, Jr, "shall publish a review of the existing literature on best practices for promoting the health of children who assert gender dysphoria, rapid-onset gender dysphoria, or other identity-based confusion."[5] That report, released May 1, 2025, portrayed PGAC as a harmful practice lacking in evidence, promoted psychotherapy to treat gender dysphoria, and included a self-conscious defense from accusations that their recommendation of psychotherapy constitutes conversion therapy.[11] In direct contrast to Murano-Kinney's review of off-label GnRHA use as safe and effective, the Department of Health and Human Services (HHS) report also reiterated arguments that off-label use of GnRHAs is dangerous, highlighting the utility and timeliness of Murano-Kinney's review to combatting misinformation and implementation of recommendations in the HHS report. The American Academy of Pediatrics (AAP)—which HHS did not consult in preparation of their report—and the Fenway Institute quickly published statements in opposition to the report, with specific concerns for its mischaracterization of existing research on PGAC and political incursions into medical practice.[12,13] Leading professional organizations, including the American Medical Association, recognize PGAC as an evidence-based standard of practice[14]; public health scientists and public health, medical, social work, and psychological professional organizations must stand with the AAP and Fenway Institute in response to misinformation in the HHS report.

Likewise, the Centers for Medicare and Medicaid Services proposed a rule to prohibit states from requiring that public insurance covers gender-affirming care, as well as coverage of Deferred Action for Childhood Arrivals recipients.[15] This is a federal attempt to gut state gender-affirming care protections and license insurance companies to discriminate against trans and migrant populations. Although data limitations inhibit precise counting of how many trans people may be affected by this proposed rule,[3] the proposed restrictions on coverage for Medicare and Medicaid enrollees would disproportionately harm impoverished and disabled trans and migrant populations. If this proposal to permit insurance discrimination is approved, state shield laws may become ineffective unless public health professionals work with insurance and pharmaceutical companies, attorneys general, and trans communities to advocate for continued coverage. To prevent ruptures in health care access, providers and clinics need assurance from their accrediting bodies and state attorneys general that they will defend their provision of evidence-based standards of care.

I also write this as, nationwide, my colleagues reel from the termination of federally funded studies, many of them specifically focused on trans youth health. Continuing research is needed to understand and respond to the needs of trans youths, their parents, and their providers. Universities have a mutual shared interest with trans communities and health researchers to resist these cuts to scientific funding to the full extent of the law. As Murano-Kinney notes, substantial evidence supports PGAC, and ongoing development of real-world evidence is necessary to support efforts to defend and expand access to care.

As Murano-Kinney emphasizes, trans communities have long fought for their right to health, including gender-affirming care and HIV prevention and treatment. The public health profession has likewise shown its mettle in resisting political attacks on care against the Affordable Care Act and the COVID-19 pandemic response. Looking to the future, the Williams Institute has noted that further federal legislative attempts to ban PGAC nationwide are likely, the Supreme Court's decision in a pending case on Tennessee's PGAC ban could have nationwide implications this summer, and litigation on PGAC will continue to shift the landscape, possibly for years to come.[3] In this long struggle for health justice, public health and trans communities need to strategize and fight in coalition to counter misinformation, defend access to care, and expand protections for trans youths. AJPH

CORRESPONDENCE

Correspondence should be sent to Rory O'Brien, 1080 S University Ave, Ann Arbor, MI 48109 (e-mail: roryobri@umich.edu). Reprints can be ordered at https://www.ajph.org by clicking the "Reprints" link.

PUBLICATION INFORMATION

Full Citation: O'Brien RP. Public health's defense of pediatric gender-affirming care. *Am J Public Health*. 2025;115(10):1602–1604.

Acceptance Date: April 29, 2025.

DOI: https://doi.org/10.2105/AJPH.2025.308185

ORCID iD:
Rory P. O'Brien https://orcid.org/0000-0002-8718-8354

ACKNOWLEDGMENTS

Thank you to Laura Ferguson, PhD, at the University of Southern California for providing feedback and support. I acknowledge and honor the contributions of trans activists past and present who inform my perspective and motivate my work.

CONFLICTS OF INTEREST

The author has no conflicts of interest to disclose.

REFERENCES

1. Turban JL, King D, Carswell JM, Keuroghlian AS. Pubertal suppression for transgender youth and risk of suicidal ideation. *Pediatrics.* 2020;145(2): e20191725. https://doi.org/10.1542/peds.2019-1725
2. Tordoff DM, Wanta JW, Collin A, Stepney C, Inwards-Breland DJ, Ahrens K. Mental health outcomes in transgender and nonbinary youths receiving gender-affirming care. *JAMA Netw Open.* 2022;5(2):e220978. :e220978-e220978. https://doi.org/10.1001/jamanetworkopen.2022.0978
3. Redfield E. *Impact of Ban on Gender Affirming Care on Transgender Minors.* Los Angeles, CA: Williams Institute, University of California, Los Angeles; 2025.
4. Georges E, Brown EC, Cohen RS. Prohibition of gender-affirming care as a form of child maltreatment: reframing the discussion. *Pediatrics.* 2024; 153(1):e2023064292. https://doi.org/10.1542/peds.2023-064292
5. Trump DJ. Protecting children from chemical and surgical mutilation. The White House. January 28, 2025. Available at: https://www.whitehouse.gov/presidential-actions/2025/01/protecting-children-from-chemical-and-surgical-mutilation. Accessed March 28, 2025.
6. Morabia A. Hank Aaron, Robert F. Kennedy Jr, and the public's health. *Am J Public Health.* 2025;115(2):108–109. https://doi.org/10.2105/AJPH.2024.307945
7. Kim H-H, Thayer N, Bernstein C, Cruz R, Roby C, Keuroghlian AS. On the frontlines: protecting and advancing gender-affirming care in a hostile sociopolitical environment. *J Gen Intern Med.* 2025;40(2):458–461. https://doi.org/10.1007/s11606-024-09080-3
8. Brandon-Friedman RA, Tabb A, Imburgia TM, et al. Perspectives of gender-diverse youth and caregivers facing gender-affirming medical intervention bans. *LGBT Health.* 2025;12(2):108–115. https://doi.org/10.1089/lgbt.2024.0079
9. Kearns S, Kroll T, O'Shea D, Neff K. Experiences of transgender and non-binary youth accessing gender-affirming care: a systematic review and meta-ethnography. *PLoS One.* 2021;16(9):e0257194. https://doi.org/10.1371/journal.pone.0257194
10. Inwards-Breland DJ, Karrington B, Sequeira GM. Access to care for transgender and nonbinary youth: ponder this, innumerable barriers exist. *JAMA Pediatr.* 2021;175(11):1112–1114. https://doi.org/10.1001/jamapediatrics.2021.2068
11. US Dept of Health and Human Services. Treatment for pediatric gender dysphoria: review of evidence and best practices. May 1, 2025. Available at: https://opa.hhs.gov/sites/default/files/2025-05/gender-dysphoria-report.pdf. Accessed May 20, 2025.
12. Kressly SJ. AAP statement on HHS report treatment for pediatric with gender dysphoria. American Academy of Pediatrics. May 1, 2025. Available at: https://www.aap.org/en/news-room/news-releases/aap/2025/aap-statement-on-hhs-report-treatment-for-pediatric-gender-dysphoria. Accessed May 20, 2025.
13. Fenway Institute. Statement in response to the report released by the US Department of Health and Human Services May 1, 2025 titled Treatment for Pediatric Gender Dysphoria Review of Evidence and Best Practices. May 1, 2025. Available at: https://fenwayhealth.org/statement-in-response-to-the-report-released-by-the-u-s-department-of-health-and-human-services-may-1-2025-titled-treatment-for-pediatric-gender-dysphoria-review-of-evidence-and-best-practices. Accessed May 20, 2025.
14. GLAAD. Medical association statements in support of health care for transgender people and youth. 2024. Available at: https://glaad.org/medical-association-statements-supporting-trans-youth-healthcare-and-against-discriminatory. Accessed April 3, 2025.
15. Patient Protection and Affordable Care Act; Marketplace Integrity and Affordability, Fed. Reg. 2025-04083 (March 19, 2025), to be codified at 45 CFR Parts 147, 155, and 156. Available at: https://www.federalregister.gov/documents/2025/03/19/2025-04083/patient-protection-and-affordable-care-act-marketplace-integrity-and-affordability. Accessed April 4, 2025.

Challenges and Best Practices Using Claims Data to Study Gender-Affirming Surgery in Transgender and Gender-Diverse Populations

Gray Babbs, MPH, Dannie Dai, BA, Elizabeth R. Boskey, PhD, MPH, MSW, Em Balkan, MSW, and Jaclyn M. W. Hughto, PhD, MPH

ABOUT THE AUTHORS

Gray Babbs, Em Balkan, and Jaclyn M. W. Hughto are with the Brown University School of Public Health, Providence, RI. Dannie Dai is with the Harvard T. H. Chan School of Public Health, Boston, MA. Elizabeth R. Boskey is with Boston Children's Hospital, Boston, MA.

See also LGBTQ+ Transgender Health, pp. 1594–1670.

Transgender and gender-diverse (TGD) people have historically been excluded from medical research. National representative surveys have collected limited data about gender and sex, often combining the concepts into a single, poorly defined term.[1] Furthermore, under the current Trump presidential administration, gender identity and modality (e.g., transgender or cisgender)[2] data have systematically been removed from federal surveys.[3] Most health-related data collected in the United States, therefore, have insufficient information to understand the health or even demographics of the TGD population in the United States, and this data gap is rapidly widening.[1]

Existing research is hard to generalize to the US-based TGD population, because to generalize, a researcher must know the characteristics of the TGD people in the United States compared with the sample.[4] In addition, much of what we know about TGD health has been derived from convenience samples in coastal cities from TGD people engaged in care in LGBTQ+ (lesbian, gay, bisexual, transgender, queer, questioning, asexual, intersex, Two-Spirit, and other nonheterosexual, noncisgender) specialized settings.[5] These surveys likely do not fully reflect the broader experience of TGD people in the United States. Additionally, the incredible diversity in the TGD population makes it difficult to generalize findings from small-scale studies.

Over the past decade, researchers have turned to administrative claims as a promising TGD health data source.[6] Claims data help overcome several limitations of traditional data sources and can provide a longitudinal sample across multiple care settings. Claims data provide more objective measures of disease incidence and health care utilization than self-reported data. Using claims reduces the risk of research fatigue among human participants.[7] These data sources offer large sample sizes and statistical power for more complex analyses. However, claims-based research on TGD populations poses unique methodological and ethical challenges that researchers must carefully address.

We use the identification of gender-affirming surgeries as a case study of the complexities that arise during claims-based research on TGD populations. We suggest best practices for navigating these complexities, including recommendations for accurately detecting gender-affirming care, designing analyses with valid comparison groups, and presenting results to advance TGD health equity. We do not outline all complexities and best practices. Instead, we highlight key pitfalls and minimum considerations for claims-based research. As the number of publications on TGD health has grown,[4,8] alongside increased national attention to TGD populations, there is a clear need for well-defined research standards.

DEFINING GENDER-AFFIRMING CARE

In general, gender-affirming care refers to social, behavioral, or medical interventions designed to support and affirm an individual's gender identity.[9] In a medical setting, gender-affirming care can refer to visits where medical gender affirmation is provided and visits where a provider respects a patient's gender (e.g., correct pronoun use) but does not provide specific gender-related medical care. Because the term

AJPH October 2025, Vol. 115, No. 10

is broad, researchers must clearly define what they mean by gender-affirming care in any project. We define medical gender-affirming care as procedures or medications that align physical gender expression with a person's intrinsic gender identity. TGD individuals' interest in medical gender-affirming care varies, as does their access to the care they need. People of all gender modalities[2] use gender-affirming care.[10]

CLAIMS DATA AND IDENTIFYING GENDER-DIVERSE PEOPLE

The central challenge to researching TGD health using claims is that insurance claims do not contain patients' self-reported gender identity or modality.[2] Researchers have developed methods to infer and categorize a person as likely TGD to address this limitation. These methods vary in complexity from using diagnosis codes associated with gender dysphoria[6,11] to hierarchical algorithms that cross-reference other diagnoses, gender-affirming procedures, and prescription drug codes.[12,13] Some methods further categorize TGD people into gender groups (e.g., transmasculine and nonbinary, transfeminine and nonbinary) using diagnoses, procedures, and drug claims.[13,14] Such algorithms have been found to have high sensitivity and specificity compared with electronic health records with self-reported gender identity.[15]

Despite their utility, claims-based methods of identifying TGD people have several limitations. Attempts to categorize people according to gender modality[2] will always underdetect TGD people, as not all TGD people receive a gender dysphoria–related diagnosis or medical gender-affirming care. Some TGD people may simply not want to receive medical gender-affirming care, whereas others may be unable to access care because of discrimination, safety concerns, or financial barriers.[16] Claims data are derived from a billing document and do not capture all subtleties of clinical care. For example, some providers may include a gender identity–related code for every service provided to a TGD patient, whereas others may include a code only when providing medicalized gender-affirming care. Finally, claims data are sensitive to hard-to-detect, systemic changes in an increasingly hostile TGD health care landscape. TGD patients may be less likely to come out to their providers, and providers might be more hesitant to bill using gender dysphoria or gender-affirming care codes.

A CASE STUDY

Classifying surgical care in claims as gender affirming poses unique challenges. Researchers must make assumptions about what surgeries occur for gender affirmation based on procedural and diagnosis codes. There are three issues we want to highlight that complicate the determination of whether a surgical claim documents gender-affirming care received by a TGD person. First, there are very few procedure codes that are specific to gender-affirming surgeries for TGD people.[17] Almost all procedures performed for gender affirmation for TGD people can be performed for other medical reasons for both TGD and cisgender people. For example, although rhinoplasties are clinically justified surgeries for gender affirmation for TGD people, they are also clinically justified for nasal injury for both TGD and cisgender people.[18] Table 1 lists the most frequent clinical justifications for several procedures that may be used for gender affirmation. (The supplementary material [available as a supplement to the online version of this article at http://www.ajph.org] details the methods used to create Table 1). Although TGD-related diagnoses appear in the top five clinical justifications for some of these procedures, they are frequently performed for other clinical reasons. In short, procedure codes alone do not typically provide enough information to determine whether a procedure is gender affirming.

Additionally, the receipt of surgical gender affirmation cannot be used to assume gender identity or modality. For example, cisgender males with gynecomastia, cisgender females, and TGD people might all use breast reduction surgery to affirm their gender (Table 1).[19] Therefore, researchers cannot use a procedure that may be gender affirming as a sole determining factor that someone is likely TGD.

Lastly, one procedure can be conducted for multiple reasons. For example, someone might seek a hysterectomy both to treat endometriosis and for gender affirmation.[20] Researchers cannot assume from claims data that all care TGD people receive, which may have been done for gender affirmation, was intended primarily or solely for gender affirmation.

RECOMMENDED APPROACH

We outline a five-step method that exemplifies the kinds of considerations required to undertake claims-based research on TGD populations, using the identification of gender-affirming surgery as a case study.

TABLE 1— Most Common Clinical Justifications for Breast Augmentation, Breast Reduction, Orchiectomy, and Oophorectomy/Hysterectomy: United States, 2019

Surgery and Clinical Justification	Claims, No. (%)
Breast augmentation (n = 2470)	
Neoplasm	1349 (54.6)
TGD gender dysphoria	485 (19.6)
Correction procedure	179 (7.2)
Other breast disorders	53 (2.1)
Cosmetic	49 (2.0)
Breast reduction (n = 41 951)	
Pain conditions	15 178 (36.2)
Neoplasm	12 007 (28.6)
Hypertrophy	6569 (15.7)
Gynecomastia	815 (1.9)
Correction procedure	724 (1.7)
Orchiectomy (n = 11 426)	
Neoplasm	3768 (33.0)
Other testicular disorder	3638 (31.8)
Undescended testicle	839 (7.3)
TGD gender dysphoria	572 (5.0)
Undescended testicle and other testicular disorders	433 (3.8)
Oophorectomy or hysterectomy (n = 119 061)	
Neoplasm	53 901 (45.3)
Endometriosis	14 798 (12.4)
Abnormal bleeding	6395 (5.4)
Prolapse	3607 (3.0)
Injury/trauma	2479 (2.1)

Note. TGD = transgender and gender diverse. The methodology is detailed in the supplement (available as a supplement to the online version of this article at http://www.ajph.org). We used *ICD-10* diagnosis codes associated with surgical claims to determine clinical justification (*International Classification of Diseases, 10th Revision*. Geneva, Switzerland: World Health Organization; 1992). When multiple diagnoses are listed, multiple diagnoses were present on the surgery claim.
Source. Data are from Inovalon Real-World Data.

Write Research Questions

Research conducted using TGD people's health data should aim to improve access, quality, safety, and the efficacy of TGD people's health care.[19] Claims-based TGD health research should be guided by TGD community input and should be conducted to maximize potential benefits and minimize potential harm to TGD communities.[8] In a moment when health care for TGD people is under attack across the United States, poorly conducted studies that reach spurious conclusions could be used to inappropriately restrict access to gender-affirming care for TGD populations. In the introduction and discussion sections of research articles, it is critical to contextualize the current evidence on the efficacy of gender-affirming care: it is lifesaving care for many TGD people. In particular, we caution against studies that posit the frequency of gender-affirming care as increasing or decreasing without providing appropriate comparison groups or contextual benchmarks because it disregards global health care trends.[21] We also caution against studies that consider the risks of gender-affirming care without discussion of the substantial evidence that barriers to accessing gender-affirming care has deleterious effects on TGD lives.[22] To ethically study gender-affirming care, researchers must consider the political context in which their research will be used.

Identify Associated Diagnoses

As we have detailed, multiple strategies can be used to identify patients as likely TGD.[11,14] When studying gender-affirming surgery, the simplest first step is to require a TGD-related diagnosis (e.g., a code in the F64 block, "gender identity disorders," among others, from the *International Classification of Diseases, 10th Revision* [Geneva, Switzerland: World Health Organization; 1992]) billed on the procedure code. This helps to ensure that the procedure may have been performed for gender affirmation.

Collate a List of Surgery Codes

There are no universally agreed-upon lists of codes used exclusively for coding gender-affirming surgery. For analyses specific to a single insurer or set of insurers, the best practice is to use the procedure codes listed in their gender-affirming care policies.[23] For other analyses, researchers should gather a list of codes from published research and insurance coverage documentation.

Determine Exclusions

Even when requiring TGD-related codes on surgery claims, researchers must determine when claims should be excluded. We recommend using a conservative approach to categorizing procedures as gender affirming, which involves compiling a list of diagnoses that could clinically justify the care being studied (e.g., cancer and other comorbidities) and using these diagnoses as exclusion criteria as appropriate for the analysis.[23] We also recommend excluding claims with intersex-related diagnosis codes. Research teams should include or consult with subject matter experts who can conduct a close case review of the gender-affirming surgeries when determining exclusion cases.

Exclusions have important methodological and ethical implications. Although exclusions do not allow researchers to determine whether someone is undergoing care for gender affirmation—a deeply personal experience—exclusions can help avoid misclassification of procedures likely being performed for other reasons. When applying the exclusions we have described to data from a national claims database in 2019 (i.e., Inovalon Real-World Data; Inovalon Holdings, Bowie, MD), we detected 17 439 claims associated with gender-affirming surgery on TGD adults. Without applying cancer, intersex, or other comorbidity-related exclusions, we identified 25 397 claims associated with gender-affirming surgery, 46% higher than with those exclusions.

Meticulous inclusion and exclusion are especially important when studying TGD populations, given the wide range of TGD people's medical histories and anatomies. One example of how these criteria may affect gender-affirming hormone research is that spironolactone, a medication used for gender affirmation, is also indicated for hypertension and heart failure; thus, researchers may choose to exclude spironolactone among TGD people with these conditions from gender-affirming hormone therapy studies.[14] Similarly, if a cohort does not include information to infer gender identity, progesterone-based medications may be misclassified as feminizing gender-affirming therapy when they are being used for contraception.[14]

Articulate Analysis Limitations

The sample of TGD individuals identifiable in claims data will always be a subset of the whole TGD population. When deciding on a study design, researchers should consider which TGD individuals can and cannot be identified through claims and assess the potential for bias in their results. For instance, if our research objective is to characterize utilization rates of gender-affirming surgery, the numerator—or number of gender-affirming surgeries—is likely to have high sensitivity given that most insurance companies require patients to have a TGD-related diagnosis for coverage of gender-affirming surgery. Determining an appropriate denominator is more difficult. Although counting the number of TGD people identified by the algorithm might be an intuitive denominator, it would likely produce a biased estimate. Individuals with more interactions with the health care system and those who have accessed gender-affirming care are the most likely to be accurately classified as TGD. This might artificially inflate the reported rate of surgical access. Given this bias alongside the inherent underdetection of TGD people in claims data, we caution against this type of TGD denominator and recommend less biased options (e.g., using a total population as the denominator[19]). Should researchers choose to use algorithmically identified TGD people as a denominator, the limitations of this approach should be enumerated in the research article's discussion.

Ensuring appropriate comparison groups is often an important component of analyses. First, to be used as a comparator, cisgender people in the data set should have at least some health care utilization (e.g., at least one outpatient visit in the study period) because health care utilization is necessary to identify TGD people via the algorithm.[23,24] Otherwise, TGD people will appear to have more utilization and a higher prevalence of disease than their cisgender counterparts. Second, when possible and reasonable, we recommend comparing similar types of care between cisgender and TGD people. Researchers should review insurance policies and ensure that studied care is similarly covered for TGD and cisgender cohorts. For instance, Dai et al. compared breast reduction utilization between TGD people and men inferred to be cisgender, as this surgery is commonly covered for TGD and cisgender adults and minors.[19]

CONCLUSIONS

The scientific nature of research on the health of TGD populations is under fire. Claims-based research offers large sample sizes, longitudinal follow-up, and comprehensive health and health care utilization data. It has enormous potential. However, using claims data for this purpose also presents methodological and ethical challenges that have yet to be comprehensively addressed in the scientific literature. Some of these methodological challenges could theoretically be addressed by the creation of more specific codes for gender-affirming procedures; however, more specific codes may make it easier for payers to deny care and make TGD individuals more identifiable to TGD-hostile administrations.[25]

We have used the identification of gender-affirming surgery as a case study to demonstrate five core considerations when constructing a methodologically robust and ethical analysis using claims-based data. First, researchers should formulate their research questions to maximize potential benefits and minimize potential harms to the TGD community, considering the context in which their work will be received. In the current political climate, in which efforts are ongoing to ban gender-affirming care and invalidate its efficacy, we recommend that all TGD health studies emphasize high-quality existing research and center new investigations on the well-established lifesaving nature of gender-affirming care. Second, claims-based research can only infer TGD identity from diagnoses and health care utilization. Researchers should be aware of existing methods of inferring TGD identity and design their analyses keeping the potential biases introduced by this inference in mind. Third, it is imperative to carefully define inclusion and exclusion criteria for identifying TGD-related care. No codes are uniquely used to bill for TGD medical utilization specifically, and inclusion and exclusion criteria should be precise and formulated based on expert clinical input. Lastly, researchers should design their studies with these data limitations and biases in mind.

Researchers looking to use claims data for TGD health research must make ethical decisions about the classification of gender-affirming care. To maximize the benefits of claims data, researchers should design analyses with thoughtful cohort selection and comparison groups, work with subject matter experts, and apply appropriate exclusions. Failure to do so risks significant harm, as can researchers' failure to explicitly consider the implications of not providing gender-affirming care in their interpretations and analyses. Researchers should evaluate whether their proposed study has the potential to benefit a marginalized group that already faces restrictions to lifesaving care. Consultations with TGD people, their health care providers, and other experts are crucial to determine the utility and health benefits of claims-based research. AJPH

CORRESPONDENCE

Correspondence should be sent to Gray Babbs, 121 S Main St, Providence, RI 02906 (e-mail: gray_babbs@brown.edu). Reprints can be ordered at https://www.ajph.org by clicking the "Reprints" link.

PUBLICATION INFORMATION

Full Citation: Babbs G, Dai D, Boskey ER, Balkan E, Hughto JMW. Challenges and best practices using claims data to study gender-affirming surgery in transgender and gender-diverse populations. *Am J Public Health*. 2025;115(10):1605–1610.

Acceptance Date: April 29, 2025.

DOI: https://doi.org/10.2105/AJPH.2025.308187

ORCID iDs:

Gray Babbs https://orcid.org/0000-0003-4060-571X

Elizabeth R. Boskey https://orcid.org/0000-0002-4982-1323

Em Balkan https://orcid.org/0009-0001-0333-9312

Jaclyn M. W. Hughto https://orcid.org/0000-0003-4722-8179

CONTRIBUTORS

G. Babbs and D. Dai drafted the article. D. Dai conducted the quantitative analysis. E. R. Boskey, E. Balkan, and J. M. W. Hughto critically revised the article for important intellectual content. All authors made substantial contributions to the conceptualization of the work and provided final approval for publication.

ACKNOWLEDGMENTS

J. M. W. Hughto was funded by the National Institute on Aging (grant 5R01AG073440) until the grant was terminated on March 21, 2025, because of its focus on gender, which is no longer a priority of the National Institutes of Health.

CONFLICTS OF INTEREST

The authors have no conflicts of interest to disclose.

HUMAN PARTICIPANT PROTECTION

The Harvard Longwood Campus institutional review board approved this research.

REFERENCES

1. Baker KE, Streed CG, Durso LE. Ensuring that LGBTQI+ people count—collecting data on sexual orientation, gender identity, and intersex status. *N Engl J Med*. 2021;384(13):1184–1186. https://doi.org/10.1056/NEJMp2032447
2. Ashley F, Brightly-Brown S, Rider GN. Beyond the trans/cis binary: introducing new terms will enrich gender research. *Nature*. 2024;630(8016):293–295. https://doi.org/10.1038/d41586-024-01719-9
3. Gaffney T. CDC will no longer process transgender data. February 25, 2025. Available at: https://www.statnews.com/2025/02/25/cdc-will-no-longer-process-transgender-data. Accessed March 9, 2025.
4. Lett E, Everhart A. Considerations for transgender population health research based on US national surveys. *Ann Epidemiol*. 2022;65:65–71. https://doi.org/10.1016/j.annepidem.2021.10.009
5. Reisner SL, Poteat T, Keatley J, et al. Global health burden and needs of transgender populations: a review. *Lancet*. 2016;388(10042):412–436. https://doi.org/10.1016/S0140-6736(16)00684-X
6. Blosnich JR, Brown GR, Shipherd JC, Kauth M, Piegari RI, Bossarte RM. Prevalence of gender identity disorder and suicide risk among transgender veterans utilizing Veterans Health Administration care. *Am J Public Health*. 2013;103(10):e27–e32. https://doi.org/10.2105/AJPH.2013.301507
7. Ashley F. Accounting for research fatigue in research ethics. *Bioethics*. 2021;35(3):270–276. https://doi.org/10.1111/bioe.12829
8. Alpert AB, Babbs G, Sanaeikia R, et al. Doing justice: ethical considerations identifying and researching transgender and gender diverse people in insurance claims data. *J Med Syst*. 2024;48(1):96. https://doi.org/10.1007/s10916-024-02111-w
9. World Health Organization. Gender incongruence and transgender health in the ICD. 2025. Available at: https://www.who.int/standards/classifications/frequently-asked-questions/gender-incongruence-and-transgender-health-in-the-icd. Accessed June 21, 2024.
10. Schall TE, Moses JD. Gender-affirming care for cisgender people. *Hastings Cent Rep*. 2023;53(3):15–24. https://doi.org/10.1002/hast.1486
11. Dragon CN, Guerino P, Ewald E, Laffan AM. Transgender Medicare beneficiaries and chronic

conditions: exploring fee-for-service claims data. *LGBT Health*. 2017;4(6):404–411. https://doi.org/10.1089/lgbt.2016.0208

12. Hughto JMW, Varma H, Babbs G, et al. Disparities in health condition diagnoses among aging transgender and cisgender Medicare beneficiaries, 2008–2017. *Front Endocrinol (Lausanne)*. 2023;14:1102348. https://doi.org/10.3389/fendo.2023.1102348
13. Jasuja GK, de Groot A, Quinn EK, et al. Beyond gender identity disorder diagnoses codes: an examination of additional methods to identify transgender individuals in administrative databases. *Med Care*. 2020;58(10):903–911. https://doi.org/10.1097/MLR.0000000000001362
14. Hughto JMW, Hughes L, Yee K, et al. Improving data-driven methods to identify and categorize transgender individuals by gender in insurance claims data. *LGBT Health*. 2022;9(4):254–263. https://doi.org/10.1089/lgbt.2021.0433
15. Streed CG, King D, Grasso C, et al. Validation of an administrative algorithm for transgender and gender diverse persons against self-report data in electronic health records. *J Am Med Inform Assoc*. 2023;30(6):1047–1055. https://doi.org/10.1093/jamia/ocad039
16. Safer JD, Coleman E, Feldman J, et al. Barriers to health care for transgender individuals. *Curr Opin Endocrinol Diabetes Obes*. 2016;23(2):168–171. https://doi.org/10.1097/MED.0000000000000227
17. Ganor O, Jolly D, Boskey ER. Nonsensical coding of gender-affirming procedures: a need for transgender-specific procedure codes. *J Am Coll Surg*. 2022;234(2):250–251. https://doi.org/10.1097/XCS.0000000000000015
18. Kim YH, Lee WS, Kim JW, Chung KJ. Cosmetic open rhinoplasty in acute nasal bone fracture with pre-existing deformity. *J Craniofac Surg*. 2023;34(4):e358–e363. https://doi.org/10.1097/SCS.0000000000009232
19. Dai D, Charlton BM, Boskey ER, et al. Prevalence of gender-affirming surgical procedures among minors and adults in the US. *JAMA Netw Open*. 2024;7(6):e2418814. https://doi.org/10.1001/jamanetworkopen.2024.18814
20. Vallée A, Feki A, Ayoubi JM. Endometriosis in transgender men: recognizing the missing pieces. *Front Med (Lausanne)*. 2023;10:1266131. https://doi.org/10.3389/fmed.2023.1266131
21. Wright JD, Chen L, Suzuki Y, Matsuo K, Hershman DL. National estimates of gender-affirming surgery in the US. *JAMA Netw Open*. 2023;6(8):e2330348. https://doi.org/10.1001/jamanetworkopen.2023.30348
22. van de Grift TC, Martens C, van Ginneken L, Mullender MG. Waiting for transgender care and its effects on health and equality: a mixed-methods population study in the Netherlands. *eClinicalMedicine*. 2024;73:102657. https://doi.org/10.1016/j.eclinm.2024.102657
23. Balkan E, Babbs G, Meyers DJ, et al. Gender-affirming surgery for transgender and gender diverse Medicare beneficiaries. *JAMA Netw Open*. 2025;8(5):e258072. https://doi.org/10.1001/jamanetworkopen.2025.8072
24. Babbs G, Hughto JMW, Shireman TI, Meyers DJ. Emergency department use disparities among transgender and cisgender Medicare beneficiaries, 2011–2020. *JAMA Intern Med*. 2024;184(4):443–445. https://doi.org/10.1001/jamainternmed.2023.8209
25. Macur J, Harmon A. Charges dropped against doctor who obtained records on minors' transgender care. *New York Times* Available at: https://www.nytimes.com/2025/01/26/us/trump-transgender-texas-doctor.html. January 27, 2025. Accessed March 10, 2025.

Beyond Prevention: How Gender-Affirming Care Can Transform HIV Outcomes for Transgender and Gender-Diverse Populations

Martha O. de la Paz, MPH, and Harry Barbee, PhD

ABOUT THE AUTHORS

At the time of this writing, Martha O. de la Paz was a student in the Bloomberg School of Public Health, Johns Hopkins University, Baltimore, MD. Harry Barbee is with the Department of Health, Behavior and Society, Bloomberg School of Public Health, Johns Hopkins University.

See also LGBTQ+ Transgender Health, pp. 1594–1670.

Transgender and gender-diverse (TGD) people, or those whose gender identities do not align with the gender typically attributed with their assigned sex at birth, are disproportionately affected by HIV, a reality that stems from complex social, legal, and structural inequities. For decades, public health efforts to address HIV have focused on prevention, treatment, and testing strategies, but many of these approaches have not considered the unique needs of TGD people.[1] A growing body of research shows that gender-affirming care for TGD individuals, including a comprehensive and personalized set of health care services that help people align their physical and mental health with their gender identity, is an essential component of achieving better health outcomes, particularly in the realm of HIV prevention and treatment.[2]

Access to gender-affirming care is crucial for improving HIV outcomes in TGD populations. Specifically, integration of gender-affirming care into HIV services can empower individuals, address long-standing health care inequities, and ultimately contribute to ending the HIV epidemic. Data overwhelmingly demonstrate that where gender-affirming care is available, HIV prevention and care outcomes improve, including stronger engagement with preexposure prophylaxis (PrEP), retention in HIV care, adherence to antiretroviral therapy (ART), and viral suppression.[2] However, major barriers such as lack of access to affirming care, discriminatory policies and practices, and insufficient health care infrastructure continue to prevent widespread adoption of this critical intervention.[3]

HIV DISPARITIES IN TRANSGENDER POPULATIONS

The global burden of HIV is acutely felt in TGD communities, particularly among transgender women.[2] For instance, one meta-analysis that examined worldwide HIV rates revealed a prevalence of 19.9% among transgender feminine individuals (i.e., people who were assigned male at birth but now identify with a feminine gender identity) and 2.56% among transgender masculine individuals (i.e., people who were assigned female at birth but now identify with a masculine gender identity).[4] Studies estimate that transgender women have 66 times the odds of reporting an HIV infection than the general population, with a global HIV prevalence rate of 19% in this group.[4] These staggering statistics reflect a constellation of risk factors that disproportionately affect TGD people, particularly transgender women, including higher rates of poverty, unemployment, homelessness, substance use, and involvement in sex work, all of which increase vulnerability to HIV exposure.[4]

Moreover, health care systems often fail to meet the needs of TGD individuals, exacerbating these vulnerabilities. Transgender people frequently face stigma and discrimination when seeking care, including being misgendered, denied services, or subjected to invasive questioning about their gender identity.[5,6] For instance, one 2022 survey of more than 92 000 TGD people in the United States showed that nearly half of all survey respondents who saw a health care provider in the preceding year experienced at least one negative interaction because of their gender identity, such as being refused care.[7] These burdens create barriers to accessing HIV prevention and treatment services such as PrEP, HIV testing, and ART.

HIV disparities are even more pronounced for TGD people of color. As an illustration, data collected by the Centers

AJPH October 2025, Vol. 115, No. 10

for Disease Control and Prevention from seven US cities revealed that the HIV prevalence was 62% among Black transgender women and 35% among Hispanic/Latina transgender women, as compared with 17% among White transgender women.[8] These statistics indicate that TGD women, particularly TGD women of color, are among the most at-risk groups for HIV infection globally.[4] This intersection of racial, gender, and health care inequities requires targeted interventions that address structural determinants of health, such as public policy and the organization of health care systems, and the individual needs of those most affected by HIV.

GENDER-AFFIRMING CARE IS MORE THAN MEDICAL INTERVENTION

At its core, gender-affirming care refers to a range of medical, social, psychological, and legal interventions that support TGD individuals in living authentically according to their gender identity.[2] These services can include hormone therapy, gender-affirming surgeries, mental health counseling, voice therapy, and legal support for name and gender marker changes on official documents. However, gender-affirming care often goes beyond medical procedures; it includes the development of health care environments where providers, practitioners, and staff treat TGD individuals with respect; where TGD people's gender identities are affirmed; and where their specific health needs are understood and addressed.

Gender-affirming care is highly relevant in the context of HIV prevention and treatment. For TGD individuals, access to gender-affirming care can be a vital entry point to the health care system, building trust and encouraging sustained engagement with HIV-related services.[9] Research consistently shows that when TGD people feel supported and affirmed in their gender identity by health care providers, they are more likely to access HIV testing, engage with PrEP, adhere to ART, and achieve viral suppression.[10–12]

Gender affirmation is not just a matter of identity; it is closely linked to health outcomes. Studies have shown that TGD individuals who receive gender-affirming care report better mental health and quality of life.[13] These psychosocial benefits, in turn, increase individuals' capacity to engage in health-promoting behaviors, including safer sex practices, consistent PrEP use, and ART adherence.[14] For many TGD patients, gender-affirming care offers a pathway to empowerment and health autonomy, helping to break the cycle of stigma and marginalization that often undermines HIV care.[2]

GENDER-AFFIRMING CARE IS INTEGRAL TO THE HIV CARE CONTINUUM

The HIV care continuum, which comprises the stages of HIV prevention, diagnosis, treatment, and viral suppression, is a useful framework for understanding how gender-affirming care can improve outcomes at each step. Across the continuum, TGD people experience disparities that are both driven by and exacerbated by inadequate access to affirming care.[1,3,7] Research indicates that access to gender-affirming care can optimize the effectiveness of the HIV care continuum by increasing PrEP uptake and adherence, encouraging regular screening, enhancing retention in care and ART adherence, and mitigating barriers to long-term health.[10–12]

Gender-affirming care plays a major role in HIV prevention, the first stage of the HIV care continuum. PrEP is a cornerstone of HIV prevention, yet many TGD individuals remain unaware of or unable to access this life-saving intervention. A 2019 study revealed that although 92% of transgender women in the United States without HIV were aware of PrEP, only 32% had used it.[8] Barriers to PrEP access include lack of knowledge, stigma, and concerns about drug interactions with gender-affirming hormone therapy.[15,16] Research has shown that when PrEP is integrated with gender-affirming care, uptake and adherence improve significantly.[2] In fact, in a focus group and interview study of transgender women living in the San Francisco Bay Area, researchers found that having a culturally competent medical provider was the most often cited facilitator of PrEP acceptability.[12] These findings suggest that by offering PrEP in a gender-affirming context, health care systems can improve both prevention and engagement in care.

Improvement of HIV testing and diagnosis, the second stage of the HIV care continuum, also goes hand in hand with greater access to gender-affirming care. Routine HIV testing is essential for early diagnosis and treatment, yet TGD individuals are less likely to be regularly tested than their cisgender counterparts.[17] Fear of discrimination and negative experiences with health care providers discourage many TGD people from seeking out testing services.[6,7] Gender-affirming care can play a pivotal role in reducing these barriers by creating environments where TGD people feel safe and respected. In fact, researchers often find that TGD patients who receive gender-affirming care are also significantly more likely to undergo regular HIV testing than those who lack access to such care.[10,18,19] This outcome demonstrates the potential of gender-affirming care to normalize HIV testing as part of routine health care for TGD populations.

Access to gender-affirming care can optimize HIV treatment, the third stage of the HIV care continuum, by enhancing retention in care and ART adherence. Retention in HIV care is important for achieving viral suppression, but many TGD individuals struggle to remain engaged in care as a result of discrimination, stigma, and competing priorities such as accessing gender-affirming hormone therapy.[1,2] Studies show that transgender women are less likely to be retained in HIV care than cisgender people with HIV.[1] However, when gender-affirming care is integrated with HIV treatment, retention rates improve.[2] By addressing the needs of the whole person, in terms of both gender identity and HIV care, integrated care models can reduce the drop off in engagement that often occurs in the HIV treatment cascade.

Achieving and maintaining viral suppression is the ultimate goal of HIV treatment, as it can improve individual health outcomes and reduce the likelihood of HIV transmission. For TGD individuals, however, achieving viral suppression can be particularly challenging, especially when access to gender-affirming care is limited.

One study of 858 transgender women of color with HIV showed that access to gender affirmation in health care mediated the relationship between experiencing transgender-related discrimination and viral suppression.[11] In other words, having access to gender-affirming care improved respondents' ability to achieve viral suppression despite other experiences of discrimination. The reasons for this outcome are multifaceted. For many TGD people, gender-affirming care is a prerequisite for overall well-being. When individuals are forced to prioritize either their gender-related health care or their HIV care, it can create a cycle of disengagement from both. Addressing this barrier requires health care models that integrate gender-affirming care with HIV services, ensuring that patients do not have to choose between the two.

EXPANDING GENDER-AFFIRMING CARE ACCESS

Despite the clear benefits of gender-affirming care for HIV prevention and treatment, many TGD individuals face significant barriers to accessing these services.[20] In the United States, discriminatory policies in many states have attempted to limit access to gender-affirming care, particularly for youths. These policies undermine the rights of TGD individuals but also represent a public health failure. To address these challenges, policymakers could take action to expand access to gender-affirming care and integrate it with HIV services. As described subsequently, specific policy developments that could expand access to gender-affirming care and, consequently, improve HIV outcomes include mandating insurance coverage, funding community-based health clinics, expanding provider training in TGD health, integrating gender-affirming care and HIV health services, and protecting TGD people against discrimination, particularly within the health care system.

Policies could require public and private insurers to cover gender-affirming care, including hormone therapy, surgeries, and mental health services, as medically necessary treatment. Many insurers currently classify gender-affirming treatments as elective, making these interventions inaccessible to many because of high out-of-pocket costs. Mandating coverage for these services as medically necessary ensures that TGD individuals can access the care they need without financial barriers. This policy also normalizes gender-affirming care within health care systems, reinforcing its legitimacy and necessity and fostering increased engagement with related health services such as HIV prevention and treatment.

Governments could also increase investments in community health centers that specialize in TGD health care. Community-based health clinics that specialize in TGD health care are uniquely positioned to address the complex needs of transgender individuals, particularly in underserved areas. These clinics often provide not only gender-affirming care but also culturally competent HIV prevention, testing, and treatment services in a welcoming environment. Expanding funding for these centers enables them to increase their reach, hire specialized staff, and offer integrated care tailored to TGD populations. In addition, investments in these clinics ensure that care is available to marginalized groups that may face barriers to accessing traditional health care systems, ultimately improving health equity and HIV outcomes.

Health care and medical organizations could implement stronger training requirements in TGD health for all providers, focusing on the principles of gender-affirming care and cultural competency. Such principles include respectful communication, use of correct names and pronouns, and an understanding of the distinct health needs of TGD populations. Equipping providers with cultural competency skills could enhance patient trust and increase the likelihood of TGD individuals seeking and remaining engaged in care. This approach is particularly crucial in HIV prevention and treatment, wherein relationships between providers and patients are foundational to long-term engagement and adherence.

Developing integrated care models that combine gender-affirming care with HIV prevention and treatment services addresses two critical health care needs of TGD populations in a single coordinated system.[2] Clinics offering integrated care create a streamlined experience for patients, reducing logistical and emotional barriers that can arise from navigating multiple providers. For example, pairing hormone therapy consultations with routine HIV testing or PrEP counseling can improve access and adherence to both gender-affirming and HIV-related care. This approach improves health outcomes and fosters a sense of community and support, making health care systems more inclusive and efficient.

Strengthening antidiscrimination laws is foundational to ensuring equitable access to health care for TGD individuals. Discrimination in medical settings not only deters TGD people from seeking care but also contributes to poorer health outcomes, including those related to HIV prevention and treatment.[2,6,7] Robust legal protections, including at the state level,[21] should prohibit health care providers from denying or delaying care on the basis of gender identity and ensure that all patients are treated with dignity and respect. These protections should be paired with mechanisms for enforcement and accountability, such as training requirements and penalties for violations, to create a health care environment where TGD individuals feel safe and valued.

CONCLUSION

HIV disparities among TGD populations are not inevitable; they are the consequence of systemic failures that can be mitigated and resolved through evidence-based interventions. Gender-affirming care is one such intervention, with the potential to transform HIV prevention and treatment among TGD individuals. By affirming identities, empowering individuals, and addressing structural barriers, gender-affirming care creates pathways to health and equity. Public health professionals, policymakers, and advocates have a responsibility to ensure that TGD people enjoy access to the care they need to thrive. Expanding access to gender-affirming care is not only a matter of justice; it is a public health imperative. AJPH

CORRESPONDENCE

Correspondence should be sent to Harry Barbee, PhD, 1812 Ashland Ave, Baltimore, MD 21205 (e-mail: hbarbee1@jh.edu). Reprints can be ordered at https://www.ajph.org by clicking the "Reprints" link.

PUBLICATION INFORMATION

Full Citation: de la Paz MO, Barbee H. Beyond prevention: how gender-affirming care can transform HIV outcomes for transgender and gender-diverse populations. *Am J Public Health*. 2025;115(10):1611–1615.

Acceptance Date: December 11, 2024.

DOI: https://doi.org/10.2105/AJPH.2024.307984

ORCID iDs:
Martha O. de la Paz https://orcid.org/0000-0002-3190-6118

Harry Barbee https://orcid.org/0000-0002-5000-0442

CONTRIBUTORS

M. O. de la Paz participated in the original conceptualization of the article, original draft writing, and revision and editing of the article. H. Barbee participated in original draft writing and revision and editing of the article.

ACKNOWLEDGMENTS

Harry Barbee was supported by the National Institutes of Health during the writing of this article (grants 1L60AG084090 and P30AG059298).

We thank the editors and anonymous reviewers for their valuable feedback throughout the peer review process.

Note. The opinions expressed in this article are the authors' own and do not reflect the view of the National Institutes of Health, the Department of Health and Human Services, or the United States government.

CONFLICTS OF INTEREST

Harry Barbee served as a public member of the Washington, DC, Board of Medicine during the time of this writing. Martha O. de la Paz has no disclosures of potential or actual conflicts of interest.

REFERENCES

1. Poteat T, Hanna DB, Rebeiro PF, et al. Characterizing the human immunodeficiency virus care continuum among transgender women and cisgender women and men in clinical care: a retrospective time-series analysis. *Clin Infect Dis.* 2020;70(6):1131–1138. https://doi.org/10.1093/cid/ciz322
2. Reisner SL, Radix A, Deutsch MB. Integrated and gender-affirming transgender clinical care and research. *J Acquir Immune Defic Syndr.* 2016;72(suppl 3):S235–S242. https://doi.org/10.1097/QAI.0000000000001088
3. Akré ERL, Barbee H, Lampe NM. Structural barriers to accessing gender-affirming care for transgender and gender diverse (TGD) individuals in the United States. Available at: https://www.tandfonline.com/doi/epdf/10.1080/26895269.2024.2431826?needAccess=true. Accessed December 20, 2024.
4. Stutterheim SE, van Dijk M, Wang H, Jonas KJ. The worldwide burden of HIV in transgender individuals: an updated systematic review and meta-analysis. *PLoS One.* 2021;16(12):e0260063. https://doi.org/10.1371/journal.pone.0260063
5. Grant JM, Mottet LA, Tanis J, Harrison J, Herman JL, Keisling M. *Injustice at Every Turn: A Report of the National Transgender Discrimination Survey.* Washington, DC: National Center for Transgender Equality and National Gay and Lesbian Task Force; 2011.
6. James SE, Herman JL, Rankin S, Keisling M, Mottet L, Anafi M. *The Report of the 2015 US Transgender Survey.* Washington, DC: National Center for Transgender Equality; 2016.
7. James SE, Herman JL, Durso LE, Heng-Lehtinen R. *Early Insights: A Report of the 2022 US Transgender Survey.* Washington, DC: National Center for Transgender Equality; 2024.
8. Centers for Disease Control and Prevention. HIV infection, risk, prevention, and testing behaviors among transgender women—national HIV behavioral surveillance, 7 US cities, 2019–2020. Available at: https://stacks.cdc.gov/view/cdc/105223. Accessed December 20, 2024.

9. Reisner SL, Poteat T, Keatley J, et al. Global health burden and needs of transgender populations: a review. *Lancet.* 2016;388(10042):412–436. https://doi.org/10.1016/S0140-6736(16)00684-X

10. McKay T, Tran NM, Barbee H, Min JK. Association of affirming care with chronic disease and preventive care outcomes among lesbian, gay, bisexual, transgender, and queer older adults. *Am J Prev Med.* 2023;64(3):305–314. https://doi.org/10.1016/j.amepre.2022.09.025

11. Sevelius J, Chakravarty D, Neilands TB, et al. Evidence for the model of gender affirmation: the role of gender affirmation and healthcare empowerment in viral suppression among transgender women of color living with HIV. *AIDS Behav.* 2021;25(suppl 1):64–71. https://doi.org/10.1007/s10461-019-02544-2

12. Sevelius JM, Keatley J, Calma N, Arnold E. "I am not a man": trans-specific barriers and facilitators to PrEP acceptability among transgender women. *Glob Public Health.* 2016;11(7-8):1060–1075. https://doi.org/10.1080/17441692.2016.1154085

13. White Hughto JM, Reisner SL. A systematic review of the effects of hormone therapy on psychological functioning and quality of life in transgender individuals. *Transgend Health.* 2016;1(1):21–31. https://doi.org/10.1089/trgh.2015.0008

14. Collins PY, Velloza J, Concepcion T, et al. Intervening for HIV prevention and mental health: a review of global literature. *J Int AIDS Soc.* 2021;24(suppl 2):e25710. https://doi.org/10.1002/jia2.25710

15. Sevelius JM, Deutsch MB, Grant R. The future of PrEP among transgender women: the critical role of gender affirmation in research and clinical practices. *J Int AIDS Soc.* 2016;19(7, suppl 6):21105. https://doi.org/10.7448/IAS.19.7.21105

16. Rael CT, Martinez M, Giguere R, et al. Barriers and facilitators to oral PrEP use among transgender women in New York City. *AIDS Behav.* 2018;22(11):3627–3636. https://doi.org/10.1007/s10461-018-2102-9

17. Pitasi MA, Oraka E, Clark H, Town M, DiNenno EA. HIV testing among transgender women and men—27 states and Guam, 2014–2015. *MMWR Morb Mortal Wkly Rep.* 2017;66(33):883–887. https://doi.org/10.15585/mmwr.mm6633a3

18. Andrzejewski J, Dunville R, Johns MM, Michaels S, Reisner SL. Medical gender affirmation and HIV and sexually transmitted disease prevention in transgender youth: results from the Survey of Today's Adolescent Relationships and Transitions, 2018. *LGBT Health.* 2021;8(3):181–189. https://doi.org/10.1089/lgbt.2020.0367

19. Lacombe-Duncan A, Kattari L, Kattari SK, et al. HIV testing among transgender and nonbinary persons in Michigan, United States: results of a community-based survey. *J Int AIDS Soc.* 2022;25(suppl 5):e25972. https://doi.org/10.1002/jia2.25972

20. Barbee H, Deal C, Gonzales G. Anti-transgender legislation—a public health concern for transgender youth. *JAMA Pediatr.* 2022;176(2):125–126. https://doi.org/10.1001/jamapediatrics.2021.4483

21. Barbee H, McKay T. Transgender youths and sanctuaries for gender-affirming care. *JAMA Health Forum.* 2023;4(12):e234244. https://doi.org/10.1001/jamahealthforum.2023.4244

Aging Amidst Anti-Trans Legislation: Strategies for Safeguarding the Mental Health of Transgender Older Adults

Nik M. Lampe, PhD, and J. E. Sumerau, PhD

See also LGBTQ+ Transgender Health, pp. 1594–1670.

This study investigates how transgender older adults manage and protect their mental health amid anti-trans stigma, discrimination, and legislation in the United States. Using semi-structured, individual interviews with 47 transgender older adults, two key strategies emerged: (1) defining transgender identities, bodies, and experiences as life-affirming; and (2) cultivating transgender-inclusive social support networks. Results from the study expand public health research by pinpointing the mental health management strategies that transgender older adults use to mitigate the negative impacts of anti-trans sociopolitical climates. (*Am J Public Health*. 2025;115(10):1616–1620. https://doi.org/10.2105/AJPH.2025.308186)

AJPH October 2025, Vol. 115, No. 10

There has been a rise in anti-transgender (hereafter, anti-trans) legislation in the United States.[1,2] Anti-trans legislation refers to laws that legalize societal exclusion and discrimination, restrict constitutional rights, and hinder access to spaces and services for transgender (hereafter, trans) people.[3] Some examples include (1) gender-affirming care bans, (2) denying trans people the use of public facilities that correspond with their gender identity, and (3) gender change bans for government documentation.[4,5] As of early 2025, such legislative patterns show no sign of slowing down.

These conditions have harmful mental health effects not only for trans people in general[1,6] but for trans older adults.[7] Trans older individuals experience significant mental health disparities compounded by sociohistorical contexts (e.g., HIV/AIDS epidemic) during which they face ongoing anti-trans discrimination.[8] Furthermore, lack of legal protections can hinder trans older adults' access to quality age-related care.[9,10] Prior research largely overlooks this population when examining the public health implications of anti-trans legislation.

STUDY OBJECTIVES

Semi-structured interviews were conducted with trans older adults in the United States (n = 47) to understand how they protect their mental health. This topic emerged thematically as respondents shared experiences.

RESEARCH QUESTION

How do transgender older adults maintain and protect their mental health amid anti-trans stigma, discrimination, and legislation in the United States?

PARTICIPANTS, SAMPLE, GEOGRAPHIC LOCATION, SETTING, AND YEAR OF STUDY

Between September 2021 and January 2022, N. M. L. conducted interviews with 47 trans older adults in the United States. Respondents were eligible if they (1) self-identified as transgender or nonbinary, (2) were aged 65 years or older, (3) resided in the United States, and (4) consented to audio-recording. Self-reported demographics are in Table 1.

To ensure participant safety during COVID-19, N. M. L. conducted 37 interviews via Zoom and 10 by telephone. Interviews lasted 1 hour and 38 minutes on average.

TABLE 1— Demographic Characteristics of Individual Interview Respondents: United States, September 2021–January 2022

Broad Demographic Category and Specific Demographic Identification	No. of Participants (%)
Gender identity	
Transgender woman[a]	27 (57.0)
Transsexual woman	1 (2.0)
Transgender man	10 (22.0)
Transgender	1 (2.0)
Nonbinary	3 (6.0)
Blended-gender	1 (2.0)
Pangenderfluid	1 (2.0)
Two-spirit	2 (4.0)
Questioning	1 (2.0)
Age, y	
65–69[a]	32 (68.0)
70–74	7 (15.0)
75–79	7 (15.0)
80–84	1 (2.0)
Sex	
Intersex	13 (28.0)
Endosex (not intersex)[a]	34 (72.0)
Sexuality	
Lesbian[a]	16 (34.0)
Bisexual	10 (21.0)
Heterosexual	6 (13.0)
Asexual	4 (9.0)
Gay	4 (9.0)
Pansexual	3 (6.0)
Queer	3 (6.0)
Flux	1 (2.0)
Race/ethnicity	
Black, non-Hispanic/Latino	6 (13.0)
White, Hispanic/Latino	3 (6.0)
Multiracial, Indigenous, non-Hispanic/Latino	1 (2.0)
Multiracial, Hispanic/Latino	1 (2.0)
Multiracial, non-Hispanic/Latino	2 (4.0)
White, non-Hispanic/Latino[a]	34 (73.0)
Social class	
Low income	8 (17.0)
Working class	7 (15.0)
Middle class[a]	29 (62.0)
Upper class	1 (2.0)
Opted not to answer	2 (4.0)

Note. The sample size was n = 47.
[a]Modal category for each self-reported demographic category.

METHODS

The study team consisted of N. M. L. and J. E. S. Respondents were recruited through social media and snowball sampling from LGBTQIA+ health clinics, aged care facilities, LGBTQIA+-affirming faith communities, and LGBTQIA+ community centers. N. M. L. developed and pretested the interview guide to ensure it was culturally appropriate. N. M. L. conducted 47 interviews where respondents discussed (1) health care, (2) end-of-life planning, and (3) health needs and management. Respondents received $40 for participation.

Interviews were audio-recorded and transcribed using NVivo Transcription software (Lumivero, Denver, CO). Transcriptions were then carefully reviewed and checked for accuracy by both authors, with all personally identifiable information removed.

Qualitative analyses were conducted by N. M. L. and J. E. S. using NVivo 15 software and thematic analysis.[11] We independently performed initial coding by reviewing a subset of transcripts to generate preliminary codes. We then compared our initial codes and collaboratively developed a coding scheme. Next, we carried out focused and thematic coding, identifying overlaps and divergences to refine and consolidate codes into broader themes. Disconfirming evidence was also identified during this phase, and we developed overall themes that highlighted patterns and connections.

We drew on analytic memos, recurring themes, and existing literature to guide our analysis in relation to the present study's research question: "If any, what are some strategies you use to manage or protect your mental health with this recent uptick in anti-trans legislation?"

KEY FINDINGS

Almost all respondents maintained and protected their mental health amid anti-trans stigma, discrimination, and legislation through two strategies: (1) defining transgender identities, bodies, and experiences as positive and life-affirming, and (2) cultivating transgender-inclusive social support networks. Box 1 provides additional examples.

Defining Trans Identities and Experiences

Many respondents reported struggling with mental health challenges (e.g., suicidal ideation) exacerbated by anti-trans messaging. Consequently, they defined being trans as a positive and satisfying way of aging—by explaining how "coming out" or otherwise "becoming or living as trans" was necessary for them to have a life worth living. Respondents explained how they continued to publicly disclose their gender identities and transition as a means of improving their mental health. Many described their trans experiences as "life-saving," "transformative," "necessary," and even "sacred." They also emphasized how access to gender-affirming care (e.g., hormone therapies) and sociolegal services (e.g., legal gender marker changes) was essential not only for their survival but also for thriving. Despite self-reported difficulties, living openly as trans fostered a sense of life fulfillment and mental clarity for respondents.

- "I had been dealing with depression most of my adult life without really recognizing it. . . . I started cross-dressing . . . and found that I felt better about myself when I did that . . . so I started doing that more . . . openly, if you will. And in doing so, I realized this was how I really wanted to live my life." —Gail
- "I'm really fortunate. You're going to hear all the negative, but even when there were issues, I needed to do this. It was like a religious thing, a rite of passage. And you get there, you realize it is positive. And then, my family accepted it. Most of my friends did, some didn't. That's too bad, but this was the right thing. It's what I needed to have a real life, so I just go about my business now." —Scott

Cultivating Trans-Inclusive Social Support

Respondents highlighted the importance of building transgender-inclusive support networks to protect their mental health and meet their own needs for age-related caregiver support. Many, especially those without quality caregiver support, turned to "families of choice" or

BOX 1— Examples of Illustrative Quotes From Interview Respondents: United States, September 2021–January 2022

Themes	Additional Illustrative Quotes
Defining transgender identities, bodies, and experiences as life-affirming	"I had to understand that transition was the right thing. . . . I needed it, I needed to be who I was supposed to be, I had to see that. . . . And that, that was a big turning point in my, my health. . . . Almost like I want to live because I want to be myself, it's all connected like that" —Fawn
	"I thought, for most of my life, I thought it was only me, which is absolutely ridiculous. It was pretty traumatic. So, how I came out of that kind of trauma was. . . . Well, I decided I needed to live a life that I love." —Bonnie
	"I've known for a long time that coming out as transgender was a possibility. It wasn't until about 5 years ago that I decided I needed to take that step. That's the process I went through. I knew from the moment I realized it was possible and that others were doing it, that it was something I could do. I knew what I was." —Gary
Cultivating transgender-inclusive social support networks	"So, you almost had the sense of paranoia every time you just stepped out on the street, [and] went out in public. Eventually, you know, get over that. . . . I did the thing that [trans] folks usually did, I changed my name first and then after surgery . . . got a birth certificate change and . . . so wonderful that I was able to accomplish that. . . . I find that most, most of my [health care] professionals are helping professionals and you know, they want to help [if you] give them the chance. . . . And that's, that's part of it, you know, you meet people, and they help you or give you recommendations . . . you have to rely on that, you need them." —Linda
	"I have a number of good friends who are certainly there for me. All of whom are . . . other trans females. . . . I always have someone there within my circle of friends." —Jane
	"I do have a trans therapist [to cope with anti-trans politics]. I've been seeing not them all the time kind of irregularly as needed. . . . She's very supportive. And outside of that . . . I can talk openly with any of my kids. And their mom is in a wonderful marriage. She married one of my closer friends and we're all still friends. . . . So it's pretty healthy. I think the world I inhabit . . . there's no open toxicity. And that's really important to me." —Yvette

Note. The sample size was n = 47.

"chosen families"—supportive individuals who are not legally or biologically related (e.g., friends and LGBTQIA+ community members). These networks were most often formed in structured settings (i.e., support groups, LGBTQIA+ community events). In such settings, respondents received invaluable emotional, logistical, and financial support (e.g., rent assistance, transportation to medical appointments), helping them cope with the mental health effects of anti-trans politics.

- "I found an online support group, and they were really helpful. . . . This past legislative session. . . . It was pretty traumatic. So, how I came out of that kind of trauma, was . . . I decided I needed to live a life that I love." —Bonnie
- "The AA [Alcoholics Anonymous] helps a lot [with coping with anti-trans stigma]. I'm involved with two groups, two trans groups that meet multiple times a week. . . . But I also go out to . . . we have a [LGBTQ+ older adult group] here that has a party every week. . . . It's a lot of fun. I get a lot of support from them." —Helen

EVALUATION, TRANSFERABILITY, AND ADVERSE EFFECTS

This study offers insight into how transgender older adults protect their mental health amid anti-trans legislation. Although we employed a thematic qualitative approach with a convenience sample, findings reveal that trans older adults maintain and protect their mental health even in suboptimal conditions. These findings can be transferable to other trans subpopulations and trans people in international contexts.[12] Furthermore, helping transgender older adults create and sustain chosen families can be a crucial buffer for them, especially in hostile times.[13] This may also be part of potential solutions to the LGBTQIA+ family caregiver availability crisis.[8]

Regarding adverse or unintended negative results, a small minority of respondents reported that anti-trans politics did not negatively affect them. They attributed this to specific anti-trans discourses (e.g., belief that trans minors are "too young" to medically transition) or social privileges (e.g., White privilege) they held. Respondents utilized similar wordings to explain these points, and we noticed the pattern when comparing interviews. It is likely that aspects of the sample, such as it being mostly White and middle-class, influenced responses. In fact, such racial and class privileges likely aided their ability to find structured social groups for support and lessened their chances of facing the worst aspects of anti-trans discrimination.[3] Future research should explore how different samples navigate these questions.

SCALABILITY

This study could be scaled to include a larger, more representative sample of transgender older adults by employing larger qualitative studies or cross-sectional and longitudinal designs. This approach could be extended to specific US regions or other countries.

PUBLIC HEALTH SIGNIFICANCE

Transgender older adults face anti-trans attitudes and policies,[14] which exacerbate mental health disparities.[6,7] Interviewees reported safeguarding their mental health by defining their trans experiences as life-affirming and cultivating trans-inclusive support networks. These strategies did not rely on traditional behavioral health care systems. Rather, these are strategies trans older adults have developed to maintain positive mental health at times when they cannot necessarily rely on behavioral health services. This study highlights how trans individuals safeguard their mental health, even in the face of sociopolitical efforts that make it significantly more challenging.

These results underscore the need for combatting anti-trans environments and for fostering mental health strategies that medically underserved populations develop outside of the normative health apparatus.[15] This may involve efforts to pass more trans-inclusive legislation at all levels of government as well as attempts to pass local and state policies capable of protecting trans populations from national anti-trans legislation. It may also involve governmental and private-sector efforts to facilitate more structured social opportunities (like support groups, online communities, book clubs, etc.) for trans older adults. Such efforts will require political mobilization capable of advocating for older trans people's health needs. AJPH

ABOUT THE AUTHORS

Nik M. Lampe is with the Department of Behavioral Health Science & Practice, University of South Florida, Tampa, Florida. J. E. Sumerau is with the Department of Sociology at the University of Tampa, Tampa, Florida.

CORRESPONDENCE

Correspondence should be sent to Nik M. Lampe, Department of Behavioral Health Science & Practice, University of South Florida, 13301 Bruce B. Downs Blvd, Tampa, FL 33612 (e-mail: nlampe@usf.edu). Reprints can be ordered at http://www.ajph.org by clicking the "Reprints" link.

PUBLICATION INFORMATION

Full Citation: Lampe NM, Sumerau JE. Aging amidst anti-trans legislation: strategies for safeguarding the mental health of transgender older adults. *Am J Public Health*. 2025;115(10): 1616–1620.

Acceptance Date: April 29, 2025.

DOI: https://doi.org/10.2105/AJPH.2025.308186

ORCID iD:

Nik M. Lampe https://orcid.org/0000-0003-1692-6740

CONTRIBUTORS

N. M. Lampe performed conceptualization, data curation, formal analysis, funding acquisition, investigation, methodology, project administration, resource acquisition, software, supervision, validation, visualization, writing the original draft, and reviewing and editing the writing. J. E. Sumerau performed conceptualization, formal analysis, investigation, methodology, resource acquisition, supervision, validation, visualization, writing the original draft, and reviewing and editing the writing.

ACKNOWLEDGMENTS

This research benefited from the financial support of the University of South Carolina Office of the Vice President for Research. N. M. Lampe was also supported by the Alzheimer's Association (N. M. Lampe, principal investigator; AARFD-23-1145127) during the manuscript preparation and submission of this article.

Note. The views expressed in this article are our own and do not necessarily represent the official views of the Alzheimer's Association or the University of South Carolina.

CONFLICTS OF INTEREST

The authors have no conflicts of interest to declare.

HUMAN PARTICIPANT PROTECTION

This research study was approved by the University of South Carolina institutional review board.

REFERENCES

1. Lee WY, Hobbs JN, Hobaica S, DeChants JP, Price MN, Nath R. State-level anti-transgender laws increase past-year suicide attempts among transgender and non-binary young people in the USA. *Nat Hum Behav*. 2024;8(11):2096–2106. https://doi.org/10.1038/s41562-024-01979-5
2. Trans Legislation Tracker. Tracking the rise of anti-trans bills in the US. Available at: https://translegislation.com/learn. Accessed December 14, 2024.
3. Lampe NM, Rodill ZE, Nowakowski ACH. "My support groups . . . have saved my life": facilitators of positive or satisfactory experiences in behavioral healthcare for transgender and gender nonconforming older adults. *Aging Ment Health*. 2025; 29(1):167–175. https://doi.org/10.1080/13607863.2024.2377261
4. Barbee H, Deal C, Gonzales G. Anti-transgender legislation—a public health concern for transgender youth. *JAMA Pediatr*. 2022;176(2):125–126. https://doi.org/10.1001/jamapediatrics.2021.4483
5. *United States v Skrmetti*. (US Supreme Court.) Available at: https://www.supremecourt.gov/search.aspx?filename=/docket/docketfiles/html/public/23-477.html. Accessed December 14, 2024.
6. Restar A, Layland EK, Hughes L, et al. Antitrans policy environment and depression and anxiety symptoms in transgender and nonbinary adults. *JAMA Netw Open*. 2024;7(8):e2431306. https://doi.org/10.1001/jamanetworkopen.2024.31306
7. Nowakowski ACH, Sumerau JE, Lampe NM. *Transformations in Queer, Trans, and Intersex Health and Aging*. Idaho Falls, ID: Lexington Books; 2020.
8. Lampe NM, Barbee H, Tran NM, Bastow S, McKay T. Health disparities among lesbian, gay, bisexual, transgender, and queer older adults: a structural competency approach. *Int J Aging Hum Dev*. 2024; 98(1):39–55. https://doi.org/10.1177/00914150231171838
9. Hiedemann B, Brodoff L. Increased risks of needing long-term care among older adults living with same-sex partners. *Am J Public Health*. 2013;103(8): e27–e33. https://doi.org/10.2105/AJPH.2013.301393
10. Perone AK. Protecting health care for transgender older adults amidst a backlash of US federal policies. *J Gerontol Soc Work*. 2020;63(8):743–752. https://doi.org/10.1080/01634372.2020.1808139
11. Charmaz K. *Constructing Grounded Theory*. 2nd ed. Thousand Oaks, CA: Sage; 2014.
12. Tanner AE, Goldenberg T, Erausquin JT, Mertus S, Jibriel MSE, Barrington C. Measuring anti-transgender stigma in low-income and middle-income countries: a scoping review protocol. *BMJ Open*. 2022;12(7):e061691. https://doi.org/10.1136/bmjopen-2022-061691
13. Flatt JD, Cicero EC, Kittle KR, Brennan-Ing M. Recommendations for advancing research with sexual and gender minority older adults. *J Gerontol B Psychol Sci Soc Sci*. 2022;77(1):1–9. https://doi.org/10.1093/geronb/gbab127
14. Bradford J, Reisner SL, Honnold JA, Xavier J. Experiences of transgender-related discrimination and implications for health: results from the Virginia Transgender Health Initiative Study. *Am J Public Health*. 2013;103(10):1820–1829. https://doi.org/10.2105/AJPH.2012.300796
15. Restar AJ, Baker K, Wang G, Ashley K, Damian AJ. Community health workers as catalysts for mental health promotion in transgender and nonbinary communities. *Am J Public Health*. 2025;115(1):34–36. https://doi.org/10.2105/AJPH.2024.307898

Addressing Transgender Erasure in HIV Clinical Trials: The Scorecard for Transgender and Gender-Diverse Inclusion

Brian Minalga, MSW, and Cindra Feuer

See also LGBTQ+ Transgender Health, pp. 1594–1670.

We sought to offer a structured framework for evaluating transgender and gender-diverse (TGD) inclusion in HIV clinical trials, with actionable criteria for trial design and conduct, and to quantify and characterize TGD inclusion in pivotal HIV studies as supporting evidence of the need for this framework.

We devised a tool (scorecard) consisting of 14 scoreable indicators for TGD-responsive HIV research with input from global TGD communities. We tested the scorecard in a cross-sectional review of 41 randomized controlled HIV biomedical efficacy trials to measure TGD responsiveness. Studies were selected to represent the spectrum of groundbreaking HIV therapeutic and prevention studies enrolling participants in countries around the world from 1991 to 2023. We found that TGD individuals represent a reported 2532 (1.4%) of 178 893 participants in the selected HIV clinical trials.

Scorecard indicators reveal a dearth of HIV research responsive to the needs of TGD communities. The lack of TGD representation in HIV clinical trials indicates a historical erasure of TGD communities with potential public health consequences. The scorecard might guide future HIV research to be more responsive to the needs of TGD people. (*Am J Public Health*. 2025;115(10):1621–1630. https://doi.org/10.2105/AJPH.2025.308134)

AJPH October 2025, Vol. 115, No. 10

Transgender and gender-diverse (TGD) people are a key population in the global HIV response. Estimates suggest that global HIV incidence is 66 times higher for transgender women (TGW), 7 times higher for transgender men (TGM), and unknown for gender nonbinary (GNB) people relative to the adult population overall.[1] Global HIV prevalence among TGD people is 9.2% on average and as high as 58% in some locations.[2] Despite these disparities, TGD people are underrepresented in HIV research. Trials conducted among cisgender people may not be generalizable to TGD people; TGD communities face unique social, biological, and epidemiological conditions, many of which remain underexplored.[3–5]

The exclusion of TGD individuals from clinical trials prevents opportunities for TGD communities to receive investigational interventions and may also hinder access to approved medical products. In the DISCOVER study, the exclusion of people assigned female at birth had the unintended consequence of limiting regulatory approval of a novel HIV prophylactic regimen to people assigned male at birth only; cisgender women, TGM, and GNB people assigned female at birth remained excluded from clinical guidelines for this HIV prevention option at the time of the writing of this article.[6] This example illustrates how a lack of diversity in clinical trials can burden medical decision-making in clinic settings where questions about managing safety and certain pharmacological interactions (e.g., approved medications and exogenous hormone therapy) may not be supported by data. Considering HIV's disproportionate impact on TGD communities, HIV research must be optimized to better respond to the needs of TGD people.

We sought to devise an evidence-based guidance tool to support the inclusion of TGD people and their priorities in the design and implementation of future HIV clinical trials. We also sought to provide further supporting evidence of the need for such a tool by measuring the extent to which a cross section of HIV clinical trials have been inclusive of and responsive to the needs of TGD communities. Here we present the HIV Research Scorecard for TGD Inclusivity (hereafter Scorecard) and findings from our review of TGD representation in 41 global HIV clinical trials conducted over the past 30 years.

METHODS

The Manifesto to Align HIV Prevention Research with Trans and Gender Diverse Realities[7] was released in 2021. This document represents the culmination of literature reviews, surveys, workshops, and interviews with more than 35 TGD individuals including communities of people with HIV, health care providers, and researchers in 27 countries around the world. Contributors were queried on research gaps and needs among TGD communities, resulting in recommendations for aligning HIV research with the lived experiences of TGD individuals and communities.

The manifesto's recommendations were recognized as a strength, but its expansive format was a potential limitation of its impact. To support the practical application of the manifesto, we removed narrative text, reduced the document to its recommendations, combined overlapping components, and ultimately synthesized it into a single-page scorecard consisting of 14 yes-or-no indicators spanning 4 domains of clinical trials: study design, study implementation, study reporting, and language. Together, these indicators constitute the Scorecard (Figure 1).

We tested the Scorecard in a cross-sectional review of HIV clinical trials. Eligibility criteria for the review included randomized controlled biomedical efficacy trials inclusive of therapeutic and prevention studies. We excluded HIV cure studies because of the lack of large, randomized efficacy studies with critical findings in this arena. Eligible studies were further narrowed down to include the most recognizable trials with breakthrough pivotal findings essential to the field, including the first trials to formally demonstrate that antiretroviral therapy regimens conferred clinical and survival benefits, the studies underpinning treatment as prevention ("undetectable equals untransmittable"), the majority of HIV vaccine efficacy studies, studies demonstrating proof of concept for broadly neutralizing antibodies for prevention, studies leading to the approval of oral and injectable preexposure prophylaxis, and a selection of additional novel preexposure prophylaxis studies incorporating a variety of microbicide and long-acting injectable formulations.

To improve the representativeness of our sample, we also chose to include studies with a variety of results (e.g., those demonstrating efficacy, futility, and superiority). On the basis of these criteria, a literature review, and database searches on ClinicalTrials.gov[8] and the clinical trials database maintained by AVAC,[9] we selected 41 studies to evaluate for TGD responsiveness using the Scorecard's 14 indicators. Table 1 presents the 41 studies included in this review; citations for the selected studies are available in the appendix (available as a supplement to the online version of this article at http://www.ajph.org). Source documents for our review included study protocols, study publications, study records hosted on ClinicalTrials.gov, conference presentations, and e-mail correspondence with investigators involved in selected trials.

RESULTS

The 41 trials included in this analysis reported a cumulative total of 178 893 study participants. We categorized participants as TGD when source documents explicitly identified TGD participation (e.g., number of "transgender women") or provided data on participants' sex assigned at birth that could be cross referenced with self-reported gender identity (e.g., participants assigned female sex at birth and identifying as male were classified as TGM). We classified cisgender participants in the same manner (i.e., the number of participants explicitly identified in source documents as "cisgender" or participants whose reported sex matched their reported gender identity). In one study, participants could select more than one gender identity; we were able to collapse multiple selections into a single category for all participants in that study (e.g., participants who selected "gender queer" and "gender variant" were categorized as gender nonbinary).

On the basis of the information available, 2532 (1.4%) participants could be categorized as TGD. Within this group, the largest percentage was made up of 2042 (80.6%) TGW, followed by 398 (15.7%) GNB individuals and 92 (3.6%) TGM. Cisgender people represent 42 905 (24.0%) of total participants, including 29 668 cisgender men and 13 237 cisgender women. The remaining 133 456 (74.6%) participants could not be categorized as TGD or cisgender because of ambiguous definitions of the study population (see the Study Design section), the studies' failure to

HIV Research Scorecard for Trans and Gender-Diverse Inclusivity

Study Design

		YES 1 pt	NO/Not Available 0 pt
1.	Eligibility criteria explicitly include gender nonbinary individuals.		
2.	Eligibility criteria explicitly include transgender men.		
3.	Eligibility criteria explicitly include transgender women.		
4.	If gender nonbinary individuals, trans men, or trans women are not included, their exclusion is explicitly justified.		
5.	Specific and measurable goals are set for the enrollment of TGD participants, either in absolute numbers or as a percentage of total participants.		
6.	Gender-affirming hormone use is accounted for as a variable (e.g., in eligibility criteria, safety monitoring, efficacy, drug-drug interactions, etc.).		

Study Implementation

7.	TGD status is ascertained in data collection using best practices (e.g., DAIDS TGD Working Group[a] or similar).		
8.	Outreach, marketing, and recruitment strategies and materials clearly exemplify TGD eligibility and inclusion.		
9.	TGD staff are included among the core study team and/or among research site staff.		
10.	Sites selected to recruit for the study have proven experience working with TGD communities.		
11.	The study includes a community engagement plan that involves partnerships with organizations serving TGD communities to foster engagement.		

Study Reporting

12.	Participant TGD status is readily ascertained in study publications, presentations, and reporting using best practices (e.g., DAIDS TGD Working Group[a] or similar).		
13.	TGD-specific safety and efficacy analyses are reported in study findings.		

Language

14.	All study-related documents, outreach materials, and study-led communications adhere to best practices in gender-inclusive language as outlined in the *NIAID HIV Language Guide*.[b]		

SCORE — TOTAL = [YES] + [NO] = [ ]

A. 11-13 points — B. 8-10 points — C. 4-7 points — D. 1-3 points — F. 0 points

FIGURE 1— HIV Research Scorecard for Transgender and Gender-Diverse (TGD) Inclusivity

[a]National Institute of Allergy and Infectious Diseases Division of AIDS Cross-Network Transgender and Gender-Diverse Working Group. Data collection: gender identity, sex assigned at birth, intersex status, and sexual orientation. https://www.hanc.info/resources/sops-guidelines-resources/community.html#trans.
[b]National Institute of Allergy and Infectious Diseases. NIAID HIV Language Guide. https://www.thebody.com/hiv/niaid-hiv-language-guide.

collect or clearly report demographic data (see the Study Reporting section), 5 ambiguous participant responses (i.e., self-reporting "female sex at birth" and "transgender male to female" gender identity or vice versa), and 30 participants who declined to report their gender identity. Focusing only on the 45 437 participants who could be categorized, TGD individuals represented 5.6% of participants, as compared with 94.4% cisgender individuals.

The first study reporting TGD enrollment was the Preexposure Prophylaxis Initiative (iPrEx) study, which began enrolling participants in 2007. Therefore, all identifiable TGD enrollment took place during the second half of the analyzed period from 2007 to 2023, when most of the studies occurred (n = 32). All 2532 TGD participants were distributed across 12 studies (Figure 2).

TABLE 1— Summary of Findings From Cross-Sectional Scorecard Review of 41 Pivotal Global HIV Clinical Trials, 1991–2023

	Score	Indicators Achieved	TGD Enrollment[a]
A-grade studies (11–13 points)			
PURPOSE 2 (2022–2023)	12/13	1, 2, 3, 5, 6, 7, 8, 9, 10, 11, 12, 14	728/3271 (209 GNB, 43 TGM, 476 TGW)
IMPOWER-024 (2021–2022)	11/13	1, 3, 4, 5, 6, 7, 8, 10, 11, 12, 14	42/494 (20 GNB, 22 TGW)
B-grade studies (8–10 points)			
HPTN 083 (2016–2020)	10/13	3, 5, 6, 8, 9, 10, 11, 12, 13, 14	570/4566 (570 TGW)
HVTN 706 (2019–2021)	10/13	1, 2, 3, 6, 7, 8, 9, 10, 11, 12	323/3887 (70 GNB, 14 TGM, 239 TGW)
HVTN 704/HPTN 085 (2016–2018)	8/13	2, 3, 6, 7, 8, 9, 10, 11	254/2699 (60 GNB, 17 TGM, 177 TGW)
C-grade studies (4–7 points)			
REPRIEVE (2015–2019)	6/13	1, 2, 3, 7, 12, 13	129/7770 (37 GNB, 7 TGM, 85 TGW)
DISCOVER (2016–2017)	5/13	3, 6, 12, 13, 14	74/5387 (74 TGW)
HVTN 702 (2016–2019)	5/13	1, 2, 3, 7, 12	21/5404 (2 GNB, 3 TGM, 16 TGW)
iPrEx (2007–2009)	5/13	3, 6, 8, 12, 13	339/2499 (339 TGW)
PARTNER 2 (2010–2017)	5/13	2, 4, 7, 12, 14	3/1564 (3 TGM)
IMPOWER-022 (2021–2022)	4/13	4, 7, 12, 14	0/730
PURPOSE 1 (2021–2023)	4/13	4, 7, 12, 14	0/5345
D-grade studies (1–3 points)			
HVTN 505 (2009–2013)	3/13	3, 6, 12	44/2496 (44 TGW)
HVTN 703/HPTN 081 (2016–2018)	3/13	4, 7, 12	0/1924
HVTN 502 (2005–2007)	2/13	2, 3	Ambiguous/3000
IPERGAY (2012–2014)	1/13	3	Ambiguous/400
HPTN 084 (2017–2020)	1/13	12	5/3224 (5 TGM)
F-grade studies (0 points)			
ACTG 175 (1991–1992)	0/13	None	Ambiguous/2467
ACTG 320 (1996–1997)	0/13	None	Ambiguous/1156
ASPIRE (2012–2015)	0/13	None	Ambiguous/2629
Bangkok Tenofovir Study (2005–2010)	0/13	None	Ambiguous/2413
CAPRISA 004 (2007–2010)	0/13	None	Ambiguous/889
FACTS 001 (2011–2014)	0/13	None	Ambiguous/2059
FEM-PrEP (2009–2011)	0/13	None	Ambiguous/2120
HPTN 052 (2005–2010)	0/13	None	Ambiguous/3526
HPTN 071 (2013–2017)	0/13	None	Ambiguous/48302
HVTN 503 (2007)	0/13	None	Ambiguous/801
HVTN 705 (2017–2019)	0/13	None	Ambiguous/2600
MTN 003 (2009–2011)	0/13	None	Ambiguous/5029
Opposites Attract (2012–2016)	0/13	None	Ambiguous/686
PARTNER 1 (2010–2014)	0/13	None	Ambiguous/1776
Partners PrEP (2008–2010)	0/13	None	Ambiguous/9494
PrEPVacc (2020–2023)	0/13	None	Ambiguous/1512
PROUD (2012–2014)	0/13	None	Ambiguous/544
Ring Study (2012–2016)	0/13	None	Ambiguous/1959
Ritonavir Study (1995)	0/13	None	Ambiguous/1090
RV 144 (2003–2005)	0/13	None	Ambiguous/16 402
SMART (2002–2006)	0/13	None	Ambiguous/5472
START (2009–2013)	0/13	None	Ambiguous/4685

Continued

TABLE 1— Continued

	Score	Indicators Achieved	TGD Enrollment[a]
TDF2 (2007–2009)	0/13	None	Ambiguous/1219
VAX 004 (1998–1999)	0/13	None	Ambiguous/5403

Note. ACTG = AIDS Clinical Trials Group; GNB = gender nonbinary; HPTN = HIV Prevention Trials Network; HVTN = HIV Vaccine Trials Network; MTN = Microbicide Trials Network; TGD = transgender and gender diverse; TGM = transgender men; TGW = transgender women. In the first column, the years in parentheses represent the study's enrollment period. Numbers in the Indicators Achieved column correspond to Scorecard indicators 1–14 shown in Figure 1. "Ambiguous" in the TGD Enrollment column represents the 133 456 (75%) participants who could not be categorized as TGD or cisgender on the basis of the information available (see Results).
[a]Number of participants identified as TGD/total number of participants enrolled.

Study Design (Scorecard Indicators 1–6)

Scorecard indicators 1 through 3 determined whether GNB individuals (indicator 1), TGM (indicator 2), and TGW (indicator 3) were discretely and explicitly included in study eligibility criteria. Most studies used ambiguous terminology, if at all, to define the study population, such as "men," "women," "females," and "males," without clarifying whether these terms referred to gender identity, sex assigned at birth, or current anatomy and without using clarifying terms such as "cisgender" and "transgender." Only 3 studies explicitly included GNB individuals, 6 studies explicitly included TGM, and 11 studies explicitly included TGW. Eligibility did not always correspond to enrollment; several studies included TGD individuals in eligibility criteria but did not report any TGD enrollment, whereas other studies did not include TGD individuals in eligibility criteria but later reported TGD enrollment.

Scorecard indicator 4 evaluated whether justification for exclusion was stated in studies that did not explicitly include TGD individuals. Five studies scored positively on this indicator, including 3 studies designed specifically for cisgender women. Each of these 3 studies had its own separate "sibling study" designed to include TGD participants as a means of addressing similar research questions. For example, the PURPOSE 1 study was designed exclusively for cisgender

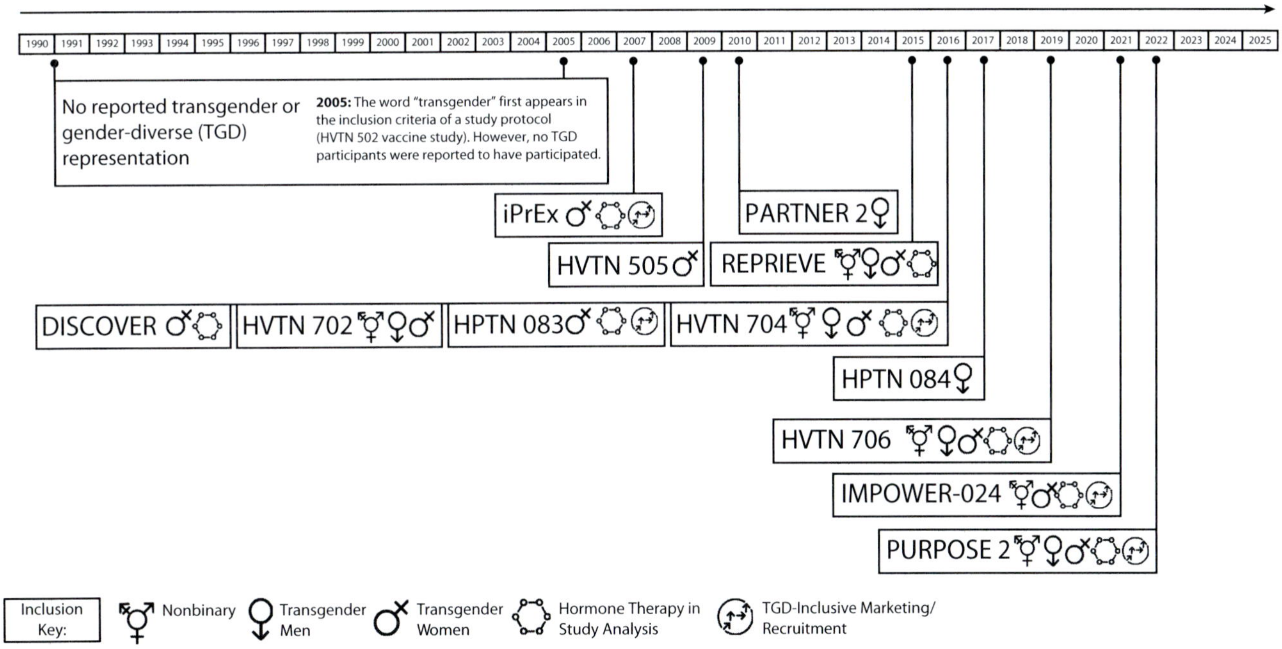

FIGURE 2— Timeline of Transgender and Gender-Diverse Representation in 41 Pivotal Global HIV Clinical Trials, 1991–2023

Note. HPTN = HIV Prevention Trials Network; HVTN = HIV Vaccine Trials Network.

women, but its sibling study, PURPOSE 2, explicitly named "cisgender men, transgender women, transgender men, and gender nonbinary people" as the study population; both studies tested the same investigational product for HIV prevention.

The fourth study that scored positively for indicator 4, IMPOWER-024, included GNB individuals and TGW but not TGM. Correspondence with the investigators revealed that planning for another study called IMPOWER-035 had been under way before a clinical hold on the investigational product halted study development. IMPOWER-035 would have included TGM and additional TGD populations, and this was the rationale for excluding TGM from IMPOWER-024. The fifth study, PARTNER 2, was designed specifically for people who identify as "gay men," with the study protocol clarifying that both cisgender and transgender gay men were eligible. We found this rationale to be reasonable for the exclusion of GNB individuals and TGW. The remaining TGD-exclusionary trials did not provide justification for excluding TGD populations, nor were "sibling studies" conducted to investigate similar research questions in TGD populations.

Scorecard indicator 5 evaluated whether studies were designed with TGD-specific enrollment goals (i.e., a number or percentage of TGD participants that the study aimed to enroll). Three studies achieved this indicator. HIV Prevention Trials Network (HPTN) 083 set a goal to enroll at least 10% TGW; 12.5% was achieved. PURPOSE 2 set a goal to enroll 20% TGW; 15% was achieved. Although PURPOSE 2 did not set an enrollment goal for GNB individuals or TGM, the study enrolled 209 (6%) and 43 (1%), respectively. IMPOWER-024 set a goal to enroll at least 100 TGW; the study enrolled 22 TGW, or 4.5% of the total enrolled participants, before it was placed on a clinical hold and subsequently discontinued. IMPOWER-024 also enrolled 20 GNB individuals, although there was no goal set for enrollment of this population.

Scorecard indicator 6 evaluated whether studies were designed to account for gender-affirming hormone use as a variable, for example in eligibility criteria, safety monitoring, efficacy, and drug–drug interactions. Eight studies achieved this indicator and did so in a variety of ways. Some studies determined the impact of hormone use on the efficacy of the investigational product under investigation, and vice versa, whereas others adjusted eligibility criteria to allow TGD participants using hormones to be clinically evaluated according to their gender identity rather than their sex assigned at birth.

Study Implementation (Scorecard Indicators 7–11)

Scorecard indicator 7 evaluated studies' use of gender-inclusive data collection practices, including measures ascertaining participants' gender identity separately from their sex assigned at birth. The Scorecard narrowly defines achievement of this indicator by referencing a 2023 best practices document based on data collection methods established in the early 2000s.[10] Among other criteria, a study's data collection practices must include options for participants to self-identify as GNB, TGM, and TGW unless a clear rationale is stated for any group's exclusion. All studies in our analysis included a measure of "sex," but the first study to consider gender as a discrete measure was HIV Vaccine Trials Network (HVTN) 502, which began enrolling in 2005; still, this study fell short of best practices in that GNB individuals were not considered.

Subsequently, many studies collected data on gender identity and sex assigned at birth, but only 10 studies in our entire analysis satisfied the Scorecard's comprehensive criteria for gender-inclusive data collection, starting with the PARTNER 2 study in 2010. Therefore, less than half of the 23 studies conducted after 2010 met the Scorecard's standards for data collection, and some studies conducted as recently as 2020 did not meet these standards. GNB exclusion was a significant barrier to achieving this indicator. Another 6 studies were found to explicitly include TGD people in study outreach, marketing, and recruitment strategies (indicator 8). Little information was available on indicators 9 through 11, but 4 studies met the criteria for employment of TGD study staff (indicator 9), 5 met the criteria for TGD-competent site selection (indicator 10), and 5 met the criteria for partnership with TGD organizations (indicator 11). Box 1 illustrates examples that explicitly met the stated criteria for indicators 8 through 11.[11–13]

Study Reporting (Scorecard Indicators 12–13)

Fourteen studies (34%) achieved Scorecard indicator 12 by clearly reporting on the gender distribution of study participants in the study results such that TGD representation could be ascertained. However, some of these studies presented only partial data. For example, 2 studies did not collect gender identity data from the first group of participants to enroll; these studies implemented TGD-inclusive data collection measures only after study enrollment had already begun, thereby missing the opportunity to screen some participants.

BOX 1— Examples of Transgender and Gender-Diverse-Responsive Study Implementation: 41 Pivotal Global HIV Clinical Trials, 1991–2023

Scorecard Indicator	Example
8. Outreach, marketing, and recruitment strategies and materials clearly exemplify TGD eligibility and inclusion	The study website and recruitment materials for the AMP study prominently featured language welcoming TGD participants and photographs of TGD models. Testing was also conducted to obtain feedback from TGD communities on the effectiveness of the imagery, language, style, and overall messaging to inform TGD-responsive marketing for studies such as AMP and HPTN 083.[11]
9. TGD staff are included among the core study team or among research site staff	The PURPOSE 2 HIV prevention study included a global community advisory group, consisting of TGD members, as an integral part of the study team. The study website also included a video stating "We also want to make sure that our sites and our site staff are representative of the communities that we're trying to recruit from so people feel comfortable and want to participate."[12]
10. Sites selected to recruit for the study have proven experience working with TGD communities	In the HVTN 706 study, research sites were expected to enroll cisgender men and transgender people. At various sites, assets included previous experience enrolling TGD study participants, participation in TGD sensitivity training for staff, involvement in trusting relationships with local TGD communities, adjustment of study visit schedules to accommodate challenges unique to TGD participants, linking of TGD participants to health services outside of the study, provision of financial support to cover participants' travel expenses, and accommodation of participants facing transphobia.[13]
11. The study includes a community engagement plan that involves partnerships with organizations serving TGD communities to foster engagement	TGD sensitivity training for staff conducting the HPTN 083 study included partnerships with individuals and organizations serving TGD communities. The study protocol also specified the expectation for each site to work with its local community advisory board and outreach teams to develop a community engagement plan that was appropriate for its local context. In addition, the study included a goal to enroll 10% transgender women; outreach and community engagement plans were expected to align with this goal.

Note. AMP = HVTN 704/HPTN 085 study; HPTN = HIV Prevention Trials Network; HVTN = HIV Vaccine Trials Network; TGD = transgender and gender diverse.

Another 2 studies failed to account for GNB participants in their data reporting (and presumably in data collection), but we classified these 2 studies as achieving indicator 12 by virtue of their reporting on the inclusion of TGM and TGW. We also identified inconsistencies with one trial's published data; we were granted approval to conduct an auxiliary study using the trial's deidentified data set to correct the trial's gender distribution and complete the analysis for our review (this study still did not earn a point for indicator 12). Three studies did not report on gender in their original journal publications, but they later published transgender-specific analyses separately from the primary study findings, thereby satisfying Scorecard indicator 12, albeit imperfectly.

Indicator 13 assessed whether studies reported TGD-specific analyses in their findings; 4 studies did so. These studies reported on a variety of safety, efficacy, and pharmacodynamic findings among TGD participants, separately from primary findings on cisgender participants. Given that several studies in our review only recently concluded, scores for indicator 13 may change as more information becomes available.

Language (Scorecard Indicator 14)

Seven studies (17%) achieved Scorecard indicator 14 by using gender-inclusive language that clearly and correctly defined the study population as operationalized by the National Institute of Allergy and Infectious Diseases (NIAID) HIV Language Guide.[14] Three of these studies predated the release of the original NIAID HIV Language Guide in 2020, demonstrating that Scorecard indicator 14 is achievable without the guide; however, this small number of studies suggests that future investigations could benefit from using the Scorecard and referencing the guide. NIAID-approved terminology included "assigned female/male at birth," "cisgender," "transgender," "gender nonconforming," "regardless of gender identity," and "participants of childbearing potential/pregnant participants." Thirty-four studies used terminology that rendered the study population ambiguous or unintentionally excluded TGD populations, as previously described.

Scores

Taking all indicators into account, only 2 studies achieved A-grade scores per the Scorecard's scoring system: PURPOSE 2 achieved 12 of 13 indicators, and IMPOWER-024 achieved 11 of 13. Three studies had B-grade scores with 8 to 10 indicators achieved, 7 studies had C-grade scores with 4 to 7 indicators achieved, 5 studies had D-grade scores with 1 to 3 indicators achieved, and 24 studies (59%) achieved zero indicators (a grade of F). Table 1 summarizes these findings.

DISCUSSION

Findings from this analysis of 41 milestone HIV clinical trials representing more than 30 years of HIV research confirm that TGD people and their priorities are critically underrepresented in HIV research despite the disproportionately high burden of HIV faced by TGD communities around the world.[1,2] Of a total of 178 893 participants, only 2042 transgender women, 398 nonbinary individuals, and 92 TGM represented TGD communities in 41 of the most influential HIV clinical trials conducted to date. The public health implications of this research gap are grave, including a dearth of HIV interventions appropriately designed, marketed, and availed to TGD communities urgently in need of these interventions as soon as they are available to other populations.

Before 2005, the word "transgender" was absent from such trials. No standard for TGD responsiveness is achievable without the recognition of the existence of TGD people. Since 2005, a trend toward greater inclusivity has been observed, owing largely to data collection practices established in the early 2000s[10] and momentum derived from a rich history of HIV activism embodied in seminal work such as The Denver Principles.[15] For example, bold activism leading up to the iPrEx study in 2007 resulted in trials that were discontinued and the lasting transformation of research ethics and the role of community involvement in research, as emblazoned in the Good Participatory Practice research guidelines.[16,17]

Research advocacy led by TGD scholars and activists has also drawn attention to the specific needs of TGD communities, a tradition that continues to this day.[4,5,18] Each of these milestones has likely contributed to the change that began in 2007 when the first TGD enrollment was reported. However, evidence suggests that some advancements have been sporadic rather than sustained. More than two thirds of studies conducted since 2007 have still failed to account for GNB people, TGM, and TGW through data collection methodologies, including studies conducted as recently as 2020; recognition of the existence of TGD communities remains a challenge.

Furthermore, very few studies have included TGD-focused research questions or study practices that directly respond to ongoing HIV-related priorities for TGD communities, such as interactions with gender-affirming hormones.[19] The extent to which these priorities are integrated in future trials will likely characterize the next era of TGD-responsive research. In our experience, the success of TGD-inclusive trials has relied heavily on the influence of investigators who specialize in TGD research—including researchers who are transgender—and a commitment to the meaningful involvement of TGD communities in the research process.

The findings outlined here support our recommendation for HIV researchers and advocates to use the Scorecard to operationalize commitment to TGD representation. Investigators, industry sponsors, study participants, community engagement staff, and advocates have a role to ensure that TGD communities are meaningfully included. When used proactively as a study design tool, the Scorecard has the potential to ensure that future HIV clinical trials either include TGD individuals or justify the rationale for their exclusion (Scorecard indicators 1–4). Researchers may also have to carefully consider safety concerns in settings with severe anti-TGD hostility where TGD enrollment could jeopardize the safety of participants and/or research staff, although these concerns must always be weighed against the harms of excluding TGD individuals. These decisions should be informed in consultation with ethicists, legal counsel, and, importantly, engagement with local TGD communities and researchers.

Researchers can use the Scorecard to ensure that, at a minimum, study populations can be accurately characterized (Scorecard indicators 7 and 12). Nearly three fourths of the participants in our analysis—133 456 individuals—could not be categorized as TGD or cisgender. TGD individuals were probably included among these participants, although they were likely assumed to be cisgender by default. This miscategorization undermines the integrity of these studies and their important findings; data that do not accurately reflect the study population compromise a study's validity and applicability to all, not just TGD communities. This vast amount of missing data highlights the need for the Scorecard to support scientific integrity, improve on the generalizability of study results, and potentially improve access to important HIV treatment and prevention measures while identifying areas for further research.

Furthermore, the failure to correctly capture demographic data erases TGD people and their contributions to science and impedes their right to benefit from science.[20] TGD individuals give their time, expertise, bodies, blood, and tissues to research. When research fails to accurately account for TGD communities, it exacerbates health disparities and diminishes TGD individuals' ability to realize scientific progress for their own communities, progress that TGD people continuously help to advance despite the erasure of their contributions. The practice of collecting TGD-inclusive participant data has only recently been established; researchers need guidance and support for the integration of these critical measures.[21] The Scorecard provides a clear and simple checklist to ensure consideration of such practices, which in turn has the potential to enhance clinical trials and their benefits for everyone, TGD and cisgender alike.

The Scorecard also supports crucial TGD-specific considerations. It encourages reflection on statistical plans, enrollment criteria, and a variety of recruitment strategies to ensure that an adequate number of TGD participants are included and that TGD-specific study objectives are reached, such as answers to important questions about interactions between investigational drugs and hormones or significant differences in safety, efficacy, adherence, acceptability, or other measures. Standards for adequate statistical power to conduct TGD-specific analyses are not well established (this is an area for further development), but the Scorecard prioritizes transparency (indicator 13). If a study lacks statistical power to test results by stratification, this information should be reported, and investigators should account for the extent to which this constitutes a study limitation. On their own, concerns about statistical power should not be used to justify exclusion of TGD communities. The previously referenced DISCOVER study illustrates how exclusion—not inclusion—can result in a lack of statistical power that undermines the basic ethical principles of research and, ultimately, public health goals.[6]

Furthermore, TGD inclusion matters even if traditional thresholds for statistical power are not feasible. Examples include studies reporting no clinically relevant interactions between the study drug and exogenous hormone use, differences in behavioral characteristics such as substance use, and differences in exploratory measures such as adherence and acceptability. Studies including TGD participants also promote trust, community awareness, and readiness to engage in research and public health initiatives. To explore TGD-specific research questions in greater detail, TGD-specific studies should be considered. For example, HPTN 091, an open-label study designed exclusively for transfeminine adults, tested the impact of co-locating gender-affirming care services with HIV prevention services.[22] (HPTN 091 was not included in our cross-sectional review because it was not an efficacy study and therefore did not meet the inclusion criteria. However, it represents an important milestone as the first study in the HIV Prevention Trials Network designed exclusively for transfeminine participants.)

Even studies without HIV-related endpoints can help in the response to conditions faced by TGD communities that are pertinent to the ecological model of HIV, such as economic hardship and psychological distress.[23] TGD-specific trials, demonstration projects, and modeling work are essential to close key knowledge gaps and answer the research questions most salient to the lived experience of TGD populations. Our cross-sectional review also justifies the need for a more comprehensive systematic review of TGD representation in clinical trials for HIV and other health conditions disproportionately affecting TGD communities, wherein an adaptation of the Scorecard could also be of use.

Finally, the last of the Scorecard's indicators, language, is integral to eliminating the exclusion of TGD people in scientific data, findings, and communications. For example, the trials leading to the approval of cabotegravir for HIV prevention, HPTN 083 and HPTN 084, included 570 TGW and 5 TGM, respectively. However, these studies are sometimes colloquially referred to as "the men's study" and "the women's study," respectively, omitting the substantial contributions of TGD people to the approval of the first long-acting injectable for HIV prevention. Furthermore, it is critical to recognize the multitude of terms describing gender diversity outside of the hegemonic understandings of gender in Europe and North America. We underscore the importance of adapting the language of HIV research to local contexts. As HIV research evolves to better respond to the epidemic, so too must our language evolve to be more gender inclusive.[24]

The lack of TGD representation in HIV clinical trials stands as a historical erasure of TGD communities with potential public health consequences. The Scorecard may guide future HIV research to be more responsive to the needs of TGD people. Importantly, use of the Scorecard during clinical trial development and implementation may enhance access to investigational HIV interventions in clinical trials and to approved products for the treatment and prevention of HIV. Inclusion of TGD people in HIV clinical trials may also provide information on differences in the safety and efficacy of interventions. The Scorecard is poised to set in motion an era of HIV research that meaningfully responds to the needs of TGD people. We invite researchers and advocates to use the Scorecard when designing and evaluating future HIV trials.

Doing so will allow the unique needs of TGM, TGW, and gender-diverse populations to be better understood and ultimately better served. *AJPH*

ABOUT THE AUTHORS

Brian Minalga is with the Office of HIV/AIDS Network Coordination, Fred Hutchinson Cancer Center, Seattle, WA. Cindra Feuer is with AVAC, New York, NY.

CORRESPONDENCE

Correspondence should be sent to Brian Minalga, MSW, 1100 Fairview Ave N, Seattle, WA 98109 (e-mail: bminalga@fredhutch.org). Reprints can be ordered at http://www.ajph.org by clicking the "Reprints" link.

PUBLICATION INFORMATION

Full Citation: Minalga B, Feuer C. Addressing transgender erasure in HIV clinical trials: the scorecard for transgender and gender-diverse inclusion. *Am J Public Health*. 2025;115(10): 1621–1630.

Acceptance Date: March 17, 2025.

DOI: https://doi.org/10.2105/AJPH.2025.308134

ORCID iD:
Brian Minalga https://orcid.org/0000-0002-8447-390X

CONTRIBUTORS

Both of the authors conceived of the project, conducted and interpreted the analyses, and wrote the article.

ACKNOWLEDGMENTS

This work was supported by the Coalition to Accelerate and Support Prevention Research and made possible by the generous support of the American people through the US President's Plan for AIDS Relief (PEPFAR) and the US Agency for International Development (USAID). Brian Minalga declares funding through National Institute of Allergy and Infectious Diseases award 2 UM1 AI068614-15 to the Fred Hutchinson Cancer Center.

We thank Leigh-Ann Van der Merwe, Richard Jefferys, Meagan O'Brien, Diana Tordoff, and Manju Chatani for contributing to this project.

Note. The contents of this work are the sole responsibility of the authors and do not necessarily reflect the official views of PEPFAR, USAID, the National Institutes of Health (NIH), or the US government.

CONFLICTS OF INTEREST

The authors have no conflicts of interest to disclose.

HUMAN PARTICIPANT PROTECTION

No human participants were included in this project.

REFERENCES

1. Stutterheim SE, van Dijk M, Wang H, Jonas KJ. The worldwide burden of HIV in transgender individuals: an updated systematic review and meta-analysis. *PLoS One.* 2021;16(12):e0260063. https://doi.org/10.1371/journal.pone.0260063.
2. Joint United Nations Programme on HIV/AIDS. HIV and transgender people. Available at: https://www.unaids.org/en/resources/documents/2024/2024-unaids-global-aids-update-transgender-people. Accessed October 31, 2024.
3. Cirrincione LR, Grieve VLB, Holloway J, Marzinke MA. Inclusion of transgender and gender diverse people in phase III trials: examples from HIV pharmacologic prevention studies. *Clin Pharmacol Ther.* 2023;113(3):557–564. https://doi.org/10.1002/cpt.2801.
4. Minalga B, Chung C, Davids JD, Matin A, Perry NL, Shook A. Research on transgender people must benefit transgender people. *Lancet.* 2022; 399(10325):628. https://doi.org/10.1016/S0140-6736(21)02806-3.
5. Restar A, Minalga BJ, Quilantang MI, et al. Mapping community-engaged implementation strategies with transgender scientists, stakeholders, and trans-led community organizations. *Curr HIV/AIDS Rep.* 2023;20(3):160–169. https://doi.org/10.1007/s11904-023-00656-y.
6. Spiegel HML. DISCOVER: much accomplished, but not yet for all. *Lancet.* 2020;396(10246):214–215. https://doi.org/10.1016/S0140-6736(20)31530-0.
7. AVAC. No data no more: manifesto to align HIV prevention research with trans and gender diverse realities. Available at: https://avac.org/project/transgender-manifesto/. Accessed October 28, 2024.
8. National Library of Medicine National Center for Biotechnology Information. ClinicalTrials.gov home page. Available at: https://clinicaltrials.gov. Accessed November 5, 2024.
9. AVAC. HIV Prevention Clinical Trials Database. Available at: https://avac.org/hiv-prevention-clinical-trials-database. Accessed November 5, 2024.
10. University of California San Francisco Center of Excellence for Transgender Health. Recommendations for inclusive data collection of trans people in HIV prevention, care, and services. Available at: https://prevention.ucsf.edu/transhealth/education/data-recs-long. Accessed January 9, 2025.
11. Gonzalez R, Hill B. Engaging transgender women and transgender men in digital spaces. Available at: https://www.hvtn.org/content/dam/hvtn/community/compass-pdf/CommunityCompass-2019-Issue1-FINAL-ENG-Web.pdf. Accessed January 5, 2025.
12. Gilead Sciences. PURPOSE 2. Available at: https://www.purposestudies.com/purpose2. Accessed January 5, 2025.
13. Pacheco D. The spectrum of transphobia experienced by student participants: observations from the MOSAICO Community and Involvement Team. Available at: https://www.hvtn.org/community/community-compass/2023/july-2023-issue/spectrum-of-transphobia.html. Accessed January 5, 2025.
14. National Institute of Allergy and Infectious Diseases. HIV Language Guide. Available at: https://www.thebody.com/hiv/niaid-hiv-language-guide. Accessed November 1, 2024.
15. Joint United Nations Programme on HIV/AIDS. The Denver Principles: 40 years on. Available at: https://www.unaids.org/en/resources/presscentre/featurestories/2023/june/20230626_denver-principles-40-years-on. Accessed January 9, 2025.
16. Folayan MO, Peterson K. HIV prevention clinical trials' community engagement guidelines: inequality and ethical conflicts. Available at: https://www.tandfonline.com/doi/full/10.1080/11287462.2020.1773061. Accessed January 9, 2025.
17. AVAC. Good participatory practice: guidelines for biomedical HIV prevention trials. Available at: https://avac.org/resource/report/good-participatory-practice-guidelines-for-biomedical-hiv-prevention-trials-second-edition. Accessed January 15, 2025.
18. Perez-Brumer A, Naz-McLean S, Huerta L, et al. The wisdom of mistrust: qualitative insights from transgender women who participated in PrEP research in Lima, Peru. Available at: https://onlinelibrary.wiley.com/doi/10.1002/jia2.25769. Accessed January 9, 2025.
19. Senneker T. Drug-drug interactions between gender-affirming hormone therapy and antiretrovirals for treatment/prevention of HIV. *Br J Clin Pharmacol.* 2024;90(10):2366–2382. https://doi.org/10.1111/bcp.16097.
20. United Nations Office of the High Commissioner for Human Rights. The right to access to and participate in science: Special Rapporteur in the field of cultural rights. Available at: https://www.ohchr.org/en/special-procedures/sr-cultural-rights/right-access-and-participate-science. Accessed November 1, 2024.
21. Tordoff DM, Minalga B, Gross BB, et al. Erasure and health equity implications of using binary male/female categories in sexual health research and human immunodeficiency virus/sexually transmitted infection surveillance: recommendations for transgender-inclusive data collection and reporting. *Sex Transm Dis.* 2022;49(2): e45–e49. https://doi.org/10.1097/OLQ.0000000000001533.
22. HIV Prevention Trials Network. HPTN 091 study shows encouraging uptake and adherence to oral PrEP among transgender women. Available at: https://www.hptn.org/news-and-events/press-releases/hptn-091-study-shows-encouraging-uptake-and-adherence-to-oral-prep. Accessed November 1, 2024.
23. Poteat TC, Reisner SL, Wirtz AL, et al. A microfinance intervention with or without peer support to improve mental health among transgender and nonbinary adults (the Creating Access to Resources and Economic Support Study): protocol for a randomized controlled trial. Available at: https://www.researchprotocols.org/2024/1/e63656. Accessed January 10, 2025.
24. Marrazzo J. Our words have power—NIAID embraces respectful, inclusive, and person-first language. Available at: https://www.niaid.nih.gov/news-events/our-words-have-power. Accessed November 1, 2024.

Community Connectedness as a Source of Adherence to HIV Prevention Behaviors and Resilience Among Transgender Women of Color in New York City, 2020–2022

Alexander Furuya, MPH, Yusuf Ransome, DrPH, MPH, Ichiro Kawachi, PhD, MBChB, Denton Callander, PhD, Asa Radix, MD, PhD, MPH, Adam Whalen, MPH, Cristina Herrera, PhD, Kim Watson, Jessica Contreras, BA, Jenesis Merriman, MPH, Krish J. Bhatt, MPH, Roberta Scheinmann, MPH, Sahnah Lim, PhD, MPH, Chau Trinh-Shevrin, DrPH, John A. Schneider, MD, MPH , Su Hyun Park, PhD, MPH, and Dustin T. Duncan, ScD

See also LGBTQ+ Transgender Health, pp. 1594–1670.

Objectives. To examine how one's community connectedness may act as a source of resilience and promote HIV prevention and care behaviors among transgender women of color.

Methods. We analyzed survey data from 313 transgender women of color living in New York City collected from August 2020 to November 2022. The Community Connectedness Scale asks participants about their baseline feelings of connection, feelings of inclusion, feelings of belonging, feelings of isolation, and feelings of being unlike in relation to the transgender community. The HIV prevention and care outcomes of interest were measured at 6-month follow-up and included consistent condom usage, recent testing for sexually transmitted infections (STIs), current preexposure prophylaxis use, and HIV viral load suppression.

Results. Those with a high (compared to low) community connectedness were 62% more likely to consistently use condoms and 16% more likely to test for STIs.

Conclusions. Community connectedness was associated with a greater likelihood of HIV prevention behaviors.

Public Health Implications. Future interventions could include strategies to strengthen community connectedness to improve HIV status neutral care continuums. (*Am J Public Health.* 2025;115(10):1631–1641. https://doi.org/10.2105/AJPH.2025.308144)

AJPH October 2025, Vol. 115, No. 10

Transgender women of color in the United States are disproportionately affected by HIV. According to the Centers for Disease Control and Prevention, HIV prevalence is 62% among Black transgender women and 35% among Latina transgender women; this is disproportionately high compared to a prevalence of 17% among White transgender women.[1] Sexual health behaviors such as consistent condom usage, regular sexually transmitted infection (STI) screening, and preexposure prophylaxis (PrEP) can effectively mitigate infections.[2] Furthermore, for those living with HIV, proper antiretroviral treatment is needed to achieve HIV viral load suppression. Upon achieving viral load suppression, people living with HIV can prevent the likelihood of transmission to other partners through "treatment as prevention," as those who maintain undetectable viral loads cannot transmit HIV to others.[3]

However, transgender women of color face barriers to engaging in HIV care and prevention behaviors because of the discrimination they face.[4] We believe it is useful to view this with an intersectionality framework, which posits that systems of oppression, such as racism, transphobia, and heteronormativity, do not operate independently, but rather intersect and operate synergistically. Transgender women of color face discriminations that operate beyond transphobia, racism, and sexism alone.[5] Systematic forms of oppression occur in nearly all aspects of life, including housing, policing, employment, health care, and interpersonal relationships.[6]

Resilience is defined as the ability to maintain physical and psychological health, even in the face of stressful events and environments.[7] According to the Minority Stress Model, the stressors that transgender women of color encounter every day can erode healthy behaviors, which can eventually lead to worse health states.[8] However, minoritized populations can cope and find ways to buffer the effects of these stressors as forms of resilience.[9] One source of resilience can come from the community. Community connectedness is the subjective feeling of belonging; more specifically, it is the "convergence of individuals' desires to belong to a larger collective, establish a mutually influential relationship with that collective, satisfy their individual needs and be rewarded through their collective affiliation, and construct a shared emotional connection."[10(p.37)]

Community connectedness can affect health in several ways. First, it can facilitate resource sharing within a community; individuals with a higher community connectedness are more likely to engage with their community and access the resources they need to improve their health.[11] Second, it can help establish beneficial norms and increase self-efficacy for healthy behaviors.[12] Third, community connectedness can motivate individuals to engage in healthy behaviors through a sense of shared responsibility.[13] For example, during the initial COVID-19 vaccine rollout, those who had a stronger community connectedness and sense of responsibility were more likely to get vaccinated.[14] The relationship between community connectedness and health, particularly mental health, has been elucidated by scientists over the years.[15]

However, it is currently unknown whether community connectedness is associated with HIV prevention and care behaviors among transgender women of color living in New York City. New York City has one of the largest transgender communities in the world, estimated at more than 90 000 individuals in 2018.[16] This has enabled the growth of a vibrant transgender community, and the active creation and participation of these communities foster community connectedness among its participants, which can protect against the negative effects of systemic oppression. However, not all transgender women of color may feel connected to their community.

In this study, we aimed to understand how differences in community connectedness affect HIV care and prevention outcomes. The findings of this study can help us identify a possible mechanism that predicts HIV prevention and care behaviors among transgender women of color, which public health practitioners can leverage when designing interventions to improve the health of this population.

METHODS

To determine whether community connectedness was associated with HIV prevention and care behaviors among transgender women of color, we analyzed baseline and 6-month data from the Trying to Understand Relationships, Networks and Neighborhoods Among Transgender Women of Color (TURNNT) cohort study. In total, 314 transgender women of color were enrolled in a 1-year prospective longitudinal cohort study from August 31, 2020, until November 4, 2022. Eligible participants (1) identified as transgender women of color, (2) were between 18 and 55 years old at enrollment, and (3) lived in the New York City metropolitan area (including northern New Jersey, Long Island, and the lower Hudson Valley). Participants spoke either English or Spanish and at enrollment planned to reside in the New York City metropolitan area for the 1-year duration of the study. We recruited participants through various channels, including social media marketing, print advertising, event-based recruitment, referrals from organizational outreach and partnership, and snowball sampling via referrals from enrolled participants.[17] An interviewer-administered survey was given to the participants, and they provided information on general health and well-being, socioeconomic characteristics, gender affirmation, social networks, social capital, neighborhood and housing characteristics, HIV prevention and care behaviors, sex work, psychological well-being, substance use, sleep health, relationships, discrimination and violence, and experiences with the COVID-19 pandemic. Participants provided responses at 3 time points: at baseline, at 6-month follow-up, and at 12-month follow-up.

HIV serostatus was self-reported at baseline as positive, negative, or unknown. Participants who reported an unknown or negative HIV status completed a point-of-care OraQuick saliva HIV test (OraSure Technologies, Bethlehem, PA) at the second interview of each wave in accordance with guidelines provided by the New York State Department of Health. Participants were mailed the HIV test between the first and second interview at each wave and completed the test over video call with an interviewer. All participants with preliminary positive test results were immediately directed to confirmatory blood testing with their primary care provider or with TURNNT partner organizations.

Although 314 individuals participated in the TURNNT cohort study, our final analytical sample size was 313 because 1 individual did not provide any information for the community connectedness measure and therefore was excluded.

Community Connectedness

We measured the construct of transgender community connectedness at baseline using the 5-item subscale from the Gender Minority Stress and Resilience Measure.[18] Using a 4-point Likert scale ("strongly disagree," "disagree," "agree," and "strongly agree"), respondents indicated the degree to which they endorsed the following 5 items:

1. "You feel connected to other people who share your gender identity" ("feel connected");
2. "You feel part of a community of people who share your gender identity" ("feel included");
3. "When interacting with members of the community that shares your gender identity, you feel like you belong" ("feel belonging");
4. "You feel isolated and separate from other people who share your gender" ("feel isolated"); and
5. "You are not like other people who share your gender identity" ("feel unlike").

In our analyses, we reverse-coded the last 2 items ("feel isolated" and "feel unlike") to be in alignment with the other items.

We assessed the reliability of our community connectedness measure to ensure that we were capturing the construct of interest reliably and validly. Through principal component analysis, we found that there were potentially 1 or 2 latent variables underlying our community connectedness measure. During the exploratory factor analysis, we compared the likelihood χ^2 statistic of a single-factor model and a 2-factor model. We found that the model with a single factor had a *P* value of less than .0047; for the model with 2 factors, the *P* value was less than .38. This indicated to us that a model with 2 factors might fit the data better. Upon examining the factor loading for the 2-factor model, we found that the item "feel unlike" was potentially unlike the other constructs. Additionally, we found that removing the item "feel unlike" resulted in a substantially higher Cronbach's α among the remaining items. Therefore, we decided to omit this item when creating our composite measure. Figures and tables of the principal component analysis and the exploratory factor analysis can be found in the Appendix (available as a supplement to the online version of this article at http://www.ajph.org).

We calculated the Cronbach's α for the 4-item measure to be 0.82; this indicated that we had good internal consistency between the items. We created a composite measure of community connectedness by taking the average score of each participant's subdomain response; this allowed us to compute a composite score even if there were item nonresponses. We examined the distribution of the composite score (Figure 1) and found that 2 groups emerged: those who had strongly endorsed every single item (33.9%) and everyone else (66.1%); we categorized them as having "high community connectedness" and "low community connectedness," respectively.

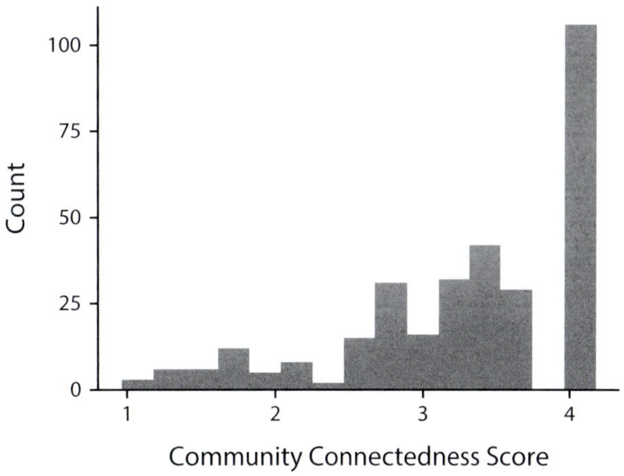

FIGURE 1— Distribution of the Community Connectedness Scores: New York City, August 2020–November 2022

Note. This histogram shows the distribution of the community connectedness score. We found that 2 groups emerged: those with a score of 4.0 (33.9% of the participants, who were categorized as having high community connectedness) and everyone else (66.1% of the participants, who were categorized as having low community connectedness).

HIV Prevention and Care Behaviors

We measured HIV prevention and care behaviors as dichotomous variables during 6-month follow-up. For condom usage, we asked participants, "In the past 6 months, about how often did you use condoms for vaginal or anal sex? Please do not include sex with people who paid you with money or other goods." Participants could respond "always," "some of the time," "never," "you did not have vaginal or anal sex in the past 6 months," "don't know," or "prefer not to answer." We chose to focus on consistent condom usage; therefore, we dichotomized participants between those who responded "always" and those who responded "some of the time" or "never."

For STI testing, we asked participants, "Have you ever been tested for sexually transmitted infections (sometimes known as STIs or STDs) other than HIV?" We purposefully excluded HIV tests as all participants who were not living with HIV needed to complete an HIV test to participate in the study. Participants could respond "yes, within the past 6 months," "yes, within the past 12 months," "yes, but not within the past 12 months," "no, never," "don't know," or "prefer not to answer." We wanted to focus on recent STI testing; therefore, we dichotomized participants between those who responded "yes, within the past 6 months" and everyone else.

For PrEP use, we asked participants who were not living with HIV, "Have you ever taken PrEP to reduce the risk of getting HIV? If so, are you taking PrEP now?" Participants could respond "yes, taking PrEP now," "yes, have taken PrEP previously but am not currently," "no, never," "don't know," or "prefer not to answer." We focused on current PrEP use, and therefore we categorized participants as current PrEP users and everyone else.

For HIV viral load suppression, we asked participants living with HIV, "Was your most recent viral load detectable or undetectable (< 200 copies/mL)?" Participants responded "undetectable," "detectable," or "don't know." We labeled those who responded "don't know" as missing data, and compared the distribution of those with undetectable viral load and those with detectable viral load.

Covariates

We anticipated confounders in our analysis between community connectedness and HIV prevention and care behaviors. We used baseline self-report measures to capture the following characteristics: annual income ("no income," "$1 to $9999," "$10 000 to $29 999," "> $30 000," and "missing"), education ("less than high school," "high school graduate or equivalent," and "more than high school"), age category in years ("18–24," "25–34," "35–44," and "45 and older"), incarceration history ("ever incarcerated" and "never incarcerated"), sex work history ("ever participated in sex work" and "never participated in sex work"), and US nativity ("born in the US" and "not born in the US").

Statistical Analysis

We performed descriptive analysis to characterize the sociodemographic composition of the study sample. We also stratified our descriptive statistics by their levels of community connectedness to assess the covariate and outcome distributions between those with high community connectedness and those with low community connectedness. To assess the association between baseline measures of community connectedness and HIV care and prevention outcomes measured at 6-month follow-up, we created Poisson regression models with a robust variance estimator; these models allowed us to interpret the exponentiated coefficient and its 95% confidence interval as an adjusted prevalence ratio, which is easier to interpret than an odds ratio.[19] We used these models to evaluate the studied association before and after controlling for potential confounders. Based on our hypothesized causal diagram, we identified the following variables to make up the minimally sufficient set of confounders: income, educational attainment, age, incarceration history, sex work history, and US nativity. We conducted all quantitative analyses using R Studio version 2024.12.0 + 467 (Posit PBC, Vienna, Austria).

RESULTS

In total, 313 participants were included in this analysis. Overall, the mean age of the study cohort was 37.0 years (SD = 9.2); 28.4% identified as Black and 46.3% identified as Latina. Of the participants, 33.5% had less than a high school education and 55.6% had an income of less than $10 000 a year. In terms of HIV prevention and care behaviors, 43.8% reported using condoms consistently, 78.6% had taken an STI test (not including an HIV test) within the past 6 months, and 42.8% of those not living with HIV were currently using PrEP; 87.7% of those living with HIV were virally suppressed. Table 1 shows these statistics, but stratified by overall community connectedness score. Of note, we found that those with a high

TABLE 1— Characteristics of the Study Population: New York City, August 2020–November 2022

	Overall, % (n = 313)	High Community Connectedness, % (n = 106)	Low Community Connectedness, % (n = 207)
Age, y			
18–24	10.2	9.4	10.6
25–34	29.7	25.5	31.9
35–44	37.7	36.8	38.2
45–55	21.1	25.5	18.8
Missing	1.3	2.8	0.5
Race and ethnicity			
Non-Hispanic Black	28.4	19.8	32.9
Non-Black Latina	46.4	62.3	38.2
Biracial/multiracial	21.4	17.9	23.2
Asian	1.9	0.0	2.8
Middle Eastern/North African	0.6	0.0	1.0
American Indian	0.3	0.0	0.5
Something else	1.0	0.0	1.4
Nativity			
US born	58.1	53.8	60.4
Non-US born	41.2	44.3	39.6
Missing	0.6	1.9	0.0
Education			
Less than high school	33.5	41.5	29.5
High school	28.5	34.0	25.6
More than high school	38.0	24.5	44.9
History of sex work			
Yes	75.4	76.4	74.9
No, never	23.6	22.6	24.1
Missing	1.0	1.0	1.0
Income status, $			
No income	16.3	20.8	14.0
1–9999	39.3	43.4	37.2
10 000–29 999	21.7	19.8	22.7
≥ 30 000	11.8	10.3	12.6
Missing	10.9	5.7	13.5
Incarceration			
Yes	27.8	21.7	31.0
No, never	71.2	78.3	67.6
Missing	1.0	0.0	1.4
HIV status			
Positive	51.8	59.4	47.8
Negative	46.3	38.7	50.2
Missing	1.9	1.9	2.0
Condom use			
Always	43.8	58.5	36.2
Never or some of the time	43.8	27.4	52.2
Missing or did not have sex	12.4	14.1	11.6

Continued

TABLE 1— Continued

	Overall, % (n = 313)	High Community Connectedness, % (n = 106)	Low Community Connectedness, % (n = 207)
STI testing			
Within past 6 months	78.6	86.8	74.4
Not within past 6 months	21.1	13.2	25.1
Missing	0.3	0.0	0.5
Current PrEP use among HIV–			
Yes	42.8	53.7	38.5
No	53.8	41.5	58.7
Missing	3.4	4.8	2.8
Viral load suppression among HIV+			
Yes	87.7	93.7	83.8
No	9.3	4.8	12.2
Missing	3.0	1.5	4.0

Note. PrEP = preexposure prophylaxis; STI = sexually transmitted infection. This table describes the demographic, socioeconomic, and sexual health characteristics of the Trying to Understand Relationships, Networks and Neighborhoods Among Transgender Women of Color (TURNNT) cohort. We also stratified these statistics by the participant's level of community connectedness.

community connectedness were less likely to have a history of incarceration (21.7% vs 31.0%). Additionally, we found that those with a high community connectedness were more likely to get tested for STIs in the past 6 months (86.8% vs 74.4%) and more likely to always use condoms (58.5% vs 36.2%). Among those not living with HIV, those with a high community connectedness were more likely to be currently on PrEP (53.7% vs 38.5%), and among those living with HIV, those with a high community connectedness were more likely to be virally suppressed (93.7% vs 83.8%). Baseline item responses regarding community connectedness are listed in Figure 2. We found that 33% of participants indicated having a strong community connectedness by our composite measure.

We found that those with a high baseline community connectedness were more likely to engage in HIV prevention and care at 6-month follow-up. Results from the bivariate analysis and multivariable analysis are shown in Table 2. Using our composite measure, we found that those who had a high community connectedness were 62% more likely to always use condoms (adjusted prevalence ratio [APR] = 1.62; 95% confidence interval [CI] = 1.17, 2.24) and 16% more likely to get an STI test (APR = 1.16; 95% CI = 1.01, 1.34) than those with a low community connectedness, adjusting for age, educational attainment, income level, US nativity, sex work history, and incarceration history. There were no associations between overall community connectedness and PrEP use or viral load suppression.

DISCUSSION

We found that community connectedness, a source of resilience, was associated with a greater likelihood of consistent condom use and frequent STI testing. Although our present study investigated the health effects of community connectedness, understanding the determinants of community connectedness is needed for potential interventions. We detailed some descriptive differences between those with high and low community connectedness; however, future research should be done to critically assess the causes of community connectedness.

Our positive findings align with those of other researchers.[20,21] A qualitative study conducted in Lima, Peru, found that communities of transgender women facilitated knowledge sharing about STI testing.[21] D'Avanzo et al. conducted a study examining the role of community belonging and attitudes towards PrEP among transgender women living in Philadelphia, Pennsylvania, and the San Francisco Bay Area of California; they found that the highest community-connected clusters were more likely to have a favorable view of PrEP.[20] Community connectedness can also affect HIV care and prevention behaviors in indirect ways. Numerous studies have found that community connectedness is positively associated with mental health and well-being.[15,22] It has also been shown that poor mental health is associated with poor

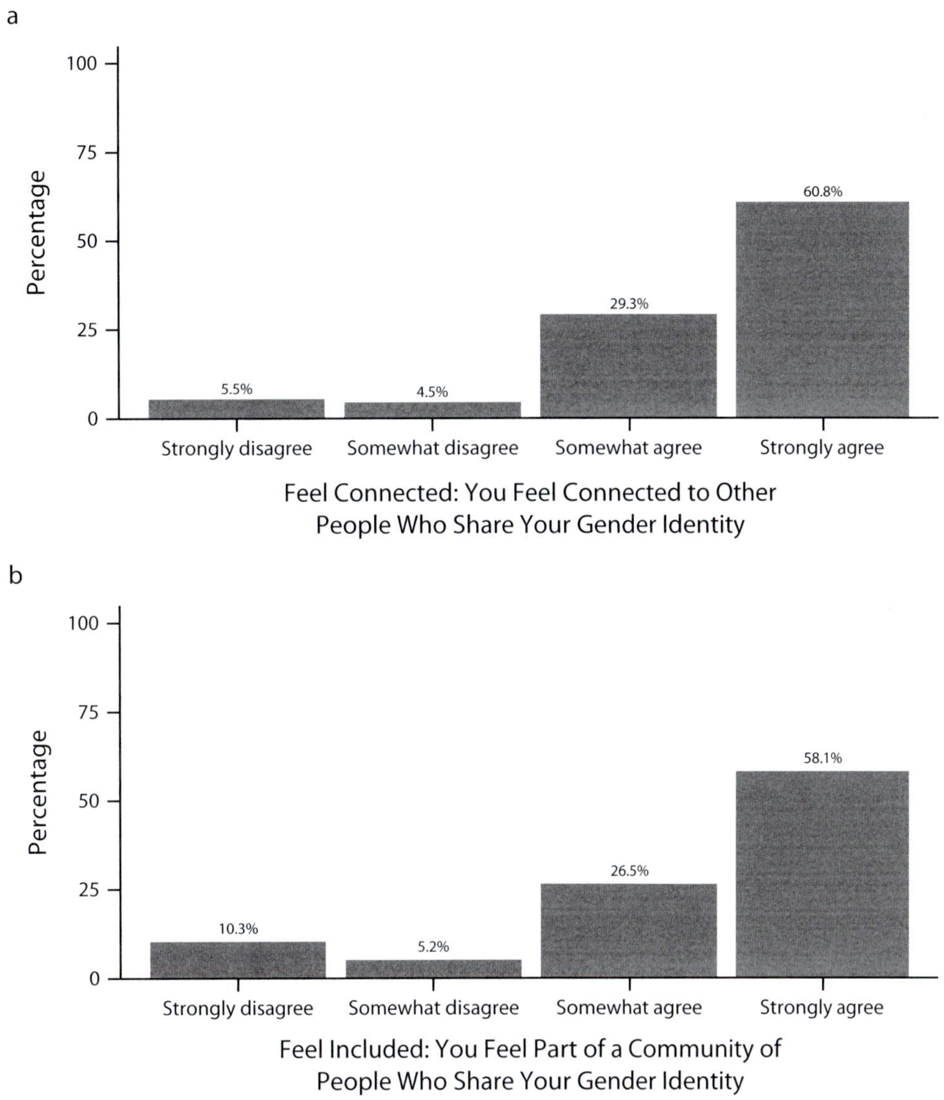

FIGURE 2— Frequency of Responses to the Community Connectedness Scale for Feeling (a) Connected, (b) Included, (c) Belonging, and (d) Isolated: New York City, August 2020–November 2022

adherence.[23] Therefore, it is possible that community connectedness affects HIV care and prevention behaviors through mental health. These studies, different in methodologies and context, help triangulate our results and suggest that community connectedness is beneficial for HIV care and prevention.

There are many ways in which community connectedness can be leveraged. Interventions involving community connectedness can focus on either the individual level (e.g., connecting individuals to supportive networks of transgender women of color) or the community level (e.g., bolstering structural resources within the transgender community). It has been suggested that sociopolitical, cultural, and individual factors may interact in complex ways to affect community connectedness.[24] Community connectedness can also be determined by objective community factors, including population density, geography of urban context, urban planning, and accessibility to public spaces.[25] The demographic composition of a neighborhood can also affect community connectedness; for example, for those who recently immigrated to the United States, the existence of ethnic and immigrant communities within a neighborhood can increase the individual's community connectedness.[26] Furthermore, community connectedness can change with age; for example, individuals in older adulthood may face a loss of social networks and feel a lesser degree of community connectedness.[27] Policies

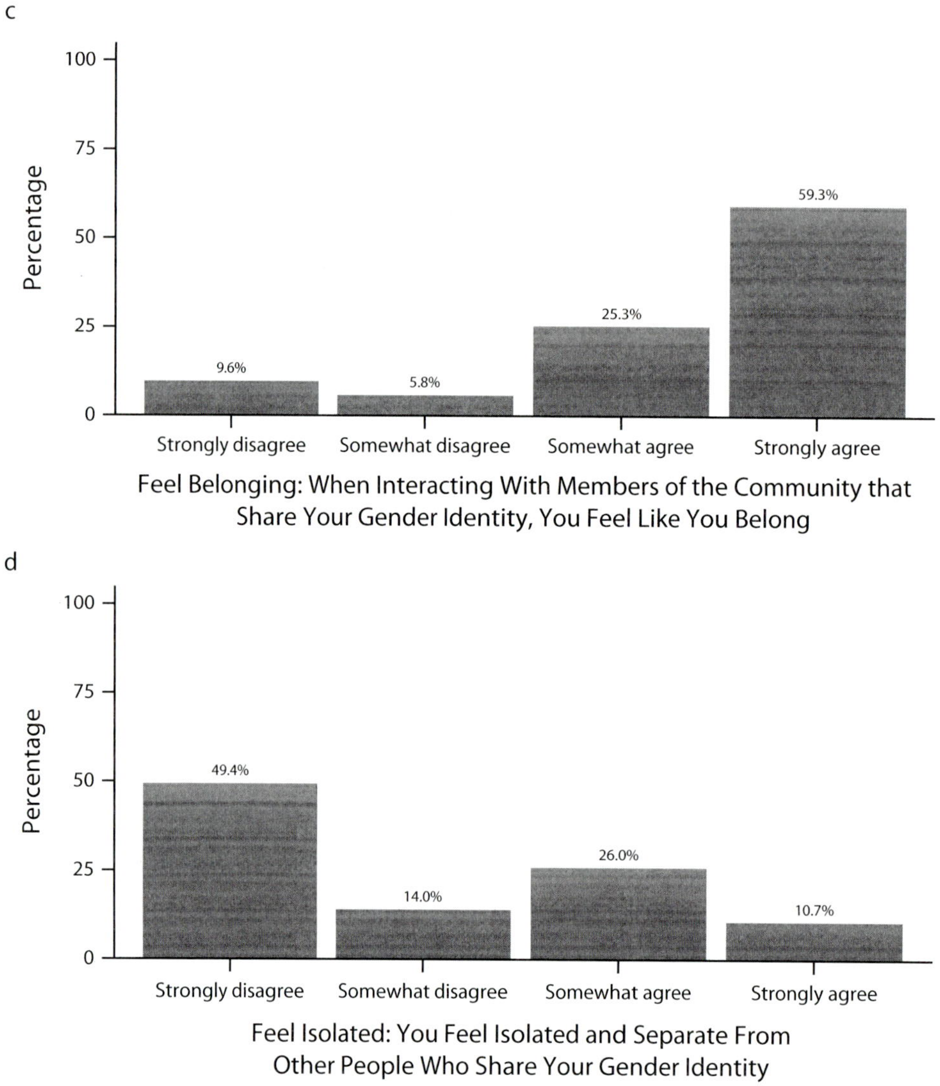

FIGURE 2— Continued.

Note. This figure details the percentage of endorsements for each community connectedness item.

can also affect community connectedness, although the effects may be heterogeneous. After the 2016 election, some transgender individuals felt disenfranchised and isolated given the anti-LGBTQ (lesbian, gay, bisexual, transgender, and queer) political administration, whereas others felt closer to their community as they leaned on their peers for support.[28] Thus, interventions involving community connectedness need to account for the complex context in which individuals live and prioritize helping those who need it most. Matsuno and Israel have proposed the Transgender Resilience Model to help identify levels of intervention that can increase community connectedness and resiliency; they provide examples of interventions including advocacy, education and training, group therapy, and online resources.[29] We hope to investigate the effectiveness of these interventions in future research.

Resiliency may be particularly powerful during unprecedented times, such as the COVID-19 pandemic. Our present study took place during that pandemic. Some may believe that this limits the transportability of our results to nonpandemic settings—for example, that COVID-19 caused a decrease in community connectedness among transgender women of color. However, during lockdown, transgender individuals were able to maintain their community connectedness through online means, and they also worked together to access HIV care and prevention resources.[30] We acknowledge, however,

TABLE 2— Crude and Adjusted Prevalence Ratios Between Community Connectedness and HIV Care and Prevention Behaviors: New York City, August 2020–November 2022

	Sample Size	Akaike Information Criterion	Prevalence Ratio (95% CI)
Consistent condom use			
Crude model	175	286.4	1.84 (1.38, 2.46)
Adjusted model	171	293.3	1.62 (1.17, 2.24)
STI testing past 6 mo			
Crude model	214	424.0	1.04 (0.91, 1.19)
Adjusted model	210	432.5	1.16 (1.01, 1.34)
Current PrEP use among HIV−			
Crude model	107	153.6	1.40 (0.80, 2.47)
Adjusted model	104	160.9	1.07 (0.62, 1.85)
Viral Load Suppression among HIV+			
Crude model	105	213.4	1.08 (0.98, 1.18)
Adjusted model	105	233.1	1.09 (0.99, 1.21)

Note. CI = confidence interval; PrEP = preexposure prophylaxis; STI = sexually transmitted infection. This table summarizes the bivariate and multivariable associations between baseline community connectedness and sexual health measured at 6-month follow-up. The prevalence ratios were calculated using regression models with Poisson distributions and robust standard errors. The adjusted model includes covariate adjustment for age, educational attainment, income level, incarceration history, sex work history, and US nativity. Each prevalence ratio includes the corresponding 95% confidence interval and the number of observations for each model building.

that the COVID-19 pandemic presented significant barriers to accessing care, particularly in HIV testing, which may have affected our outcome measures and study results.[31,32] Although this issue is complex, we believe that the findings presented here are relevant today; according to Friedman et al.'s theory of Big Events, we are still experiencing the long-term effects of the COVID-19 pandemic today.[33] We believe that the resilience of the transgender women of color community was exemplified during this time period.

Limitations

Although we controlled for income, education, age, incarceration history, sex work history, and US nativity, there may be unmeasured confounding that could affect both community connectedness and HIV prevention and care behaviors. Specific to our target population, racism, transphobia, sexism, and the unique forms of discrimination that transgender women of color face may affect both community connectedness and engagement with healthy behaviors. Although we did our best to create exchangeability between those with high and low community connectedness by controlling for confounders, there may be unobserved confounding that can explain the associations.

We note that the TURNNT cohort was sampled using convenience sampling methods such as recruitment from sexual health clinics. This may explain why we observed higher-than-expected PrEP use and viral load suppression. Currently, there are no sources of demographic information that are representative of all transgender women of color living in New York City to assess the representativeness of our cohort. When we compared the demographics of the TURNNT cohort and those of people enrolled in the Transgender Women Engagement and Entry of Care Project, however, the demographic distributions were similar.[34] We still acknowledge the limitations in external validity. Additionally, because TURNNT utilized some snowball sampling, there may be clusters of participants who are more similar to each other than others. In our analyses, we assumed that participants were independent of each other, and therefore our standard errors may be incorrect. We also note, on the other hand, that representative sampling of transgender women of color is challenging because of structural barriers and issues with sampling coverage. The TURNNT cohort is one of the largest study populations of transgender women of color, and we have prioritized creating findings with high internal validity.

Public Health Implications

Community connectedness was associated with a higher likelihood of HIV prevention behaviors among transgender women of color. Community connectedness can be thought of as a manifestation of resilience—a construct that enables marginalized individuals to practice healthy behaviors and maintain good health statuses in spite of encountering interlocking systems of oppression on a daily basis. To inform future interventions, additional research is needed to identify the determinants of community connectedness and the mechanisms of how community connectedness affects health. AJPH

ABOUT THE AUTHORS

Alexander Furuya, Asa Radix, Adam Whalen, Jessica Contreras, Jenesis Merriman, Krish J. Bhatt, Roberta Scheinmann, and Dustin T. Duncan are with the Department of Epidemiology, Columbia University Mailman School of Public Health, New York, NY. Yusuf Ransome is with the Department of Social and Behavioral Sciences, Yale School of Public Health, New Haven, CT. Ichiro Kawachi is with the Department of Social and Behavioral Science, Harvard School of Public Health, Boston, MA. Cristina Herrera is with the Trans Latina Network, New York, NY. Denton Callander is with the Kirby Institute, University of New South Wales, Australia. Kim Watson is with CK Life, New York, NY. Sahnah Lim and Chau Trinh-Shevrin are with the Callen-Lorde Community Health Center, New York, NY. John A. Schneider is with the Department of Medicine, University of Chicago, Chicago, IL. Su Hyun Park is with the Saw Swee Hock School of Public Health, National University of Singapore and National University Health System, Singapore.

CORRESPONDENCE

Correspondence should be sent to Alexander Furuya, MPH, Department of Epidemiology, Columbia University Mailman School of Public Health, 722 West 168th St, 7th Floor, Room 720.1, New York City, NY 10032 (e-mail: ahf2128@cumc.columbia.edu). Reprints can be ordered at https://www.ajph.org by clicking the "Reprints" link.

PUBLICATION INFORMATION

Full Citation: Furuya A, Ransome Y, Kawachi I, et al. Community connectedness as a source of adherence to HIV prevention behaviors and resilience among transgender women of color in New York City, 2020–2022. *Am J Public Health*. 2025;115(10):1631–1641.

Acceptance Date: March 31, 2025.

DOI: https://doi.org/10.2105/AJPH.2025.308144

ORCID iDs:

Alexander Furuya https://orcid.org/0009-0008-4596-9014

Yusuf Ransome https://orcid.org/0000-0003-4170-2001

Denton Callander https://orcid.org/0000-0002-4116-4250

Asa Radix https://orcid.org/0000-0001-9611-4181

Adam Whalen https://orcid.org/0000-0003-0235-1341

Jenesis Merriman https://orcid.org/0009-0008-7950-5701

Krish J. Bhatt https://orcid.org/0000-0002-0007-5470

Dustin T. Duncan https://orcid.org/0000-0001-8586-8711

CONTRIBUTORS

A. Furuya contributed to the primary analysis, drafting of the article, revision of the article, and approval of the final version. Y. Ransome, I. Kawachi, and A. Radix contributed to the concept of the study, interpretation of results, revision of the article, and approval of the final version. D. Callander contributed to the survey development, design of the Community Connectedness Scale, drafting of the article, revision of the article, and approval of the final version. A. Whalen contributed to the analytical plan, revision of the article, and approval of the final version. C. Herrera, K. Watson, S. Lim, C. Trinh-Shevrin, and J. A. Schneider contributed to the revision of the article and approval of the final version. R. Scheinmann, J. Contreras, and K. J. Bhatt contributed to the quantitative research interviews, managing survey assessments and data collection, engaging in participant recruitment and retention, the revision of the article, and approval of the final version. J. Merriman contributed to the quantitative research interviews, the revision of the article, and approval of the final version. S. H. Park contributed to the code review, the revision of the article, and approval of the final version. D. T. Duncan contributed to securing funding, the concept and design of the study, the drafting of the article, the revision of the article, and approval of the final version.

ACKNOWLEDGMENTS

The Trying to Understand Relationships, Networks and Neighborhoods Among Transgender Women of Color (TURNNT) Cohort Study was funded through grants from the National Institute on Minority Health and Health Disparities (grant numbers R01MD013554, 3R01MD013554-02S1, and 3R01MD013554-05S1; principal investigator: Dustin T. Duncan, ScD). Research reported in this publication was supported by the National Institute of Allergy and Infectious Diseases of the National Institutes of Health (award number T32AI114398) and the National Institute of Environmental Health Sciences (award number T32ES007322).

We thank the Community Advisory Board members: Cristina Herrera of TransLatinx Network, Ceyenne Doroshow of GLITS (Gay and Lesbian in a Transgender World), Kim Watson of Community Kinship Life, Kiara St. James of New York Transgender Advocacy Group, BianeyGarcia of Make the Road NY, Morticia Godiva of Black Trans Travel Fund, Xoai Pham of Transgender Law Center, Egyptt LaBeija of the House of LaBeija, and Nala Toussaint. We also thank our Scientific Advisory Board members: Sari Reisner, ScD, of Harvard Medical School, Tonia Poteat, PhD, of the University of North Carolina Chapel Hill, Rachel Bluebond-Langner, MD, of New York University School of Medicine, Robert Garofalo, MD, of Northwestern University, Walter Bockting, PhD, of Columbia University, and Jae Sevelius, PhD, of Columbia University. We additionally thank TURNNT study staff, including Krish J. Bhatt, MPH, Jessica Contreras, BA, Roberta Scheinmann, MPH, Jenesis Merriman, MPH, Magdalena Palavecino, MPH, Laura Staeheli, MPH, Kobe Pereira, MPH, Mia N. Campbell, MHS, Elias Preciado, MPH, Astrea Villarroel-Sanchez, MPH, and Kevalyn Bharadwaj, MPH. We also thank Callen-Lorde Community Health Center staff that contributed to this project. We further thank the following colleagues for their thoughtful input on coding racial and ethnic categories for our data: Renee M. Johnson, PhD, MPH, of Johns Hopkins University, Paris "AJ" Adkins-Jackson, PhD, of Columbia University, Carlos Rodriguez-Diaz, PhD, of The George Washington University, as well as Howard Shih, MSE, and Ryan Vinh from AAPI Data. We also thank the participants for engaging in this research.

Note. The contents are solely the responsibility of the authors and do not necessarily represent the official views of the National Institutes of Health.

CONFLICTS OF INTEREST

The authors of this article have no conflicts to disclose.

HUMAN PARTICIPANT PROTECTION

The study was approved by the Institutional review board at Columbia University Irving Medical Center (IRB-AAAS8164).

REFERENCES

1. Centers for Disease Control and Prevention. HIV infection, risk, prevention, and testing behaviors among transgender women—National HIV Behavioral Surveillance: 7 US Cities, 2019–2020. 2021. HIV Surveillance Special Report 27. Available at: https://www.cdc.gov/hiv/library/reports/hiv-surveillance.html. Accessed September 30, 2024.
2. Lake JE, Clark JL. Optimizing HIV prevention and care for transgender adults. *AIDS*. 2019;33(3):363–375. https://doi.org/10.1097/QAD.0000000000002095
3. Centers for Disease Control and Prevention. HIV treatment as prevention. August 9, 2023. Available at: https://www.cdc.gov/hiv/risk/art/index.html. Accessed October 7, 2024.
4. White Hughto JM, Reisner SL, Pachankis JE. Transgender stigma and health: a critical review of stigma determinants, mechanisms, and interventions. *Soc Sci Med*. 2015;147:222–231. https://doi.org/10.1016/j.socscimed.2015.11.010

5. Bowleg L. The problem with the phrase women and minorities: intersectionality—an important theoretical framework for public health. *Am J Public Health.* 2012;102(7):1267–1273. https://doi.org/10.2105/AJPH.2012.300750

6. Wesp LM, Malcoe LH, Elliott A, Poteat T. Intersectionality research for transgender health justice: a theory-driven conceptual framework for structural analysis of transgender health inequities. *Transgend Health.* 2019;4(1):287–296. https://doi.org/10.1089/trgh.2019.0039

7. Morton MJ, Lurie N. Community resilience and public health practice. *Am J Public Health.* 2013; 103(7):1158–1160. https://doi.org/10.2105/AJPH.2013.301354

8. Frost DM, Meyer IH. Minority stress theory: application, critique, and continued relevance. *Curr Opin Psychol.* 2023;51:101579. https://doi.org/10.1016/j.copsyc.2023.101579

9. Meyer IH. Resilience in the study of minority stress and health of sexual and gender minorities. *Psychol Sex Orientat Gend Divers.* 2015;2(3): 209–213. https://doi.org/10.1037/sgd0000132

10. Frost DM, Meyer IH. Measuring community connectedness among diverse sexual minority populations. *J Sex Res.* 2012;49(1):36–49. https://doi.org/10.1080/00224499.2011.565427

11. Kim ES, Kawachi I. Perceived neighborhood social cohesion and preventive healthcare use. *Am J Prev Med.* 2017;53(2):e35–e40. https://doi.org/10.1016/j.amepre.2017.01.007

12. Ramirez-Valles J, Brown AU. Latinos' community involvement in HIV/AIDS: organizational and individual perspectives on volunteering. *AIDS Educ Prev.* 2003;15(1 suppl A):90–104. https://doi.org/10.1521/aeap.15.1.5.90.23606

13. Nowell B, Boyd NM. Sense of community responsibility in community collaboratives: advancing a theory of community as resource and responsibility. *Am J Community Psychol.* 2014;54(3-4):229–242. https://doi.org/10.1007/s10464-014-9667-x

14. Wakefield JRH, Khauser A. Doing it for us: community identification predicts willingness to receive a COVID-19 vaccination via perceived sense of duty to the community. *J Community Appl Soc Psychol.* 2021;31(5):603–614. https://doi.org/10.1002/casp.2542

15. Kertzner RM, Meyer IH, Frost DM, Stirratt MJ. Social and psychological well-being in lesbians, gay men, and bisexuals: the effects of race, gender, age, and sexual identity. *Am J Orthopsychiatry.* 2009; 79(4):500–510. https://doi.org/10.1037/a0016848

16. Sexual orientation and gender identity: selected demographics and health indicators; New York State adults, 2014–2016. Behavioral Risk Factor Surveillance System Brief Number 1806. July 19, 2018. Available at: https://www.health.ny.gov/statistics/brfss/reports/docs/1806_brfss_sogi.pdf. Accessed October 17, 2024.

17. Callander D, Schneider JA, Radix A, et al. Longitudinal cohort of HIV-negative transgender women of colour in New York City: protocol for the TURNNT ("Trying to Understand Relationships, Networks and Neighbourhoods Among Transgender Women of Colour") study. *BMJ Open.* 2020;10(4):e032876. https://doi.org/10.1136/bmjopen-2019-032876

18. Testa RJ, Habarth J, Peta J, Balsam K, Bockting W. Development of the Gender Minority Stress and Resilience Measure. *Psychol Sex Orientat Gend Divers.* 2015;2(1):65–77. https://doi.org/10.1037/sgd0000081

19. Zou G. A modified Poisson regression approach to prospective studies with binary data. *Am J Epidemiol.* 2004;159(7):702–706. https://doi.org/10.1093/aje/kwh090

20. D'Avanzo PA, Bass SB, Kelly PJ, Brajuha J, Gutierrez-Mock L, Sevelius J. Community belonging and attitudes towards HIV pre-exposure prophylaxis (PrEP) among transgender women. *AIDS Behav.* 2021;25(9):2728–2742. https://doi.org/10.1007/s10461-021-03183-2

21. Temelkovska T, Moriarty K, Huerta L, et al. Social networks play a complex role in HIV prevention knowledge, attitudes, practices, and the uptake of PrEP through transgender women communities centered around three "casas trans" in Lima, Peru: a qualitative study. *J Int Assoc Provid AIDS Care.* 2023;22:23259582231196705. https://doi.org/10.1177/23259582231196705

22. Ramirez-Valles J, Fergus S, Reisen CA, Poppen PJ, Zea MC. Confronting stigma: community involvement and psychological well-being among HIV-positive Latino gay men. *Hisp J Behav Sci.* 2005;27(1):101–119. https://doi.org/10.1177/0739986304270232

23. Hennessy F, Turner L, Higgins V, Piercy J, Holbrook T. 1539. Presence of mental health concerns is associated with poor adherence in people taking pre-exposure prophylaxis in real-world clinical practice in the United States. *Open Forum Infect Dis.* 2023;10(suppl 2):ofad500.1374. https://doi.org/10.1093/ofid/ofad500.1374

24. Cramm JM, Nieboer AP. Relationships between frailty, neighborhood security, social cohesion and sense of belonging among community-dwelling older people. *Geriatr Gerontol Int.* 2013;13(3):759–763. https://doi.org/10.1111/j.1447-0594.2012.00967.x

25. Mannarini T, Rochira A, Ciavolino E, Salvatore S. Individual and perceived community determinants of sense of community: the role of universalistic values. *J Community Psychol.* 2020;48(2):623–637. https://doi.org/10.1002/jcop.22255

26. Salami B, Salma J, Hegadoren K, Meherali S, Kolawole T, Diaz E. Sense of community belonging among immigrants: perspective of immigrant service providers. *Public Health.* 2019; 167:28–33. https://doi.org/10.1016/j.puhe.2018.10.017

27. Michalski CA, Diemert LM, Helliwell JF, Goel V, Rosella LC. Relationship between sense of community belonging and self-rated health across life stages. *SSM Popul Health.* 2020;12:100676. https://doi.org/10.1016/j.ssmph.2020.100676

28. Pulice-Farrow L, Gonzalez KA, Lefevor GT. LGBTQ rumination, anxiety, depression, and community connection during Trump's presidency. *Psychol Sex Orientat Gend Divers.* 2023;10(1):80–90. https://doi.org/10.1037/sgd0000497

29. Matsuno E, Israel T. Psychological interventions promoting resilience among transgender individuals: Transgender Resilience Intervention Model (TRIM). *Couns Psychol.* 2018;46(5):632–655. https://doi.org/10.1177/0011000018787261

30. Zubizarreta D, Trinh MH, Reisner SL. COVID-19 risk and resilience among US transgender and gender diverse populations. *Am J Prev Med.* 2022;62(2):299–303. https://doi.org/10.1016/j.amepre.2021.07.017

31. Poteat TC, Reisner SL, Miller M, Wirtz AL, American Cohort To Study HIV Acquisition Among Transgender Women (LITE). Letter to the editor: vulnerability to COVID-19-related harms among transgender women with and without HIV infection in the eastern and southern US. *J Acquir Immune Defic Syndr 1999.* 2020;85(4):e67–e69. https://doi.org/10.1097/QAI.0000000000002490

32. DiNenno EA, Delaney KP, Pitasi MA, et al. HIV testing before and during the COVID-19 pandemic—United States, 2019–2020. *MMWR Morb Mortal Wkly Rep.* 2022;71(25):820–824. https://doi.org/10.15585/mmwr.mm7125a2

33. Friedman SR, Mateu-Gelabert P, Nikolopoulos GK, et al. Big events theory and measures may help explain emerging long-term effects of current crises. *Glob Public Health.* 2021;16(8-9): 1167–1186. https://doi.org/10.1080/17441692.2021.1903528

34. Hirshfield S, Contreras J, Luebe RQ, et al. Engagement in HIV care among New York City transgender women of color: findings from the peer-led, TWEET intervention, a SPNS trans women of color initiative. *AIDS Behav.* 2021;25(suppl 1):20–30. https://doi.org/10.1007/s10461-019-02667-6

Antitransgender Legislation and Needs of Transgender Floridians, 2018–2024

Callan Hummel, PhD, Kim-Phuong Truong-Vu, PhD, Kathryn Nowotny, PhD, Ashley Mayfaire, BA, Beaux Ramos, BS, BA, Jasmine McKenzie, Charlton Copeland, JD, and Tiffany R. Glynn, PhD

See also LGBTQ+ Transgender Health, pp. 1594–1670.

Objectives. To document transgender Floridians' service needs before and after antitransgender state legislation.

Methods. We conducted descriptive and change point analyses of intake survey data collected by a transgender-led community-based organization in Florida from 701 clients who requested services between 2018 and 2024.

Results. Findings show enrollment for services increased during the rise in antitransgender legislation, with pressing needs for legal and financial support for name changes and gender-affirming health care. The percentage of clients requesting sexual health resources increased, especially among Black clients.

Conclusions. Findings underscore the urgency of (1) understanding the impact of antitransgender legislation on service needs, and (2) understanding the sequelae, including the ability for organizations to meet needs and the impact on psychosocial health outcomes. Findings emphasize the crucial role of community-based organizations in supporting transgender people in a discriminatory environment and generating data to inform policy.

Public Health Implications. Antitransgender legislation constitutes a public health crisis by restricting life-saving care and exacerbating health disparities. Community-based organizations can resist these laws and act as a protective buffer for affected individuals. (*Am J Public Health*. 2025;115(10):1642–1651. https://doi.org/10.2105/AJPH.2025.308171)

AJPH October 2025, Vol. 115, No. 10

Discrimination is a social determinant of health, especially for transgender people (people are transgender if they experience incongruence between gender identity and gender assigned at birth).[1–3] Transphobia interacts with other forms of discrimination (e.g., racism, sexism, homophobia), including legal discrimination enacted through legislation, and is syndemic with other social determinants of health such as access to health services and socioeconomic status.[4–6] Legislation that discriminates against lesbian, gay, bisexual, transgender, and queer (LGBTQ) people decreases well-being and increases depression and anxiety.[1,7] Antitransgender legislation increased across the United States after 2020,[7] and Florida passed some of the most restrictive antitransgender legislation.[8] According to the American Civil Liberties Union, Florida state legislators proposed 36 antitransgender bills and passed 7 between 2020 and 2024 (Table 1).[9]

One prominent Florida bill—HB 1557 (2022), popularized as the "Don't Say Gay or Trans" bill—prohibited discussions of gender and sexual identity in elementary schools, which later expanded to grades K–12 in 2023. Another bill, SB 254 (2023), banned gender-affirming care for minors, made providing such treatments a first-degree misdemeanor, and allowed state courts to issue warrants to take temporary custody of children receiving gender-affirming care. SB 254 restricted transgender adults' transition-related care by requiring an in-person physician's approval rather than approval by nurse practitioners or via telehealth. SB 254 disrupted up to

TABLE 1— Major Antitransgender Legislation Passed in Florida: 2018–2024

Introduced	Passed	Bill Name (Nickname)	Policy Area	Antitransgender Content
March 2021	June 2021	SB 1028: Fairness in Women's Sports Act	Education, sports	Bars transgender children from school sports
January 2022	March 2022	HB 1467	Education	Allows books to be challenged in schools
January 2022	March 2022	HB 1557: Parental Rights in Education Act (Don't Say Gay)	Education	Prohibits teachers from discussing gender identity and sexual orientation in grades K–3
February 2023	May 2023	HB 1069 (Don't Say Gay or Trans)	Education	Prohibits teachers from discussing gender identity and sexual orientation in grades K–12
March 2023	May 2023	SB 254 (Gender-Affirming Care Ban)	Health care	Bans gender-affirming surgeries and medications for minors, restricts adult care, imposes criminal penalties for doctors
March 2023	May 2023	SB 1438 (Drag Ban)	Public space	Prohibits minors from attending some performances, targets drag shows
March 2023	May 2023	HB 1521: Safety in Private Spaces Act (Bathroom Bill)	Public space	Requires bathrooms to align with gender assigned at birth, states that gender is immutable, lists potential criminal penalties

80% of transition-related health care for adults in Florida.[10]

Research documents that antitransgender laws that inhibit transgender people's right to openly exist and receive health care exacerbate the extreme disparities in suicidality and mental health issues between transgender and cisgender individuals.[3,11–15] Almost half of transgender people report suicidal ideation and 26% have attempted suicide.[16] People who do not receive gender-affirming care have double the risk of experiencing moderate to severe depression and a fourfold likelihood of experiencing anxiety than do those who receive appropriate health care.[17] Thus, antitransgender laws endanger the lives and well-being of transgender people and create greater health inequities.[7,11,12]

Further challenging transgender people's right to openly exist, HB 1521 (2023, the "Bathroom Bill") criminalized using a public bathroom designated for a gender that differs from one's gender assigned at birth. A January 2024 memo from the Florida Department of Highway Safety and Motor Vehicles ended gender marker changes on driver's licenses in Florida and caused widespread fear by declaring that "misrepresenting one's gender . . . on a driver's license constitutes fraud" and is subject to criminal penalties.[18] Transgender individuals who do not have gender-affirming identification report higher levels of psychological distress and suicidal ideation.[19–20] Aligned with allostatic load theory, research finds that sweeping discriminatory legislation and accumulated adversities increase chronic stress that leads to "wear and tear" on the body over time with subsequent higher rates of disability and morbidity.[21]

Research finds that discriminatory legislation increases health disparities across minority groups.[5–7] An estimated 111 100 transgender people aged 13 years and older live in Florida.[14,22] Transgender people in Florida are overpoliced, are denied basic rights, and face exclusion from health-monitoring systems (i.e., informational and institutional erasure).[1,23] The 2018 Human Rights Watch report on transgender women and human rights found a uniquely high-risk environment for transgender women and concluded that in South Florida transgender women face a fragmented landscape for health care that fails to ensure that effective care is available. Research about transgender people greatly benefits from academic–community partnerships.

Our study is a collaboration between university researchers and activists at TransSOCIAL, a grassroots transgender-led community-based organization (CBO) in Florida. We examined the potential impact of antitransgender legislation on the health and well-being of transgender people. We examined the service needs of transgender people in Florida over time and compared results from before and after the increase in antitransgender legislation.

METHODS

We analyzed de-identified administrative intake data from transgender clients in Florida ($n = 701$; aged ≥ 18 years) who enrolled in services with TransSOCIAL from April 2018 to August 2024. Clients learned about TransSOCIAL's services through their social networks or at LGBTQ community outreach events in Florida and autonomously sought the CBO's services. This is a nonprobability sample, and we did not cluster respondents. The intake form stated that anonymized responses may be used for research and that no identifying information would be shared outside TransSOCIAL.

Trained advocacy personnel from TransSOCIAL conducted an intake to connect new clients with services and referrals. This quantitative survey included demographic questions, a checklist of service needs from the organization, and additional assessments on need for legal assistance with name changes and gender markers, housing, and employment. The intake survey has been administered to new clients since 2018. English-speaking clients completed the survey online; Spanish- and Haitian Creole–speaking clients completed the survey over the telephone or in person with advocacy personnel fluent in those languages. Advocacy personnel then shared the de-identified intake data with us in August 2024.

Measures and Variables

Sociodemographics. Age, race, ethnicity, gender, and economic status as indicated by employment status, annual income (income added in 2021; n = 427), and housing status (housing added in 2021; n = 507) were self-reported. We grouped gender into (1) feminine, (2) masculine, or (3) nonbinary gender based on responses to multiple response items and an open-ended item. It is important to note that most clients endorsed and reported multiple gender, racial, and ethnic identities. These responses were reported in multiple groups to represent the array of nonmutually exclusive self-reported identities; therefore, the percentage of responses does not add to 100%. Such operationalization of identities as not mutually exclusive is crucial for studying the health of the transgender population because it accounts for the variability and multiple dimensions of gender, race, and ethnicity.[24]

Service needs. We categorized TransSOCIAL's service offerings into 4 domains: legal assistance, health services and referrals, employment services, and basic need services. Clients self-reported each service needed. For legal assistance, clients selected from legal name change, legal gender marker change, obtaining or updating identity documents, and fees required for the identity documents (the fees question was added in 2019; n = 596). Other legal assistance included immigration services and help with filing a discrimination complaint, but because of the small number of these requests, we do not discuss them in this study. For health services and referrals, clients selected from help getting insurance, letter of support for gender-affirming surgery or other gender-affirming care, referral for primary care, mental health provider, hormone replacement therapy or gender-affirming surgery, and sexual health needs (i.e., condoms, lubricant, counseling, sexually transmitted infection [STI] testing, and referral for preexposure prophylaxis [PrEP]). For employment needs, clients selected whether they needed assistance finding employment.

Statistical Analysis

The primary investigator (C. H.) cleaned and analyzed the anonymized data. First, we used R version 4.4 (RStudio, Boston, MA) to calculate proportions for dichotomous and categorical variables and means and SDs for continuous variables. Next, we conducted a change point analysis in a Bayesian regression framework on the daily intake data using R's mcp package.[25] Change point analysis identifies data points that shift trends in a time series and returns reliable estimates for medium (e.g., n = 500) to large samples.[26] Change point analysis is used to suggest when a change in a trend may come from a change in policy.[25,26] We used change point analysis to examine whether client intake patterns shifted after Florida implemented antitransgender legislation across the state. The mcp package estimates posterior distributions for change points using Markov chain Monte Carlo simulations. Given a number of change points, the mcp package automatically detected where a change point most likely occurred.

RESULTS

From April 18, 2018, to August 1, 2024, 701 clients aged 18 years and older and living in Florida completed TransSOCIAL's client intake. The study included 49% feminine, 32% masculine, and 25% nonbinary clients. The clients were racially and ethnically diverse, consisting of 54% (382) White, 46% (320) Latinx, and 31% (217) Black/African American clients, among others. The mean age was 28 years (SD = 10.24), with most clients aged between 18 and 30 years. Among the clients, 28% (195) reported being unemployed, and 32% (225) reported being uninsured.

Appendix Tables A and B (available as a supplement to the online version of this article at http://www.ajph.org) summarize clients' sociodemographic characteristics, including gender identity, race, age, annual income, housing status, and financial ability to afford name change fees. A majority (286; 67%) of transgender clients who were asked about income (n = 427) reported making less than

$25 000 in the previous year. Of clients who were asked about housing (n = 507), 22% (113) reported not having stable housing, being unhoused, or feeling unsafe in their housing. Additionally, more than half (357) of the respondents could not afford the $400 court fee for a legal name change.

Trends in Transgender Client Intake

Overall, 37 clients sought TransSOCIAL services in 2018, 64 in 2019, 81 in 2020, 129 in 2021, 76 in 2022, 154 in 2023, and 160 in the first 8 months of 2024. Several factors likely affected intake trends, including CBO outreach, CBO staffing, the COVID-19 pandemic, and employment opportunities for transgender people. For example, CBO personnel point to a temporary reduction in paid staff for several months in 2022 and a website outage in October 2022 to explain the decrease in intakes in 2022. Figure 1 illustrates TransSOCIAL's client daily intake numbers from April 2018 to August 2024.

We suggest that antitransgender policy is a major driver of CBO intake. Although the CBO has recorded an uptick in new clients in most years, there was a substantial increase during the years and months that the Florida legislature pursued antitransgender legislation. Advocacy personnel reported that they saw a spike in requests for help when antitransgender policies were in the news, specifically on social media, and discussed in their informal networks. News coverage of antitransgender policies in Florida are highest during the state legislative session, which runs from January to March in even-numbered years and March to May in odd-numbered years.

Using Bayesian change point analysis, we identified a large shift in the daily intake trend between the end of 2022 and the beginning of 2023. We selected a model with 1 change point and 2 segments with autoregressive errors after comparing R-hat convergence diagnostics across models with 1 to 5 change points and selecting the model with R-hat values closest to 1. The R-hat convergence diagnostic compares the within- and between-chain estimates for parameters from the Markov chain Monte Carlo simulations; an R-hat of 1 means those estimates converge.

Figure 1 plots the daily number of intakes from 2018 to 2024. The peaked lines along the x-axis are the posterior distributions of the estimated change point. The highest peak in the posterior distributions—the area the algorithm identified as the most likely to contain a fundamental shift in the data—occurred in January 2023, when an unprecedented number of antitransgender bills were introduced in Florida and in statehouses around the country.[9] After this turning point, the number of daily intakes continued to increase.

Service Need Requests

Table 2 presents the requested service needs. Although clients requested a wide array of service needs, some were more prominent. First, legal services were the most requested, especially legal name changes—TransSOCIAL's primary service; 92% requested help with legally changing their names, updating their identification documents, or both. Half (353; 50%) of the clients requested health care services or referrals, many for sexual health resources (217; 31%), followed by hormone replacement therapy (74; 11%) and gender-affirming surgeons (63; 9%). About one fifth (130; 19%) requested help with employment, and 22% (113) of clients who were asked about housing reported that they needed stable housing.

To understand the top 3 service areas that TransSOCIAL offers (i.e., legal assistance, health care services and referrals, and employment assistance), we analyzed the requests by year (we excluded housing, which was not asked about in all years). As shown in Figure 2, the number and percentage of clients requesting these services increased almost annually after the Florida legislature started passing antitransgender laws. In 2024, 155 (97%) incoming clients sought legal aid compared with 33 (89%) in 2018. In the same year, 83 (52%) clients requested health care assistance compared with 10 (27%) in 2018.

Requests for employment assistance displayed a different pattern, which may reflect the COVID-19 pandemic's impact on employment. The proportion of people requesting employment assistance peaked in 2020 (30% of clients). These requests eased as the job market improved and then increased again in 2023 (30%) before dipping slightly, to 27% in 2024.

Requests for health care services and referrals increased overall and in the proportion of clients requesting them. This growth was driven by a surge in requests for sexual health resources (e.g., condoms, lubricant, STI testing, and PrEP referrals; plotted by type in Appendix Figure A, available as a supplement to the online version of this article at http://www.ajph.org). In 2024, 29% (61) of clients asked for sexual health resources compared with 11% (5) in 2018. Similarly, requests for PrEP and STI testing increased significantly. In 2024, 11% (18) and 12% (19) of clients requested PrEP referrals and STI testing, respectively, compared with

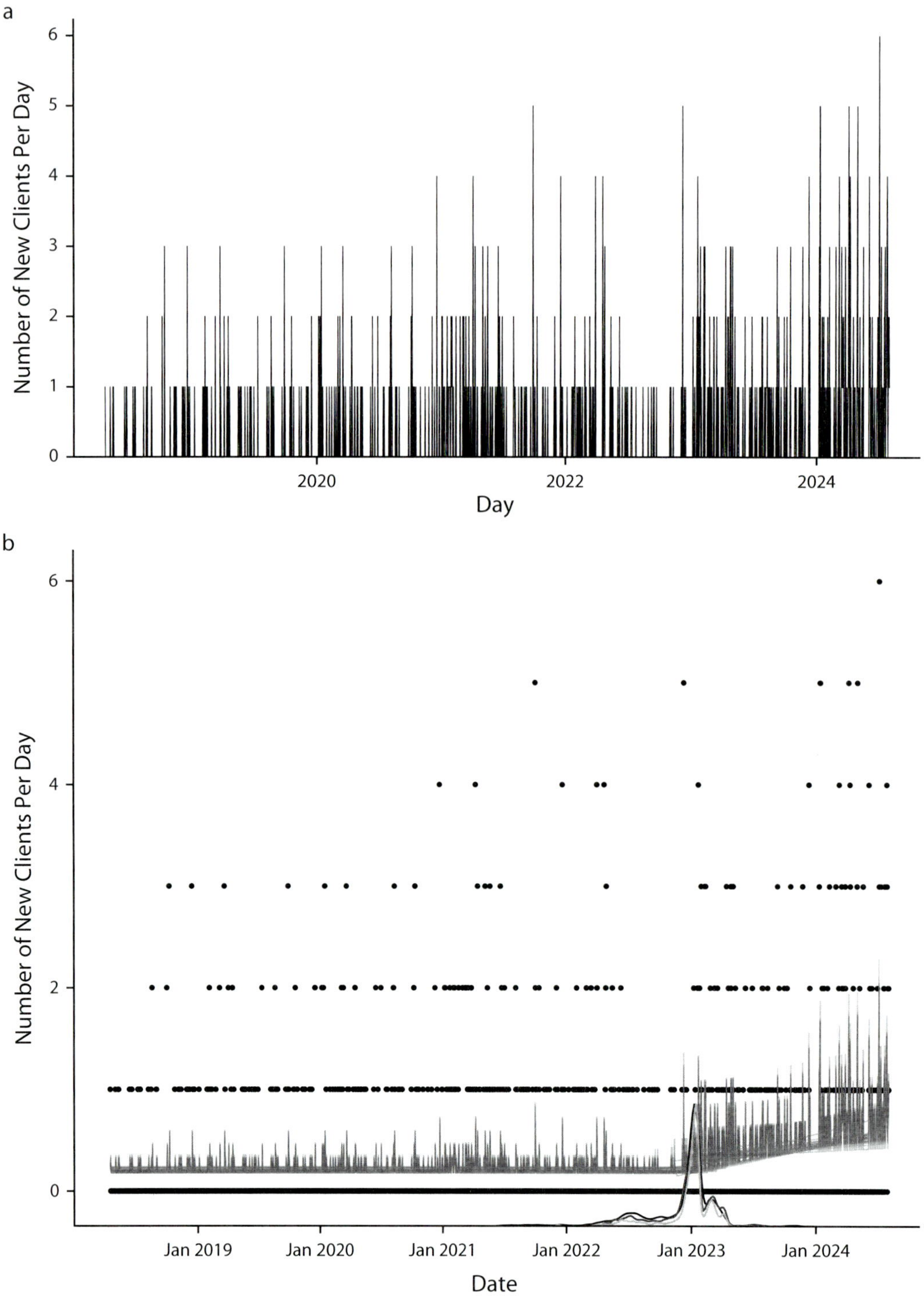

FIGURE 1— **Transgender Clients Enrolled With TransSOCIAL by (a) Number of Daily New Client Intakes, and (b) Number of Daily New Client Intakes With Bayesian Change Point Detection: Florida, 2018–2024**

1 client requesting PrEP and STI testing in 2018.

PrEP and STI testing requests doubled between 2022 and 2024. This contrasts with other health care service and referral requests, which either stayed constant or decreased. The increase in requests for sexual health resources is largely driven by an increase in requests from Black clients (Appendix Figure B, available as a supplement to the online version of this

TABLE 2— Requested Services Among Transgender Floridians Enrolled With TransSOCIAL: 2018–2024

Statistic	No. (%)
Need legal assistance	662 (94)
Need assistance in name change process	646 (92)
Need immigration services	18 (3)
Need to file a discrimination claim	17 (2)
Need health care referrals or services	353 (50)
Need condoms, lubricants, or safer sex counseling	217 (31)
Need HRT referral	74 (11)
Need gender-affirming surgeon	63 (9)
Need PrEP	62 (9)
Need STI testing	58 (8)
Need insurance	59 (8)
Need mental health provider	52 (7)
Need primary care doctor	49 (7)
Need letter of support for gender-affirming care	43 (6)
Need stable housing[a]	113 (22)
Need employment assistance	130 (19)

Note. HRT = hormone replacement therapy; PrEP = preexposure prophylaxis; STI = sexually transmitted infection. The study population was n = 701.
[a]For this question, n = 507.

article at http://www.ajph.org). Black clients requested sexual health resources at higher rates than did clients with other racial and ethnic identities across all years. Latinx clients requesting sexual health resources contributed to the overall increase in requests in later years.

Black clients requested STI testing and PrEP referrals at higher rates than did other clients. However, the absolute numbers were not as large as those requesting condoms and lubricant. By contrast, White clients requested notably fewer sexual health services than did other clients. For example, 12% (19) of Black clients, 9% (22) of Latinx clients, and 6% (9) of White clients requested PrEP referrals, whereas 12% (19) of Black clients, 10% (24) of Latinx clients, and 3% (5) of White clients requested STI testing. There were no sustained and substantial racial or ethnic differences in other service area requests (Appendix Figures C, D, and E, available as a supplement to the online version of this article at http://www.ajph.org).

DISCUSSION

We found that the number of transgender people requesting services from a CBO shifted dramatically in January 2023 and continued to increase as Florida implemented antitransgender measures. These findings suggest that antitransgender legislation prompts transgender people to seek support, resources, and protection from advocacy groups, which are an important source of resistance to these laws. These patterns emphasize the importance of advocacy groups in providing access to supportive resources and crucial information about legal rights and how to navigate new laws.

Many transgender people in this study reported considerable economic vulnerabilities, in line with other studies on transgender demographics.[14–15] Compared with other needs assessment data on the cisgender population, the intake survey data demonstrate that transgender Floridians reported fewer socioeconomic status resources and higher needs than did the cisgender population. For example, in our study, 28% (195) of transgender people reported being unemployed, 32% (225) reported being uninsured, and 22% (113) reported having unstable housing, compared with 3.8%, 12%, and about 1% of cisgender national populations, respectively.[15,27] Additionally, requests for sexual health resources (e.g., condoms, STI testing, and PrEP referrals) increased more than other service requests over time and during the antitransgender legislative period.

A high number of individuals sought legal aid across all years, even in years with no antitransgender legislation. This may be unique to our study because of TransSOCIAL's name change program, which is the largest in Florida. The high prevalence of legal service requests is likely a ceiling effect—requests started high and went higher but cannot exceed 100%—rather than a null effect of antitransgender legislation.

The majority of clients requested help with changing their names and accessing health care. Legal name changes are critical for the social determinants of health among transgender individuals.[28–29] Legal name changes provide social and legal affirmation of one's gender identity and foster a sense of acceptance, which is important in health care settings.[20,30] Gender affirmation, which includes legal name changes, is associated with reductions

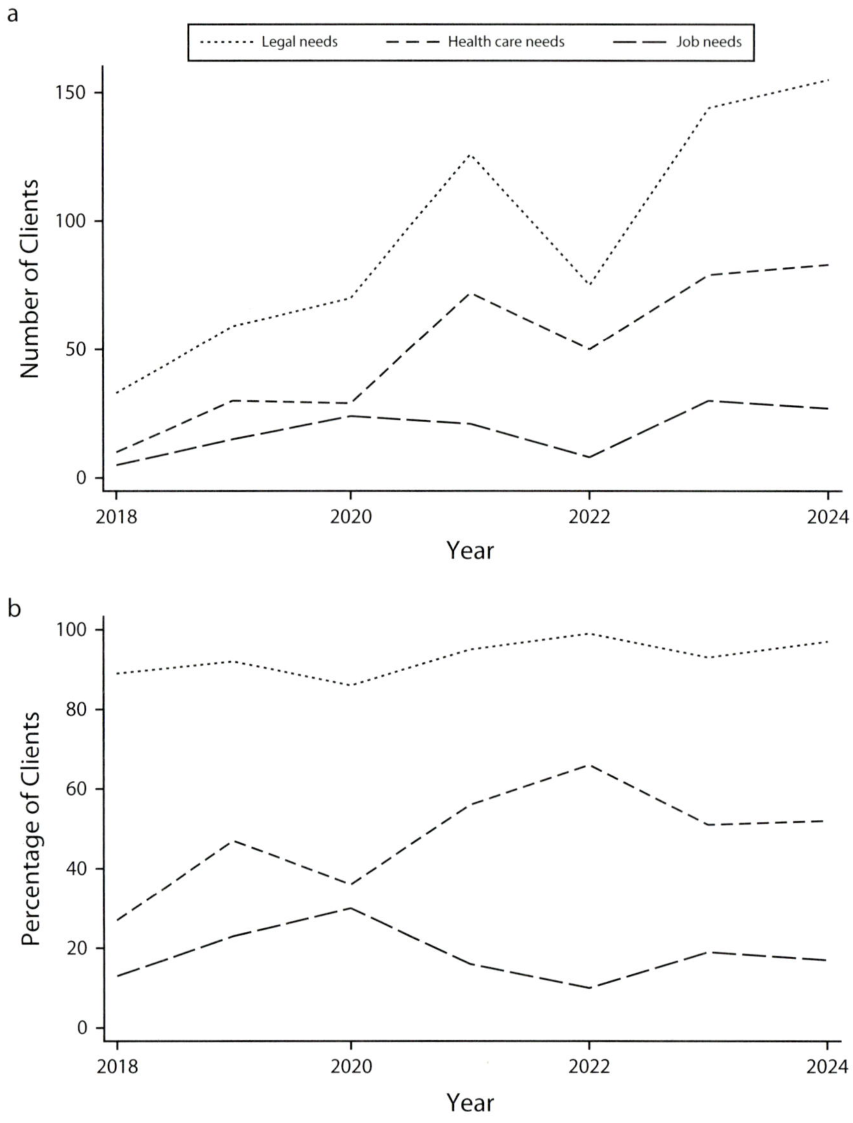

FIGURE 2— TransSOCIAL Clients Requesting Legal, Health Care, and Employment Services by Type of Service (a) Numbers, and (b) Percentages: Florida, 2018–2024

Note. The 3 peaked lines along the x-axis are the posterior distributions of the estimated change point.

in depression, anxiety, and suicidal ideation.[19,31,32] Additionally, legal name changes may increase safety by decreasing discrimination in medical, occupational, and housing settings.[28]

Limitations

Limitations of this study include the nonprobability sample of transgender Floridians seeking TransSOCIAL services and the observational analysis. The data and our analyses suggest that antitransgender legislation precedes an increase in intakes and that intakes increased as Florida implemented more antitransgender policies. However, observational analyses on a nonprobability sample cannot demonstrate a causal relationship between policy and intakes. Similarly, we expect that other factors also influence intake trends, but we do not have the data to statistically estimate or control for the influence of other factors. These findings cannot be generalized to all transgender people, including transgender people who do not seek TransSOCIAL services in Florida. Additionally, TransSOCIAL is physically located in South Florida, and clients from South Florida are overrepresented in the data set.

TransSOCIAL's most developed service is assistance with name changes, which means that the need for legal assistance may be overrepresented in this sample.[33] Other services (e.g., gender-affirming health care, employment, and housing) may be a top priority for transgender individuals in Florida who seek assistance elsewhere. Despite these limitations, this study provides important insights into the needs of the transgender population in an antitransgender legislative period.

Public Health Implications

There has been an acute and rapid increase in antitransgender legislation at the state and federal levels. As reported by the Trans Legislation Tracker, 2024 was the fifth consecutive record-breaking year for antitransgender legislation: 587 antitransgender bills were introduced across 43 states along with 87 national bills. In the first 100 days of 2025, 854 bills were under consideration across 49 states, including 36 at the national level.[34] These bills reinforce harmful medical practices and discriminatory societal attitudes; therefore, they lead to negative health outcomes.[2,13,23]

Discriminatory policy actions are linked to severe physical and mental health morbidities, as well as increased mortality, in transgender populations.[7,11,12] Transgender youths reported an increase in victimization and suicidality during the rise of antitransgender legislation.[12,17] To avoid anticipated discrimination, many transgender individuals of all ages avoid or delay seeking necessary health care and treatments, leading to poorer health outcomes, chronic health issues, and downstream consequences from unaddressed health issues.[1,2,13,23] Antitransgender legislation will further exacerbate health disparities and barriers to health care, including but not limited to pathologization of gender nonconformity, restricting access to necessary medical care, and increasing stress and stigma, which may lead to an increase in health-harming behaviors used as coping mechanisms.[2,7,11–13]

Anti-LGBTQ legislation is associated with national economic negative consequences,[35] including increasing unemployment, housing instability, and poverty, as well as limiting resources and support, which is associated with poor health among the entire population. Thus, antitransgender legislation is a public health crisis for all, as it endangers the lives and well-being of this population and the communities in which they work, live, and age.

Multifaceted strategies are required to combat inequalities driven by antitransgender legislation. One way is to increase funding for advocacy groups who help transgender clients resist legal discrimination, such as Trans-SOCIAL. With increased resources, advocacy groups can provide or facilitate access to gender-affirming health care services, mental health support, crisis intervention, and other essential health services. Increased funding to advocacy groups also helps reduce homelessness, housing instability, economic instability, and survival sex work by allowing advocacy groups to offer housing assistance programs, job training programs, and employment placement services. Furthermore, funding can support research initiatives that provide evidence-based data to highlight the negative impacts of antitransgender legislation, which can be used to advocate policy changes.

Addressing these pressing needs and increasing health equity require collaboration between CBOs, scholars, health professionals, legal systems, and policymakers.[3,5,24,28,33] This unique data set illustrates the needs of a marginalized population during a period in which legislators specifically targeted transgender people. The size and insights of the data set demonstrate the role of CBOs in collecting vital data on the experiences and needs of marginalized populations, which can directly inform policy, social programs, and health care. This administrative data set is relatively large and covers a long period compared with many other data sets of transgender respondents in public health research. CBOs can reach populations that researchers and health departments struggle to contact. Collaborating with CBOs helps public health officials, health care professionals, and researchers address the social determinants of health and serve transgender communities. AJPH

ABOUT THE AUTHORS

Callan Hummel is with the Department of Political Science, University of British Columbia, Vancouver, BC, and was with the Department of Political Science, University of Miami, Coral Gables, FL, at the start of the study. Kim-Phuong Truong-Vu and Kathryn Nowotny are with the Department of Sociology, University of Miami, Coral Gables, FL. Ashley Mayfaire and Beaux Ramos are with Trans-SOCIAL, Miami, FL. Jasmine McKenzie is with the McKenzie Project, Inc, Miami, FL. Charlton Copeland is with the School of Law, University of Miami, Coral Gables, FL. Tiffany R. Glynn is with the Department of Psychiatry, Massachusetts General Hospital, and Harvard Medical School, Boston, MA.

CORRESPONDENCE

Correspondence should be sent to Callan Hummel, Buchanan C422, 1866 Main Mall, University of British Columbia, Vancouver, BC, V6T 1Z1 Canada (e-mail: callan.hummel@ubc.ca). Reprints can be ordered at http://www.ajph.org by clicking the "Reprints" link.

PUBLICATION INFORMATION

Full Citation: Hummel C, Truong-Vu K-P, Nowotny K, et al. Antitransgender legislation and needs of transgender Floridians, 2018–2024. *Am J Public Health*. 2025;115(10):1642–1651.

Acceptance Date: April 16, 2025.

DOI: https://doi.org/10.2105/AJPH.2025.308171

ORCID iDs:

Callan Hummel https://orcid.org/0000-0003-3673-0657

Kim-Phuong Truong-Vu https://orcid.org/0000-0001-9344-9584

Kathryn Nowotny https://orcid.org/0000-0002-6899-1440

Ashley Mayfaire https://orcid.org/0009-0008-4925-5844

Tiffany R. Glynn https://orcid.org/0000-0002-0305-1976

CONTRIBUTORS

C. Hummel analyzed and interpreted the data. C. Hummel and K-P. Truong-Vu designed the study and drafted the article. C. Hummel, K. Nowotny, and A. Mayfaire acquired funding. K-P. Truong-Vu interpreted the data. K. Nowotny and T. R. Glynn conceptualized the study. A. Mayfaire, B. Ramos, and J. McKenzie acquired, curated, and interpreted the data. All authors revised and approved the final version of the article.

ACKNOWLEDGMENTS

We thank the University of Miami, Laboratory for Integrative Knowledge initiative for funding the preliminary research for this project and the University of Miami, Center for AIDS Research and the National Institutes of Health (NIH) for funding (award 5P30AI073961-17) ongoing data collection and writing for C. Hummel, K. Nowotny, A. Mayfaire, and J. McKenzie. C. Hummel's work is supported by a Hampton New Faculty grant from the University of British Columbia. T. R. Glynn's work is supported by the NIH, including the National Institute on Drug Abuse (awards K23DA060719 and L60DA059128).

We gratefully acknowledge the participation of transgender Floridians in the design and implementation of this research during a difficult time for transgender communities across the state. We thank Cameron Riopelle and Avery Everhart for feedback.

Note. The content of this article is solely the responsibility of the authors and does not necessarily represent the official views of their employers or the NIH.

CONFLICTS OF INTEREST

A. Mayfaire is a founder and board member of TransSOCIAL. B. Ramos is an employee of TransSOCIAL. J. McKenzie is the executive director of the McKenzie Project, Inc, which works with TransSOCIAL to provide name changes.

HUMAN PARTICIPANT PROTECTION

The University of Miami institutional review board determined the study to be exempt from review. The University of British Columbia Behavioral Research Ethics Board approved the study under minimal risk.

REFERENCES

1. Johnson AH, Hill I, Beach-Ferrara J, Rogers BA, Bradford A. Common barriers to healthcare for transgender people in the US Southeast. *Int J Transgend Health.* 2019;21(1):70–78. https://doi.org/10.1080/15532739.2019.1700203
2. Kcomt L, Gorey KM, Barrett BJ, McCabe SE. Healthcare avoidance due to anticipated discrimination among transgender people: a call to create trans-affirmative environments. *SSM Popul Health.* 2020;11:100608. https://doi.org/10.1016/j.ssmph.2020.100608
3. Restar AJ, Layland AK, Davis B, Thompson H, Streed C. The public health crisis state of transgender health care and policy. *Am J Public Health.* 2024;114(2):161–163. https://doi.org/10.2105/AJPH.2023.307523
4. Bailey ZD, Krieger N, Agénor M, Graves J, Linos N, Bassett MT. Structural racism and health inequities in the USA: evidence and interventions. *Lancet.* 2017;389(10077):1453–1463. https://doi.org/10.1016/S0140-6736(17)30569-X
5. Bailey ZD, Feldman JM, Bassett MT. How structural racism works—racist policies as a root cause of US racial health inequities. *N Engl J Med.* 2021;384(8):768–773. https://doi.org/10.1056/NEJMms2025396
6. Biello KB, Hughto JMW. Measuring intersectional stigma among racially and ethnically diverse transgender women: challenges and opportunities. *Am J Public Health.* 2021;111(3):344–346. https://doi.org/10.2105/AJPH.2020.306141
7. Barbee H, Deal C, Gonzales G. Anti-transgender legislation—a public health concern for transgender youth. *JAMA Pediatr.* 2022;176(2):125–126. https://doi.org/10.1001/jamapediatrics.2021.4483
8. Garcia Gutiérrez JM, Dusic E, Bambilla AJK, Restar AJ. A narrative synthesis review of legislation banning gender-affirming care. *Curr Pediatr Rep.* 2024;12(3):44–51. https://doi.org/10.1007/s40124-024-00320-y
9. American Civil Liberties Union. Mapping attacks on LGBTQ rights in US state legislatures in 2024. 2023. Available at: https://www.aclu.org/legislative-attacks-on-lgbtq-rights-2024. Accessed September 5, 2024.
10. Reed E. Trans patients being dropped as Florida law bans "up to 80%." *Los Angeles Blade.* May 11, 2023. Available at: https://www.losangelesblade.com, 2023/05/11/trans-patients-being-dropped-as-florida-law-bans-up-to-80. Accessed September 5, 2024.
11. Cunningham GB, Watanabe NM, Buzuvis E. Anti-transgender rights legislation and Internet searches pertaining to depression and suicide. *PLoS One.* 2022;17(12):e0279420. https://doi.org/10.1371/journal.pone.0279420
12. Lee WY, Hobbs JN, Hobaica S, DeChants JP, Price MN, Nath R. State-level anti-transgender laws increase past-year suicide attempts among transgender and non-binary young people in the USA. *Nat Hum Behav.* 2024;8(11):2096–2106. https://doi.org/10.1038/s41562-024-01979-5
13. Hughto JM, Meyers DJ, Mimiaga MJ, Reisner SL, Cahill S. Uncertainty and confusion regarding transgender non-discrimination policies: implications for the mental health of transgender Americans. *Sex Res Social Policy.* 2022;19(3):1069–1079. https://doi.org/10.1007/s13178-021-00602-w
14. Meerwijk EL, Sevelius JM. Transgender population size in the United States: a meta-regression of population-based probability samples. *Am J Public Health.* 2017;107(2):e1–e8. https://doi.org/10.2105/AJPH.2016.303578
15. Thomeer MB, Patterson B. Using administrative data to assess transgender health and mortality disparities. *Am J Public Health.* 2022;112(10):1365–1367. https://doi.org/10.2105/AJPH.2022.307046
16. Adams NJ, Vincent B. Suicidal thoughts and behaviors among transgender adults in relation to education, ethnicity, and income: a systematic review. *Transgend Health.* 2019;4(1):226–246. https://doi.org/10.1089/trgh.2019.0009
17. Tordoff DM, Wanta JW, Collin A, Stepney C, Inwards-Breland DJ, Ahrens K. Mental health outcomes in transgender and nonbinary youths receiving gender-affirming care. *JAMA Netw Open.* 2022;5(2):e220978. https://doi.org/10.1001/jamanetworkopen.2022.0978
18. Ellenborgen R. Transgender Floridians face new challenges with driver's license ID changes. *Tampa Bay Times.* January 30, 2024. Available at: https://www.tampabay.com/news/florida-politics/2024/01/30/transgender-florida-drivers-license-id-gender-sex-trans. Accessed August 7, 2024.
19. Scheim AI, Baker KE, Restar AJ, Sell RL. Health and health care among transgender adults in the United States. *Annu Rev Public Health.* 2022;43:503–523. https://doi.org/10.1146/annurev-publhealth-052620-100313
20. Restar A, Jin H, Breslow A, Reisner SL, Mimiaga M, Cahill S, Hughto JMW. Legal gender marker and name change is associated with lower negative emotional response to gender-based mistreatment and improve mental health outcomes among trans populations. *SSM Popul Health.* 2020;11:100595. https://doi.org/10.1016/j.ssmph.2020.100595
21. Delozier AM, Kamody RC, Rodgers S, Chen D. Health disparities in transgender and gender expansive adolescents: a topical review from a minority stress framework. *J Pediatr Psychol.* 2020;45(8):842–847. https://doi.org/10.1093/jpepsy/jsaa040
22. Herman JL, Flores AR, O'Neill KK. How many adults and youth identify as transgender in the United States? 2022. Available at: https://williamsinstitute.law.ucla.edu/publications/trans-adults-united-states. Accessed July 1, 2025.
23. Seelman KL, Colón-Diaz MJP, LeCroix RH, Xavier-Brier M, Kattari L. Transgender noninclusive healthcare and delaying care because of fear: connections to general health and mental health among transgender adults. *Transgend Health.* 2017;2(1):17–28. https://doi.org/10.1089/trgh.2016.0024
24. Kronk CA, Everhart AR, Ashley F, et al. Transgender data collection in the electronic health record: current concepts and issues. *J Am Med Inform Assoc.* 2022;29(2):271–284. https://doi.org/10.1093/jamia/ocab136
25. Lindeløv JK. mcp: an R package for regression with multiple change points. 2020. Available at: https://osf.io/preprints/osf/fzqxv. Accessed July 1, 2025.
26. White SR, Muniz-Terrera G, Matthews FE. Sample size and classification error for Bayesian change-point models with unlabelled sub-groups and incomplete follow-up. *Stat Methods Med Res.* 2018;27(5):1476–1497. https://doi.org/10.1177/0962280216662298
27. US Bureau of Labor Statistics. Labor force statistics from the current population survey. Available at: https://www.bls.gov/web/empsit/cpseea10.htm. Accessed September 18, 2024.
28. Hill BJ, Crosby R, Bouris A, et al. Exploring transgender legal name change as a potential structural intervention for mitigating social

determinants of health among transgender women of color. *Sex Res Social Policy.* 2018;15(1):25–33. https://doi.org/10.1007/s13178-017-0289-6

29. Malta M, LeGrand S, Turban J, Poteat T, Whetten K. Gender-congruent government identification is crucial for gender affirmation. *Lancet Public Health.* 2020;5(4):e178–e179. https://doi.org/10.1016/S2468-2667(20)30054-2
30. Glynn TR, Gamarel KE, Kahler CW, Iwamoto M, Operario D, Nemoto T. The role of gender affirmation in psychological well-being among transgender women. *Psychol Sex Orientat Gend Divers.* 2016;3(3):336–344. https://doi.org/10.1037/sgd0000171
31. King WM, Gamarel KE. A scoping review examining social and legal gender affirmation and health among transgender populations. *Transgend Health.* 2021;6(1):5–22. https://doi.org/10.1089/trgh.2020.0025
32. Hsieh N, Shuster SM. Health and health care of sexual and gender minorities. *J Health Soc Behav.* 2021;62(3):318–333. https://doi.org/10.1177/00221465211016436
33. Mayfaire A, Mayfaire M, Glynn T. The vital role of trans-led CBOs in public health research and efforts: an example from TransSocial, Inc. *HPHR.* 2021;43:10.54111/0001/QQ3. https://doi.org/10.54111/0001/QQ3
34. Trans Legislation Tracker. Anti-trans bills tracker. Available at: https://translegislation.com. Accessed April 14, 2025.
35. Badgett MVL, Waaldijk K, van der Meulen Rodgers Y. The relationship between LGBT inclusion and economic development: macro-level evidence. *World Development.* 2019;120:1–14. https://doi.org/10.1016/j.worlddev.2019.03.011

Discrimination and Sleep Health Among Transgender Women of Color in New York City: Cross-Sectional and Longitudinal Associations From the TURNNT Cohort Study

Adam M. Whalen, MPH, Alexander Furuya, MPH, Jessica Contreras, BA, John A. Schneider, MD, MPH, Sahnah Lim, PhD, MPH, Chau Trinh-Shevrin, DrPH, Asa Radix, MD, PhD, MPH, and Dustin T. Duncan, ScD

See also LGBTQ+ Transgender Health, pp. 1594–1670.

AJPH October 2025, Vol. 115, No. 10

Objectives. To determine whether discrimination is associated with sleep health among transgender women of color.

Methods. We included 269 participants from the Trying to Understand Relationships, Networks, and Neighborhoods Among Transgender Women of Color (TURNNT) Cohort Study in New York City in a cross-sectional analysis and 179 in a longitudinal analysis of the association between discrimination and sleep duration, quality, and latency.

Results. Median sleep duration was 6 hours per night, with 65% of participants reporting poor sleep in the past month. Nearly two thirds experienced moderate or high levels of discrimination. Cross sectionally, high discrimination was associated with a 14% greater risk of poor sleep quality relative to low discrimination (prevalence ratio [PR] = 1.14). Longitudinally, high discrimination was associated with a 15% higher risk of poor sleep (PR = 1.15) and an average of 43 minutes less per night.

Conclusions. Transgender women of color generally do not receive an adequate amount of sleep, and that sleep is often of poor quality. Those who experience higher rates of discrimination are particularly vulnerable to poor sleep health.

Public Health Implications. Effort should be focused on reducing antitransgender discrimination and developing interventions to mitigate the negative impact of discrimination on sleep health among transgender populations. (*Am J Public Health*. 2025;115(10):1652–1661. https://doi.org/10.2105/AJPH.2025.308208)

Sleep is essential for human health. Adults 18 to 60 years of age should sleep at least 7 hours each night to support optimal health, although individual sleep needs may vary according to genetic, medical, behavioral, and environmental factors.[1] Insufficient sleep duration is associated with an elevated risk of cardiovascular disease, immune dysfunction, poor general health, depression, anxiety, and mortality.[1,2] Conversely, good sleep—sufficient in duration and quality to feel well rested in the morning—enhances physical, mental, and social health.[3] Despite its importance, more than one third of adults in the United States report insufficient sleep, and nearly 40% of primary care patients report significant sleep disturbances, an early indicator of insomnia.[2,4]

Limited—although growing—research suggests that transgender and other gender minority groups sleep worse than cisgender individuals.[3,5] In comparison with their cisgender peers, US and Canadian transgender college students have 2 times higher odds of insomnia and sleep disorders,[6] transgender and gender nonconforming youths have 5 times higher odds of insomnia,[7] and gender minority and gender questioning youths 10 to 14 years of age have higher odds of short sleep duration and long sleep latency.[8] Furthermore, a German study of transgender women and transgender men identified poor sleep quality as the strongest predictor of poor quality of life, with about 80% of respondents across both groups reporting poor sleep quality.[9]

Transgender and gender nonconforming people experience a greater burden of stress, anxiety, and depression than cisgender people, potentially as a result of discrimination.[6,10,11] In 2024, 65% of transgender and nonbinary young people experienced gender identity discrimination.[12] Repeated exposure to discrimination contributes to mistrust of authorities—including medical care providers—cardiovascular disease, and other physical and mental health problems such as impaired or insufficient sleep.[11,13,14]

Minority stress theory suggests that transgender women of color (TWOC) face higher risks of discrimination than their peers (e.g., cisgender White women) because of intersecting systems of transphobia, racism, and heterosexism.[5,15] These compounded oppressions contribute to chronic psychosocial stressors and subsequent mental health problems.[11,15] Discrimination against TWOC likely differs from the discrimination experienced by other groups, such as White transgender women, transgender men, and cisgender people of color.[11]

Transgender women, particularly TWOC, face a disproportionately high risk for social and behavioral risk factors associated with both discrimination and poor sleep, including high HIV prevalence and very low socioeconomic resources.[3,7,16–19] Transgender women frequently face housing instability or homelessness[11,19]; more than 40% of transgender women experience at least 1 night of homelessness annually, and 31% experience homelessness for at least 30 nights.[16,17] Sex hormones such as estrogen and estradiol influence sleep patterns in cisgender populations and are commonly used among transgender women, but the evidence surrounding gender-affirming hormone therapy and sleep is mixed.[7,18] Gender-affirming hormone therapy may affect sleep through the mental health effects of improved gender congruence or through reduced discrimination by passing—blending into public life without being identified as transgender—although more evidence is needed.[7]

Discrimination and sleep health have been examined in racial and ethnic minority groups,[10,14] but research is limited in transgender populations.[3,5,17] Gender minority populations (e.g., transgender people) are often conflated with sexual minority populations (e.g., gay, lesbian, or bisexual people). However, given the diverse and intersectional nature of these identities, it is crucial to examine transgender people separately from sexual minority groups to better understand their unique sleep health outcomes.[3] Only 3 studies to our knowledge have explored discrimination and sleep among transgender adults, generally finding that higher discrimination is associated with worse sleep quality and shorter sleep duration.[20–22]

Most existing studies of sleep in transgender populations are descriptive or exploratory.[6,23] Many do not focus on the role of discrimination as an exposure[7,9,18] or fail to isolate the effects of transgender or racial/ethnic minority identity.[10,20,21] The only study to explore the intersection of racial/ethnic and gender minority identity was limited by low statistical power.[22] To address these gaps and develop a more precise understanding of how intersecting minority stressors contribute to sleep disparities, we assessed the cross-sectional and longitudinal relationships between everyday experiences of intersectional discrimination and sleep outcomes among TWOC.

METHODS

To explore the association between everyday discrimination against TWOC and sleep outcomes, we used baseline and 6-month follow-up data from the Trying to Understand Relationships, Networks, and Neighborhoods Among Transgender Women of Color (TURNNT) Cohort Study.[19] In total, 315 participants were enrolled in a 1-year prospective cohort study from August 31, 2020, until November 4, 2022. Eligible participants identified as TWOC, were between 18 and 55 years old at enrollment, spoke English or Spanish, lived in the New York City metropolitan area (including northern New Jersey, Long Island, and the lower Hudson Valley), and planned to reside in the study region for at least 1 year. We recruited participants through various channels including social media marketing, print advertising, event-based recruitment, referrals from organizational outreach and partnership, and snowball sampling. A total of 314 participants completed the baseline survey in its entirety; 218 participants also completed the 6-month follow-up survey, yielding a 69.5% retention rate.

Participants were included in our analysis if they had complete data on exposures, outcomes, and key covariates. At baseline, 21 participants were missing exposure data, 3 were missing outcome data, and 21 were missing covariate data, resulting in an analytic sample of 269. At 6 months, 96 participants were missing outcome data and 15 were missing covariate data, yielding an analytic sample of 179.

Measures

We measured baseline self-reported discrimination, our main exposure, using a modified version of the 5-item Everyday Discrimination Scale (EDS).[13] Whereas the original EDS assesses perceived day-to-day discrimination without a specific time frame, our modification limited responses to the previous 6 months. Participants were asked, "In the past 6 months, how often have any of the following things happened to you: you are treated with less courtesy or respect than other people; you receive poorer service than other people at restaurants or stores; people act as if they think you are not smart; people act as if they are afraid of you; or you are threatened or harassed?" Responses ranged from 1 to 4 (never, a few times a month, at least once a week, or almost every day). Refusals were coded as missing and excluded (see the Appendix, available as a supplement to the online version of this article at http://www.ajph.org). Scores were summed (range: 5–20), and participants were categorized as experiencing low (EDS score below 7), moderate (EDS score of 7–9), or high (EDS score of 10 or above) discrimination on the basis of a previous condensed 5-level EDS categorization.[13,24]

For each discrimination item reported as occurring "a few times a month" or more, participants were asked to identify the main reason(s) for these experiences. Potential responses included being a woman, being transgender, race or ethnicity, age, religion, physical appearance, sexual orientation, disability, and immigration status. Interviewers coded multiple reasons if a participant offered more than one.

Our primary outcomes were sleep duration, sleep quality, and sleep latency, as measured via the Pittsburgh Sleep Quality Index.[25] Sleep duration and quality (index items 4 and 6) were assessed at baseline and 6-month follow-up, whereas sleep latency (index item 5a) was assessed only at follow-up. Sleep duration was measured by asking, "In the past month, on average, how many hours of actual sleep did you get at night?" Sleep quality (categorized as very/fairly good or very/fairly poor) was assessed by asking, "During the past month, how would you rate your sleep overall?" Sleep latency (dichotomized as occurring at least 3 times weekly or less frequently) was measured by asking, "During the past month, how often have you not been able to fall asleep within 30 minutes?"[4] In this analysis, sleep latency should not be considered synonymous with insomnia. Insomnia is typically characterized as difficulty falling asleep, trouble remaining asleep throughout the night, or waking up too early and being unable to fall back asleep; here we measured only the former.[4]

We identified theoretical confounders including continuous age, HIV serostatus (positive or negative),[3,19] current hormone therapy use (yes or no),[18] educational level (less than high school, high school diploma or equivalent, or more than high school), annual income (less than $10 000 per year, $10 000 per year or more, or missing),[26] racial/ethnic identity (Black, Latina, or multiethnic/other),[10,14] and housing stability (stable housing or residence in a shelter/temporary housing/institutional care).[16,17,26] All covariates were self-reported at the baseline visit.

Statistical Analysis

We initially assessed baseline sociodemographic characteristics of the study sample by discrimination score category. We then examined the reasons for EDS item endorsement descriptively. In our regression analysis, we examined the cross-sectional associations between EDS and sleep quality and duration at baseline and then separately studied the longitudinal associations between baseline EDS and sleep quality, sleep duration, and sleep latency after 6 months of follow-up. We used linear regression to model sleep duration outcomes and a Poisson regression with robust standard errors to model dichotomous sleep quality and latency. We fit 2 models for each outcome: (1) a model adjusted only for EDS and (2) a model adjusted for theoretical confounders including age, HIV status, hormone therapy use, education, income, racial/ethnic identity, and housing stability. To assess the impact of baseline sleep health, we fit a third model for the longitudinal analysis, adjusting for theoretical confounders and baseline sleep outcome. Sleep latency was measured only at the follow-up visit, so baseline adjustment was not possible.

We conducted our analyses using R/R Studio version 4.3.2 (R Foundation for Statistical Computing, Vienna, Austria). All statistical tests were 2-sided at the 5% level of significance.

RESULTS

Table 1 presents descriptive characteristics for the study sample, stratified

TABLE 1— Descriptive Characteristics of the Study Sample at Baseline, Stratified by Everyday Discrimination Scale: TURNNT Cohort Study, 2020–2022

		Everyday Discrimination Scale		
	Overall	Low	Moderate	High
Total, no. (%)	269 (100)	102 (38)	101 (37)	66 (25)
Age, y, median (IQR)	37 (31, 44)	39 (33, 48)	37 (30, 43)	35 (31, 40)
Race/ethnicity, no. (%)				
Black	72 (27)	31 (30)	21 (21)	20 (30)
Latina	136 (51)	56 (55)	50 (50)	30 (45)
Multiethnic/other	61 (23)	15 (15)	30 (30)	16 (24)
HIV serostatus, no. (%)				
Positive	146 (54)	57 (56)	56 (55)	33 (50)
Negative	123 (46)	45 (44)	45 (45)	33 (50)
Hormone therapy use, no. (%)				
Yes	238 (88)	93 (91)	87 (86)	58 (88)
No	31 (12)	9 (9)	14 (14)	8 (12)
Annual income, $, no. (%)				
Less than $10 000	161 (60)	60 (59)	60 (59)	41 (62)
$10 000/y or more	88 (33)	32 (31)	36 (36)	20 (30)
Missing	20 (7)	10 (10)	5 (5)	5 (8)
Education, no. (%)				
Less than high school	95 (35)	40 (39)	35 (35)	20 (30)
High school or equivalent	78 (29)	35 (34)	26 (26)	17 (26)
More than high school	96 (36)	27 (26)	40 (40)	29 (44)
Housing status, no. (%)				
Stable housing	228 (85)	91 (89)	82 (81)	55 (83)
Shelter, institutional care, temporary	41 (15)	11 (11)	19 (19)	11 (17)
Average sleep per night, hours, median (IQR)	6 (5, 8)	7 (6, 8)	6 (5, 8)	6 (5, 8)
Average sleep quality, no. (%)				
Very or fairly good	94 (35)	26 (26)	40 (40)	28 (42)
Very or fairly poor	175 (65)	76 (75)	61 (60)	38 (58)

Note. IQR = interquartile range; TURNNT = Trying to Understand Relationships, Networks, and Neighborhoods Among Transgender Women of Color.

according to EDS score. Most participants identified as Latina (51%), were living with HIV (54%), were on hormone therapy (88%), lived in stable housing (85%), and had an annual income below $10 000 (60%). Among the 269 participants included at baseline, 37% reported moderate everyday discrimination and 25% reported high levels of discrimination. In comparison with those who experienced low discrimination, a higher proportion of TWOC who experienced high discrimination earned less than $10 000 annually (62% vs 59%), were educated beyond high school (44% vs 26%), and were not living with HIV (50% vs 44%). Median nightly sleep duration was 6 hours (interquartile range: 5–8), with 46% sleeping at least 7 hours, and 65% reporting very or fairly poor sleep quality.

Table 2 contains descriptive results related to EDS item endorsement. More than two thirds of the sample endorsed at least one form of discrimination (69%). The items with the highest overall endorsement were being treated with less respect than others (54%), being treated as if one is not smart (45%), and being threatened or harassed (41%). Of all possible reasons for experiencing discrimination, the overwhelming majority of participants reported their transgender identity (range across items: 72%–89%). The next most frequent reasons were physical appearance (range: 36%–48%), race or ethnicity (32%–45%), sexual orientation (23%–31%), and being a woman

TABLE 2— Response Frequencies and Reasons for Endorsement of Each Item of the Everyday Discrimination Scale Among Respondents at Baseline: TURNNT Cohort Study, 2020–2022

	Everyday Discrimination Scale Item[a]				
	Item 1: Less Respect, No. (%)	Item 2: Poor Service, No. (%)	Item 3: Not Smart, No. (%)	Item 4: Afraid, No. (%)	Item 5: Threatened, No. (%)
Frequency					
Almost every day	18 (7)	12 (4)	25 (9)	25 (9)	15 (6)
At least once a week	19 (7)	12 (4)	6 (2)	15 (6)	12 (4)
A few times a month	107 (40)	76 (28)	90 (34)	55 (20)	84 (31)
Never	125 (47)	169 (63)	148 (55)	174 (65)	158 (59)
Any endorsement	144 (54)	100 (37)	121 (45)	95 (35)	111 (41)
Specific reasons[b]					
You're a woman	19 (13)	13 (13)	21 (17)	10 (11)	22 (20)
You're transgender	128 (89)	84 (84)	87 (72)	79 (83)	95 (86)
Your race or ethnicity	48 (33)	45 (45)	44 (36)	36 (38)	36 (32)
Your age	10 (7)	6 (6)	16 (13)	5 (5)	6 (5)
Your religion	5 (3)	3 (3)	6 (5)	8 (8)	4 (4)
Your physical appearance	53 (37)	38 (38)	44 (36)	46 (48)	43 (39)
Your sexual orientation	33 (23)	27 (27)	28 (23)	29 (31)	33 (30)
Your education or income	12 (8)	7 (7)	18 (15)	12 (13)	11 (10)
A disability	11 (8)	3 (3)	9 (7)	4 (4)	5 (5)
Your immigration status	12 (8)	9 (9)	12 (10)	9 (9)	11 (10)
Don't know	3 (2)	1 (1)	4 (3)	2 (2)	3 (3)
Multiple reason endorsement[c]	86 (58)	68 (68)	79 (65)	68 (72)	72 (65)

Note. TURNNT = Trying to Understand Relationships, Networks, and Neighborhoods Among Transgender Women of Color. The sample size was 269. Respondents do not include those who answered "don't know" or "prefer not to answer" for any of the items.
[a]Item prompt: In the past 6 months, how often did the following things happen to you: (1) you were treated with less courtesy or respect than other people, (2) you received poorer service than other people at restaurants or stores, (3) people acted as if they thought you were not smart, (4) people acted as if they were afraid of you, or (5) you were threatened or harassed.
[b]Percentages for response frequencies refer to total responses (n = 269). Percentages for reasons for endorsement refer to the total count of endorsements per item, and totals could exceed 100%.
[c]Count and percentage of respondents who reported more than one reason for experiencing the specific item. Percentages refer to the total count of endorsements per item.

(11%–20%). Roughly 60% of participants or more consistently provided more than one reason across EDS items.

Cross-Sectional Analysis

Table 3 presents the modeling results. In the unadjusted model, TWOC who experienced moderate discrimination had 1.11 times the risk of reporting very or fairly poor sleep at baseline (95% confidence interval [CI] = 1.01, 1.23) relative to individuals with low discrimination, and those experiencing high discrimination had 1.14 times the risk (95% CI = 1.03, 1.27). After adjustment for potential confounders, TWOC experiencing moderate discrimination had 1.10 times the risk of reporting very or fairly poor sleep (95% CI = 1.00, 1.21) relative to the low discrimination group, and those experiencing high discrimination had 1.14 times the risk (95% CI = 1.12, 1.27). Discrimination was not significantly associated with sleep duration at baseline.

Longitudinal Analysis

In the unadjusted model, TWOC who reported moderate discrimination at baseline had a 24% higher risk of very or fairly poor sleep quality at follow-up (prevalence ratio [PR] = 1.24; 95% CI = 1.12, 1.38) than those with low discrimination, and those reporting high discrimination had a 19% higher risk (PR = 1.19; 95% CI = 1.05, 1.35). After adjustment for potential confounders, TWOC with moderate discrimination at baseline had a 21% higher risk of very

TABLE 3— Results of Multivariable Linear and Robust Poisson Regressions for Sleep Health–Related Outcomes by Everyday Discrimination Scale Category: Cross-Sectional and Longitudinal Analyses, TURNNT Cohort Study, 2020–2022

	Sleep Duration,[a] b (95% CI)	Sleep Quality,[b] PR (95% CI)	Sleep Latency, PR (95% CI)
Cross sectional[c]			
Model 1[d]			
Low (ref)	0	1	
Moderate	−0.43 (−0.91, 0.06)	1.11 (1.01, 1.23)	
High	−0.47 (−1.02, 0.07)	1.14 (1.03, 1.27)	
Model 2[e]			
Low (ref)	0	1	
Moderate	−0.42 (−0.92, 0.08)	1.10 (1.00, 1.21)	
High	−0.55 (−1.11, 0.01)	1.14 (1.12, 1.27)	
Longitudinal[f]			
Model 1			
Low (ref)	0	1	1
Moderate	−0.42 (−0.95, 0.11)	1.24 (1.12, 1.38)	1.01 (0.98, 1.24)
High	−0.72 (−1.34, −0.10)	1.19 (1.05, 1.35)	1.08 (0.94, 1.24)
Model 2			
Low (ref)	0	1	1
Moderate	−0.44 (−1.00, 0.12)	1.21 (1.08, 1.36)	1.04 (0.92, 1.16)
High	−0.71 (−1.34, −0.07)	1.15 (1.01, 1.30)	0.99 (0.88, 1.13)
Model 3[g]			
Low (ref)	0	1	
Moderate	−0.38 (−0.89, 0.13)	1.18 (1.06, 1.32)	
High	−0.48 (−1.07, 0.11)	1.09 (0.98, 1.23)	

Note. CI = confidence interval; EDS = Everyday Discrimination Scale; PR = prevalence ratio; TURNNT = Trying to Understand Relationships, Networks, and Neighborhoods Among Transgender Women of Color.
[a]Sleep duration was modeled with linear regression.
[b]Sleep quality and latency were modeled with modified (robust) Poisson regression.
[c]The cross-sectional analysis included baseline EDS score and baseline sleep quality and duration (n = 269).
[d]Model 1 included only EDS score as an independent variable.
[e]Model 2 included EDS score, age, HIV status, hormone therapy use, education, income, racial/ethnic identity, and housing stability as covariates.
[f]The longitudinal analysis included baseline EDS score and sleep quality, duration, and latency after 6 months of follow-up (n = 179).
[g]Model 3 included baseline EDS score, age, HIV status, hormone therapy use, education, income, racial/ethnic identity, housing stability, and baseline sleep outcomes as covariates.

or fairly poor sleep (PR = 1.21; 95% CI = 1.08, 1.36) than the low discrimination group, and those with high discrimination had a 15% higher risk (PR = 1.15; 95% CI = 1.01, 1.30). After adjustment for baseline sleep outcomes, TWOC experiencing moderate discrimination at baseline had an 18% higher risk of very or fairly poor sleep (95% CI = 1.06, 1.32) than those with low discrimination. High discrimination was no longer associated with sleep quality.

In the unadjusted model, TWOC who reported high levels of discrimination at baseline slept an average of 43.2 minutes less per night at follow-up than those who reported low discrimination (b = −0.72; 95% CI = −1.34, −0.10). After adjustment for potential confounders, TWOC with high discrimination slept an average of 42.6 minutes less per night (b = −0.71; 95% CI = −1.34, −0.07) than the low discrimination group. Moderate discrimination was not associated with sleep duration, and, after adjustment for baseline sleep duration, high discrimination was no longer associated with sleep duration. Baseline discrimination was not associated with sleep latency.

DISCUSSION

In this study, discrimination was associated with sleep health among TWOC, both cross sectionally and longitudinally. TWOC who experienced discrimination were more likely to have poorer and shorter sleep than those who did not experience discrimination. TWOC generally had poor-quality sleep, and more than half did not have the recommended 7 hours of sleep each night. Nearly two thirds of the sample reported moderate or high discrimination, and 69% reported at least one form of discrimination in the 6 months preceding the baseline assessment. Participants noted that being transgender, physical appearance, racial/ethnic identity, sexual orientation, and womanhood may have motivated the discrimination they faced, highlighting the importance of an intersectional approach.

To our knowledge, this is the first study to investigate intersectional discrimination and sleep specifically among TWOC. Our results build on previous evidence linking discrimination to poor sleep health in transgender and gender minority groups. In one study, transgender adults in South Korea who experienced transgender identity discrimination were 48% more likely to have sleep problems than those who did not.[20] Similarly, in another study gender minority individuals with high stigma consciousness and gender-related discrimination scores experienced greater sleep disturbance and shorter sleep duration than those with low scores.[21] Both studies focused exclusively on gender-related discrimination, potentially overlooking other salient forms of discrimination, such as racism and heterosexism, that may affect sleep. In addition, they were unable to disentangle gender identity–specific effects, potentially conflating individuals with diverse gender expressions who may experience discrimination in distinct ways (e.g., transgender women and nonbinary people assigned male at birth).[20,21]

Belloir et al., using both self-report and objective sleep measures, found that sexual and gender minority people of color who experienced day-to-day intersectional discrimination had greater same-night sleep disturbance than those who did not.[22] However, this study was limited by a small sample size (n = 43) and was unable to disentangle gender identity–specific effects. A recent scoping review showed that although research into sleep health in sexual and gender minority populations has expanded in recent years, most studies fail to disentangle identity-specific outcomes or do not assess intersectional discrimination and its effects on sleep health in multiply vulnerable groups.[27]

Our study addressed several of these limitations by including multiple sleep outcomes in both cross-sectional and longitudinal analyses, using an intersectional measure of discrimination, employing validated assessments for discrimination and sleep outcomes,[13,25] and examining this association in a well-characterized sample of TWOC. By avoiding collapsing of gender and sexual minority identities into a single category, our work provides a more nuanced understanding of the ways in which intersectional discrimination affects sleep health in this population.[3]

Intersectional discrimination may affect sleep through psychosocial stress and rumination pathways. Gender identity rumination—persistent negative thought patterns about one's gender identity—may be exacerbated by gender-related discrimination.[20,28] In a qualitative study of 40 transgender people in New York City, one third of the participants attributed their poor sleep to gender dysphoria–related stress and anxiety.[23] TWOC are particularly vulnerable because of the intersection of transphobia with racism and heterosexism.[11,15]

Sentiment against lesbian, gay, bisexual, transgender, and queer (LGBTQ+) individuals, particularly transphobia, is rising across the United States.[12] Familial and social support may buffer the effects of discrimination on sleep health, highlighting the importance of building affirming communities for transgender people and cisgender allies.[3,20] Epidemiologists, public health practitioners, and public health professional societies should collaborate with transgender support organizations, such as the New York Transgender Advocacy Group, to amplify transgender voices in biomedical research and support legislation to protect the health of transgender and gender nonconforming individuals nationwide.[29] The Health Equity Research Production Model emphasizes involving research participants in study development, with community advisory boards playing a key role; we encourage their early and frequent engagement.[30]

Interventions that promote sleep health may buffer the effects of anti-transgender discrimination on overall health. However, most existing sleep interventions are highly individualistic, do not address structural causes of poor sleep such as discrimination, and often show mixed effectiveness in the general population.[14,31] Effective sleep interventions, such as cognitive behavioral therapy, should be adapted for marginalized populations such as TWOC.[22,31] For example, sleep tracking through mHealth applications or consumer wearables may mitigate the impact of discrimination on sleep health when paired with coping, resiliency, or sleep hygiene interventions delivered through just-in-time adaptive intervention.[10,32] In addition, gender-affirming care may enhance sleep via improved passing and reduced discrimination or improved gender congruence and reduced rumination to the extent that such care supports each person's unique transition goals.[7,18,28] Therefore, combating provider-based discrimination and increasing affordable and sustainable access to gender-affirming care should be an active priority for public health.[7,11,21]

Future research should aim to replicate our results with diverse measures of discrimination and objective sleep data.[14,22] Differences between self-reported and objective sleep measures may vary by racial/ethnic group and educational level; psychometric properties of established sleep measures should be assessed in diverse populations.[33] Stress, substance use, familial support, and clinical sleep disorders such as obstructive sleep apnea may mediate this relationship and therefore deserve additional investigation.[10,20,22] Our analysis was designed specifically to examine intersectional discrimination and sleep in TWOC. Although we recognize the importance of comparing our results with those from other gender minority populations to clarify intersectional health disparities, such an analysis is beyond the scope of the present work. Future research should prioritize longer prospective follow-ups, increased power, and representative sampling to investigate discrimination and sleep health in other racial/ethnic and gender minority groups.

Despite its strengths, this study has several limitations. The nonrandom sampling design of the TURNNT study may limit the generalizability of our findings as a result of selection bias. Recruitment through neighborhood partners including transgender support organizations may have led to a sample of TWOC who are engaged in their communities and actively seek peer support, potentially underestimating the relationship between discrimination and sleep outcomes because discrimination in this cohort is mediated by social support and resiliency. However, these populations are often underrepresented in probability-based samples, and the TURNNT cohort is similar to other gender minority populations in terms of sociodemographic characteristics including income, education, and HIV burden.[12,16] Furthermore, our findings align with existing research, reinforcing the likelihood of a generalizable underlying effect.[14,20–22,27] Although specific mechanisms may vary across marginalized populations, we anticipate that our findings will be replicated in other socially marginalized groups.

Our results could be biased by missing data (Table A, available as a supplement to the online version of this article at http://www.ajph.org). Roughly 30% of the participants were lost to follow-up at 6 months, although those lost did not differ significantly from retained participants on baseline characteristics other than age (Table B, available as a supplement to the online version of this article at http://www.ajph.org). Data on additional sleep outcomes—medication use and hypersomnia—were available at 6 months, but we decided against pursuing these analyses because of low power.[25] We encourage future consideration of these important aspects of sleep health. As with all observational studies, our findings are subject to unmeasured confounding, although we adjusted for a theoretically informed set of confounders.

Finally, our exposure measure captured discrimination over 6 months, whereas our outcome measures assessed sleep in the past month, potentially introducing measurement bias. However, we used validated scales to measure both exposures and outcomes, supporting the construct validity of our variables.[13,25] Self-reported sleep tends to overestimate objective sleep, and single-night measures including sleep diaries provide only marginal improvements in accuracy over habitual measures.[34] Therefore, although self-reported estimates of habitual sleep may be slightly inflated, recall time frames should not have a substantial impact on measurement error.

The original EDS measured perceived discrimination without a time frame, whereas we restricted responses to the past 6 months.[13] Participants may recall discrimination less accurately over time[35]; although a limitation, our modification improves temporal precision relative to the original EDS.[13,33] Individuals with sleep disturbances may have remembered discrimination more accurately, but our longitudinal analysis employing baseline EDS to predict 6-month sleep would not be affected by this bias. The consistency of our cross-sectional and longitudinal results further supports the robustness of our observed associations.

PUBLIC HEALTH IMPLICATIONS

Sleep is a fundamental determinant of health, yet most US adults do not sleep enough. Sleep disparities are particularly pronounced among transgender individuals, who experience poorer sleep than their cisgender peers, and such inequities are shaped by anti-transgender discrimination. In a cohort of TWOC, experiences of everyday discrimination were associated with poorer sleep quality and shorter sleep duration. Transphobia, racism, and heterosexism intersect to exacerbate health inequities, reinforcing structural oppression. Our study advances the growing body of research on intersectional discrimination and sleep health among transgender populations of color. Public health authorities and professional societies should collaborate with transgender advocacy groups to mitigate the harmful effects of anti-transgender discrimination and develop interventions to improve sleep health and overall well-being in transgender communities of color. AJPH

ABOUT THE AUTHORS

Adam M. Whalen, Alexander Furuya, Jessica Contreras, Asa Radix, and Dustin T. Duncan are with the Department of Epidemiology, Mailman School of Public Health, Columbia University, New York, NY. Asa Radix is also with the Callen-Lorde Community Health Center, New York, NY. John A. Schneider is with the Department of Public

AJPH October 2025, Vol. 115, No. 10

Health Sciences, University of Chicago, Chicago, IL. Sahnah Lim and Chau Trinh-Shevrin are with the Department of Population Health, Grossman School of Medicine, New York University, New York, NY, and the Callen-Lorde Community Health Center, New York, NY.

CORRESPONDENCE

Correspondence should be sent to Adam M. Whalen, MPH, 722 W 168th St, Room 720, New York, NY 10032 (e-mail: amw2275@cumc.columbia.edu). Reprints can be ordered at https://www.ajph.org by clicking the "Reprints" link.

PUBLICATION INFORMATION

Full Citation: Whalen AM, Furuya A, Contreras J, et al. Discrimination and sleep health among transgender women of color in New York City: cross-sectional and longitudinal associations from the TURNNT Cohort Study. *Am J Public Health*. 2025;115(10):1652–1661.

Acceptance Date: May 25, 2025.

DOI: https://doi.org/10.2105/AJPH.2025.308208

ORCID iDs:

Adam M. Whalen https://orcid.org/0000-0003-0235-1341

Asa Radix https://orcid.org/0000-0001-9611-4181

Dustin T. Duncan https://orcid.org/0000-0001-8586-8711

CONTRIBUTORS

A. M. Whalen contributed to the writing of the original draft and to review and editing. A. Furuya, J. A. Schneider, S. Lim, C. Trinh-Shevrin, and A. Radix contributed to review and editing. J. Contreras contributed to project administration and resource provision. D. T. Duncan contributed to review, editing, and supervision.

ACKNOWLEDGMENTS

The Trying to Understand Relationships, Networks, and Neighborhoods Among Transgender Women of Color (TURNNT) Cohort Study was funded through grants from the National Institute on Minority Health and Health Disparities (grants R01MD013554, 3R01MD013554-02S1, and 3R01MD013554-05S1). Adam M. Whalen was supported by grant T32ES007322 from the National Institute for Environmental Health Sciences. Alexander Furuya was supported by grant T32AI114398 from the National Institute of Allergy and Infectious Diseases of the National Institutes of Health (NIH).

We thank the Community Advisory Board members: Cristina Herrera of the TransLatinx Network, Ceyenne Doroshow of Gay and Lesbian in a Transgender World, Kim Watson of Community Kinship Life, Kiara St. James of the New York Transgender Advocacy Group, Bianey Garcia of Make the Road NY, Morticia Godiva of the Black Trans Travel Fund, Xoai Pham of the Transgender Law Center, Egyptt LaBeija of the House of LaBeija, and Nala Toussaint. We also thank the Scientific Advisory Board members: Sari Reisner of Harvard Medical School, Tonia Poteat of the University of North Carolina at Chapel Hill, Rachel Bluebond-Langner of the New York University School of Medicine, Roberta Garofalo of Northwestern University, Walter Bockting of Columbia University, and Jae Sevelius of Columbia University. In addition, we thank the TURNNT study staff, including Krish J. Bhatt, Roberta Scheinmann, Jenesis Merriman, Magdalena Palavecino, Laura Staeheli, Kobe Pereira, Mia N. Campbell, Elias Preciado, Astrea Villarroel-Sanchez, and Kevalyn Bharadwaj. We also thank the Callen-Lorde Community Health Center staff who contributed to this project. We further thank the following colleagues for their thoughtful input on coding racial and ethnic categories for our data: Renee M. Johnson of Johns Hopkins University, Paris "AJ" Adkins-Jackson of Columbia University, and Carlos Rodriguez-Diaz of The George Washington University, as well as Howard Shih and Ryan Vinh from AAPI Data. We acknowledge Roberta Scheinmann and Cristina Herrera for their input on a previous version of this analysis presented at the World Professional Association for Transgender Health 28th Scientific Symposium in Lisbon, Portugal. Finally, we thank the participants for engaging in this research.

Note. The work described herein is the sole responsibility of the authors and does not represent the official views of NIH or its institutes.

CONFLICTS OF INTEREST

The authors have no conflicts of interest to disclose.

HUMAN PARTICIPANT PROTECTION

This study was approved by the institutional review board at the Columbia University Irving Medical Center. At the initial enrollment interview, a consent form describing the study background, requirements, timeline, confidentiality procedures, and participant rights was reviewed with interested individuals. Participants gave consent voluntarily by agreeing to the terms of the study and signing the consent form. Participants were also asked to sign an optional release of information form to allow for sharing of sexually transmitted infection and HIV testing information with the study team.

REFERENCES

1. Watson NF, Badr MS, Belenky G, et al. Recommended amount of sleep for a healthy adult: a joint consensus statement of the American Academy of Sleep Medicine and Sleep Research Society. *Sleep*. 2015;38(6):843–844. https://doi.org/10.5665/sleep.4716
2. Liu Y, Wheaton AG, Chapman DP, Cunningham TJ, Lu H, Croft JB. Prevalence of healthy sleep duration among adults—United States, 2014. *MMWR Morb Mortal Wkly Rep*. 2016;65(6):137–141. https://doi.org/10.15585/mmwr.mm6506a1
3. Millar BM, Goedel WC, Duncan DT. Sleep health among sexual and gender minorities. In: Duncan DT, Kawachi I, Redline S, eds. *The Social Epidemiology of Sleep*. Oxford University Press; 2019:187–204. https://doi.org/10.1093/oso/9780190930448.003.0008
4. Morin CM, Jarrin DC. Epidemiology of insomnia: prevalence, course, risk factors, and public health burden. *Sleep Med Clin*. 2022;17(2):173–191. https://doi.org/10.1016/j.jsmc.2022.03.003
5. Butler ES, McGlinchey E, Juster RP. Sexual and gender minority sleep: a narrative review and suggestions for future research. *J Sleep Res*. 2020;29(1):e12928. https://doi.org/10.1111/jsr.12928
6. Hershner S, Jansen EC, Gavidia R, Matlen L, Hoban M, Dunietz GL. Associations between transgender identity, sleep, mental health and suicidality among a North American cohort of college students. *Nat Sci Sleep*. 2021;13:383–398. https://doi.org/10.2147/NSS.S286131
7. Gavidia R, Whitney DG, Hershner S, Selkie EM, Tauman R, Dunietz GL. Gender identity and transition: relationships with sleep disorders in US youth. *J Clin Sleep Med*. 2022;18(11):2553–2559. https://doi.org/10.5664/jcsm.10158
8. Leonard SI, Liu J, Jackman KB, Bruzzese JM. Sexual and gender minority sleep health disparities and minority stress in early adolescence. *J Adolesc Health*. 2024;75(3):471–478. https://doi.org/10.1016/j.jadohealth.2024.05.022
9. Auer MK, Liedl A, Fuss J, et al. High impact of sleeping problems on quality of life in transgender individuals: a cross-sectional multicenter study. *PLoS One*. 2017;12(2):e0171640. https://doi.org/10.1371/journal.pone.0171640
10. Slopen N, Lewis TT, Williams DR. *Discrimination and sleep: a systematic review. Sleep Med*. 2016;18:88–95. https://doi.org/10.1016/j.sleep.2015.01.012
11. Wesp LM, Malcoe LH, Elliott A, Poteat T. Intersectionality research for transgender health justice: a theory-driven conceptual framework for structural analysis of transgender health inequities. *Transgend Health*. 2019;4(1):287–296. https://doi.org/10.1089/trgh.2019.0039
12. Trevor Project. 2024 US National Survey on the Mental Health of LGBTQ+ Young People. Available at: https://www.thetrevorproject.org. Accessed October 20, 2024.
13. Williams DR, Yu Y, Jackson JS, Anderson NB. Racial differences in physical and mental health: socioeconomic status, stress, and discrimination. *J Health Psychol*. 1997;2(3):335–351.
14. Lewis TT, McKinnon II. Exposure to discrimination and sleep. In: Duncan DT, Kawachi I, Redline S, eds. *The Social Epidemiology of Sleep*. Oxford University Press; 2019:257–324. https://doi.org/10.1093/oso/9780190930448.003.0011
15. Hatzenbuehler ML. How does sexual minority stigma "get under the skin"? A psychological mediation framework. *Psychol Bull*. 2009;135(5):707–730. https://doi.org/10.1037/a0016441
16. Marcus R, Trujillo L, Olansky E, et al. Transgender women experiencing homelessness—national HIV behavioral surveillance among transgender women, seven urban areas, United States, 2019–2020. *MMWR Suppl*. 2024;73(1):40–50. https://doi.org/10.15585/mmwr.su7301a5
17. Duncan DT, Schneider JA, Radix A, Harry-Hernandez S, Callander D. Sleep health among transgender women of color in New York City: preliminary analyses of interim baseline data from the TURNNT study cohort. *Sleep Health*. 2021;7(2):153–154. https://doi.org/10.1016/j.sleh.2021.01.005

18. Morssinkhof MWL, van der Werf YD, van den Heuvel OA, et al. Influence of sex hormone use on sleep architecture in a transgender cohort. *Sleep.* 2023;46(11):zsad249. https://doi.org/10.1093/sleep/zsad249
19. Duncan DT, Park SH, Dharma C, et al. Neighborhood safety and neighborhood police violence are associated with psychological distress among English- and Spanish-speaking transgender women of color in New York City: finding from the TURNNT Cohort Study. *J Urban Health.* 2024;101(3):557–570. https://doi.org/10.1007/s11524-024-00879-3
20. Eom YJ, Lee H, Kim R, Choo S, Yi H, Kim SS. Discrimination keeps transgender people awake at night: a nationwide cross-sectional survey of 583 transgender adults in South Korea. *Sleep Health.* 2022;8(6):580–586. https://doi.org/10.1016/j.sleh.2022.06.012
21. Caceres BA, Jackman KB, Belloir J, et al. Examining the associations of gender minority stressors with sleep health in gender minority individuals. *Sleep Health.* 2022;8(2):153–160. https://doi.org/10.1016/j.sleh.2021.10.006
22. Belloir JA, Ensari I, Jackman K, et al. Day-to-day associations of intersectional minority stressors with sleep health in sexual and gender minority people of color. *Health Psychol.* 2024;43(8):591–602. https://doi.org/10.1037/hea0001372
23. Harry-Hernandez S, Reisner SL, Schrimshaw EW, et al. Gender dysphoria, mental health, and poor sleep health among transgender and gender nonbinary individuals: a qualitative study in New York City. *Transgend Health.* 2020;5(1):59–68. https://doi.org/10.1089/trgh.2019.0007
24. Oh H, Glass J, Narita Z, Koyanagi A, Sinha S, Jacob L. Discrimination and multimorbidity among Black Americans: findings from the National Survey of American Life. *J Racial Ethn Health Disparities.* 2021;8(1):210–219. https://doi.org/10.1007/s40615-020-00773-z
25. Buysse DJ, Reynolds CF, Monk TH, Berman SR, Kupfer DJ. The Pittsburgh Sleep Quality Index: a new instrument for psychiatric practice and research. *Psychiatry Res.* 1989;28(2):193–213. https://doi.org/10.1016/0165-1781(89)90047-4
26. Duncan DT, Park SH, Chen YT, et al. Sleep characteristics among Black cisgender sexual minority men and Black transgender women during the COVID-19 pandemic: the role of multi-level COVID-19-related stressors. *Sleep Health.* 2022;8(5):440–450. https://doi.org/10.1016/j.sleh.2022.06.006
27. Leonard SI, Castiblanco MR, Chang A, et al. Sleep health among sexual and gender minority people in the United States: a scoping review. *Sleep Med.* 2025;128:12–21. https://doi.org/10.1016/j.sleep.2024.12.033
28. Bauerband LA, Galupo MP. The Gender Identity Reflection and Rumination Scale: development and psychometric evaluation. *J Couns Dev.* 2014;92(2):219–231. https://doi.org/10.1002/j.1556-6676.2014.00151.x
29. New York Transgender Advocacy Group. NYTAG home page. Available at: https://www.nytag.org. Accessed October 20, 2024.
30. Duncan DT. Composing authorship teams for health equity: an introduction to the health equity research production model. Available at: https://equityhealthj.biomedcentral.com/articles/10.1186/s12939-025-02524-0. Accessed October 20, 2024.
31. Albakri U, Drotos E, Meertens R. Sleep health promotion interventions and their effectiveness: an umbrella review. *Int J Environ Res Public Health.* 2021;18(11):5533. https://doi.org/10.3390/ijerph18115533
32. Jackson CL, Powell-Wiley TM, Gaston SA, Andrews MR, Tamura K, Ramos A. Racial/ethnic disparities in sleep health and potential interventions among women in the United States. *J Womens Health (Larchmt).* 2020;29(3):435–442. https://doi.org/10.1089/jwh.2020.8329
33. Robbins R, Quan SF, Barger LK, et al. Self-reported sleep duration and timing: a methodological review of event definitions, context, and timeframe of related questions. *Sleep Epidemiol.* 2021;1:100016. https://doi.org/10.1016/j.sleepe.2021.100016
34. Lauderdale DS, Knutson KL, Yan LL, Liu K, Rathouz PJ. Sleep duration: how well do self-reports reflect objective measures? The CARDIA Sleep Study. *Epidemiology.* 2008;19(6):838–845. https://doi.org/10.1097/EDE.0b013e318187a7b0
35. Dyke MEV, Kramer MR, Kershaw KN, Vaccarino V, Crawford ND, Lewis TT. Inconsistent reporting of discrimination over time using the Experiences of Discrimination Scale: potential underestimation of lifetime burden. *Am J Epidemiol.* 2022;191(3):370–378. https://doi.org/10.1093/aje/kwab151

Analogous Analogs: Considerations Regarding Off-Label Use of Gonadotropin-Releasing Hormone Analogs Among Transgender Adolescents

Sinéad Murano-Kinney, MFA

See also LGBTQ+ Transgender Health, pp. 1594–1661.

Although gonadotropin-releasing hormone (GnRH) analogs have been the gold-standard treatment for adolescents with gender dysphoria for more than 3 decades, they continue to be categorized as an off-label use of the same drugs often prescribed to cisgender adolescents.

Off-label provision of these medications is one of the many arguments deployed to frame legislative restrictions on pediatric gender-affirming care as an effort to "protect" adolescents from experimental drugs.

Here I not only problematize such politicization but use these claims as an entry point to further consider how prospective and historically rooted public health policies could support approval of supplemental indications for certain GnRH analog products for gender dysphoria among adolescents.
(*Am J Public Health*. 2025;115(10):1662–1670. https://doi.org/10.2105/AJPH.2025.308130)

AJPH October 2025, Vol. 115, No. 10

As of June 2025, 27 states had passed laws either banning or restricting pediatric transition-related health care for adolescents, including puberty-pausing medications. These laws have jeopardized the health and safety of more than 110 000 adolescents,[1] a vulnerable subpopulation of an already vulnerable and medically underserved community. Many justifications have been made to frame these restrictions as measures to protect adolescents. This article addresses claims that off-label provision of these drugs to transgender adolescents represents "experimental" prescribing practices by clinicians.[2]

The issue of label indication has been invoked by lawmakers, government officials, and the media, and has been a key topic in discussions of legal challenges of some of these laws.[3] However, such governmental restrictions are exceedingly rare for other off-label uses of medications,[4] suggesting that ideological control rather than scientific caution guides these lawmakers. Gonadotropin-releasing hormone (GnRH) analogs are prescribed "off label" to transgender adolescents to pause incongruent pubertal development. The United States Food and Drug Administration (FDA) currently approves several GnRH analogs as treatments for precocious puberty: leuprolide acetate (Lupron Depot-Ped), leuprolide acetate (Fensolvi), nafarelin (Synarel), histrelin (Supprelin LA), and triptorelin (Triptodur).

After demonstrating efficacy among adolescents with precocious puberty in the 1980s,[5,6] GnRH analogs became the gold-standard treatment for adolescents with gender dysphoria in the 1990s to pause pubertal development.[6–8] As early as 1993, products from this drug class were approved by the FDA as a treatment for precocious puberty.[6] Despite similarities in use, population, quality of evidence, and historicity, no GnRH analogs have been approved to treat gender dysphoria. Yet, their safety and efficacy are so well established that their use constitutes the standard of care.[9,10]

GnRH analogs are provided to adolescents between 12 and 14 years of age as an intervention to prevent pubertal development that would exacerbate a patient's gender dysphoria. Gender dysphoria is the primary diagnostic framework for the provision of transition-related health care in the United States. It describes the clinically significant distress or impairment that individuals might experience as a result of misalignment or incongruence between their gender identity and how others perceived them or how their anatomy and physiology endogenously manifested.[10] Untreated dysphoria is associated with an increased risk of negative psychiatric outcomes such as disordered eating, depression, anxiety, and suicidality.[11–15] When transgender adolescents are both socially and medically affirmed, psychological well-being improves.[12,16–21] Because of this inverse association, many describe this form of care as lifesaving and therefore medically necessary health care.[22] Thus, gender dysphoria could be considered a potentially life-threatening condition if left untreated.

Here I examine the prevalence of off-label pediatric use of GnRH analogs as well as the safety and efficacy of these medications. Also, I assess the evidence base supporting the provision of the drugs to transgender, nonbinary, and gender-diverse (hereafter "transgender") adolescents. I conclude by considering frameworks rooted in current US policies to address inequities in the use of these medications.

However, given the current administration's hostility toward the transgender community and the field of transgender medicine,[23] these frameworks remain largely theoretical. Since the initial drafting of this article, the Trump administration has taken escalating measures against transgender people across the United States. Within the first weeks of President Trump's second term, multiple executive orders were introduced attacking the rights and personhood of transgender adolescents, including an order seeking to definitionally erase transgender people and another to prohibit the use of federal funds to research hormonal transition-related health care or provide it to people younger than 19 years.[24,25] It is likely that there will be more alarming attacks on transgender health care. We have already begun to see targeted attacks on agencies that have historically contributed to improvements in transgender health such as the National Institutes of Health, the FDA, and the Centers for Disease Control and Prevention.[26]

One of the most dangerous attacks so far is the day one executive order Defending Women From Gender Ideology Extremism and Restoring Biological Truth to the Federal Government.[24] This order and its definitions are left intentionally broad. As described in the order, "The following definitions shall govern all Executive interpretation of and application of Federal law and administration policy."[24] The impact is clear from the rigid definitions of sex and broad definition of "gender ideology" presented within. The order's lack of coherent definitions and broad scope are intended to provide the widest possible interpretations to justify as many targeted attacks as possible on transgender, intersex, and nonbinary people throughout the United States. The order creates a standard of exclusion targeting individuals whose gender is inconsistent with their assigned gender at birth and individuals whose sexual development naturally diverges from established definitions.

Under this executive order, any number of restrictions on transition-related health care can be justified by government agencies, including negative determinations of coverage, cessation of state Medicaid matching funds, and Hyde Amendment–like restrictions of federal funding that supports the provision of this health care, and more. Nonetheless, advocacy in the face of systemic governmental apathy (and outright oppression) is a consistent thread throughout the history of transgender health advocacy.

There is no better example of uphill advocacy yielding policy advancements than the actions of ACT-UP (a coalition of HIV/AIDS activists) and its application of sustained political pressure against the torpidity of the FDA's drug approval process relative to that of other countries.[27] Many attribute the accelerated and expanded access to HIV/AIDS drugs to ACT-UP's consistent pressure on the Department of Health and Human Services, such as its 1988 protest outside the FDA's headquarters. ACT-UP's relentless advocacy was also pivotal in if not responsible for the reduction in cost of the early antiretroviral medication azidothymidine by manufacturer Burroughs Wellcome.[28] Although the Trump administration will continue to attack the rights of transgender adolescents, contemporary activists possess the same raw potentiality to compel this administration as ACT-UP did the Reagan administration. Fortunately for advocates, the drug approval process is such that transgender patients and their advocates may be on the same side as pharmaceutical companies in this struggle.

OFF-LABEL DRUG USE AND SUPPLEMENTAL INDICATIONS

Seeking approval from the FDA for drugs is a long, complicated, and expensive process, particularly for brand-name drugs. Depending on the drug and its treatment population, the review process may take between 6 and 12 months.[29] Before the FDA reviews a new drug application, a significant and costly volume of research must be conducted, primarily by drug sponsors. During this process, sponsors develop evidentiary data about their drug's effects, which will be key to its future safety profile. Typically, this process starts with preclinical in vitro or in vivo testing to establish a baseline understanding of the drug's molecular potential.

To conduct further research on the drug, the drug sponsor will need to submit an investigational new drug application containing evidence produced from animal testing, toxicity data, outlines for further study design, and manufacturing information. These data are reviewed by an interdisciplinary panel that scrutinizes the data it receives within a 30-day window. If approved, sponsors advance testing in 4 progressive phases of human trials, each increasing in size and duration, which may take up to 6 years to complete.

In phase 1, the drug is tested for safety, dosage, absorption, distribution, metabolism, elimination, and administration. Phase 2 tests pharmacodynamics, that is, the therapeutic physiological effect of the drug. Phase 3 tests the new drug against another competitor used for the same purpose. If no such drug exists, other forms of controls may be used. Phase 4 trials are "postmarket safety trials" conducted after approval to ensure that the medication remains safe and effective. Generic versions of an existing drug require fewer studies than brand-name drugs. However, manufacturers must demonstrate that their generic can be safely and effectively used in place of the original drug.

This process ensures that a drug's therapeutic and potential adverse effects are proportionally appropriate. A drug's safety is a balance of the harm it remedies and the harm it may cause. Subjecting patients to headaches or fatigue would be considered harmful on its own, but these effects are within tolerable margins of safety for a drug such as duloxetine, which has been approved for use among adolescents 7 to 17 years of age.[30] A drug's safety is not solely determined by its label indication, nor is "off label" synonymous with "experimental." As asserted by Furey and Wilkins, "Off-label drug use is not the same as experimental or research use,"[31(p588)] a sentiment that has been affirmed by the American Academy of Pediatrics.[32]

At the time of initial application, sponsors cannot foresee every potential use for a drug, nor can they efficiently pursue applications for all potential uses because of the burden of time and costs associated with the approval process. Off-label use is therefore a common and necessary part of pediatric care, as many drugs are tested only among adults.[33,34] An estimated 38% of pediatric prescriptions are off label.[33] This led to the development of policies to address the unmet health needs of adolescents such as the Best Pharmaceuticals for Children Act and the Pediatric Research Equity Act.

With off-label prescription being common, pharmaceutical companies are not incentivized to seek approval for supplemental indications.[35] From a cynically capitalistic perspective, if money can be made from a drug's off-label use, why expend substantial resources seeking supplemental approval? Public health agencies must therefore seek out novel measures to address the growing public health crisis facing transgender adolescents in the United States. As of January 2025, however, the Trump administration was directing federal agencies to enforce discriminatory policies targeting transgender and intersex Americans and disrupting the operations of agencies including the National Institutes of Health. This political climate creates major obstacles to creating such policies.

Via supplemental applications, drug sponsors can make labeling changes for approved drugs including dosages, clinical indications, manufacturing processes, and patient populations. Supplemental indications are a common part of drug development.[35] One study revealed that, in the past 10 years, 48% of drugs had at least 1 supplemental indication and 20% had 2 or more.[36] However, there is less incentive for companies to seek supplemental indication approval once a drug is available for off-label use. Seeking approval can be costly, with costs measured in the tens of millions.[37] Because precocious puberty is an orphan condition affecting fewer than 200 000 people annually, companies are incentivized to develop drugs to treat the disease under the Orphan Drug Act of 1983. Such incentives may be necessary to encourage companies to seek approvals for drugs associated with transgender medicine.

SAFETY AND EFFICACY

A drug is not "safe" because there is no risk of adverse effects. Few legitimate treatments are without risks or side effects. The FDA under previous administrations maintained such a realistic standard:

> No drug is absolutely safe; all drugs have side effects. "Safe" in this sense

AJPH October 2025, Vol. 115, No. 10

means that the benefits of the drug appear to outweigh the known risks. If the FDA decides the benefits of a drug outweigh the known risks, the drug will receive approval.[38]

Safety

There is evidence that the effects of these medications are reversible[6,8,39–41] and are well tolerated, with common adverse effects no more severe than those associated with other pediatric drugs.[8,41–43] The most common adverse effects are becoming flushed and experiencing headaches, weight gain, and fatigue.[39] The adverse effects invoked to defend legislative restrictions are those on bone development, fertility, and cognitive function.

Bone development. Sex hormones play an important role in bone maturation and development. Pubertal pause has been shown to arrest adolescent bone development across metrics of length, mineralization, and cortical and trabecular growth.[44] Hormonal factors are not the only determinants of bone health, however; key factors such as age, medical history, nutrition, environment, and physical activity play significant roles in bone development.

Providers may mitigate these adverse effects through dietary changes, exercise regimens, and prescription of supplemental vitamins such as vitamin D and calcium.[6] Importantly, impacts on bone health are not assured, with systemic reviews identifying both studies reporting minimal changes in bone health and studies detailing more substantial impacts.[45] Bone development often improves once sex hormones are reintroduced, either from cessation of pubertal pause or from subsequent initiation of hormone replacement therapy.[46–51]

Reproductive capacity. Puberty-pausing medications arrest the development of reproductive capacity during treatment, but long-term reproductive capacity is not permanently impaired by pubertal pause alone.[52–55] In the case of patients resuming endogenous puberty and not receiving subsequent hormonal treatment, this capacity will return. Depending on how early in development pubertal pause begins, future fertility preservation options may be limited, and individuals may need to consider delaying initiation of hormonal treatment of certain fertility preservation methods if these methods are to be effective.

Cognitive function. Fewer studies have addressed the cognitive effects on humans, and there is even less evidence from studies of participants receiving these drugs for gender dysphoria.[56] Impacts on neurocognitive development require additional study. Evidence in this domain is often conflicting, impacted by methodological limitations, and at times rooted in normative values placed on abstract performance metrics.[42] These effects are notable but do not paint a definitive picture. There are no data to suggest that such effects manifest in any way that would measurably influence the life chances, career goals, academic achievement, or social navigation of transgender adolescents or adults.

It would also behoove us to weigh these potential effects with the negative psychological effects of gender dysphoria, including effects on cognition and social functioning. Other compelling evidence shows that these medications are associated with improved psychoemotional functioning among patients.[16,21,57–59]

Efficacy

The medications described here are indisputably effective at safely pausing pubertal development in adolescents.[41,42,59–62] Similarly, a compelling body of evidence has consistently noted their safety and reversibility.[39,43,62–64] Although some research has shown that dysphoria may be reduced by pubertal pause, such interventions are preventive.[65] These medications are expected not to eliminate gender dysphoria but to prevent escalations in severity from pubertal development. Although primarily preventive, pubertal pause can have immediate and long-term benefits for transgender people such as improving mental health and reducing the burden and cost of transition.

Pubertal pause can have a positive impact on a transgender person's embodiment goals, rendering aspects of adult transition less invasive, less costly, or unnecessary altogether, and it is associated with greater satisfaction with one's transition.[8,39,42,45,60,66] Patients seeking gender-affirming hormone therapy may not require supraphysiological doses, which are often necessary for those who did not undergo pubertal pause and can increase unwanted or adverse effects.[10,67] Inversely, endogenous puberty can substantially attenuate a person's embodiment goals and reduce satisfaction with transition. Pubertal pause is also associated with reduced anxiety, depression, and suicidality and improves overall psychological functioning.[16,19–21,43,59,64]

Quality of the Evidence

Although off-label use is not objectionable, gender dysphoria may be an appropriate supplemental indication for these medications. Use of GnRH analogs is supported by a quality and volume of evidence comparable to historically approved initial or supplemental indications.[45,68,69] This evidence is not generally classified as "high quality," but it is important to properly contextualize this term. Rarely is evidence graded high quality without it being associated with a randomized controlled trial. However, the valorization of randomized trials ignores many other means of studying drugs and producing scientific knowledge.[70,71]

There are limitations that researchers and drug sponsors must contend with when studying these drugs.[72,73] Given the drugs' pharmacodynamic efficacy and the psychiatric risks of unimpeded gender dysphoria, randomization is logistically and ethically inappropriate. Logistically, participant retention and blinding protocols would be undermined because of the drugs' efficacy. Ethically, transgender adolescents in the placebo arm would be willfully exposed to psychologically distressing pubertal development. The FDA acknowledges that when randomization or placebo control may not be ethically or logistically appropriate, other forms of evidence may be sufficient to demonstrate efficacy.[74] The FDA itself has suggested that placebo controlled trials impose ethical burdens on the study of gender-affirming treatments.[4]

Use of GnRH analogs among transgender patients may satisfy the evidentiary and safety standards for supplemental indication without a randomized trial. A substantial body of research has scrutinized and affirmed their safety, efficacy, benefits, and potential risks.[43,45,75] As Wang and Kesselheim found, a diverse range of evidence has been used to support supplemental indications, including in the case of pediatric drugs.[68] In an ideal world, all medicine would be supported by swaths of "high-quality literature." As pointed out by Reed, "low-quality evidence" supports many treatments without stoking controversy.[76] A recent study by van der Zanden et al. seeking to understand the evidence base in support of off-label prescribing in pediatrics showed that only 14% of the more than over 750 drugs included were "supported by high quality evidence (4% meta-analysis or systematic reviews, 10% [randomized controlled trials] of high quality)."[77(p1243)] On the basis of their findings, van der Zanden et al. concluded:

> Many have advocated that off-label use is only justified when supported by a high level of evidence. We show that this prerequisite would seriously limit available drug treatment for children as the underlying evidence is low across ages and drug classes.[77(p1243)]

These findings seem to confirm Howick and colleagues' analysis of evidence indicating that few treatments are supported by the type of high-quality evidence demanded of transgender medicine.[78] This double standard has been raised in critiques of a British report, the *Cass Review*.[79] Despite its own methodological carelessness, the review applies a uniquely critical lens to the evidence base supporting GnRH analogs. In many of the peer-reviewed critiques of this report, critics note that in addition to anonymous and biased authors, lack of peer review, and methodological flaws, the level of scrutiny applied in the review is an unrealistic standard that many treatments we depend on today could not withstand.[80,81]

van der Zanden et al. caution us against such standards. The findings suggest that the evidence base supporting puberty-pausing medications is similar to that of many pediatric drugs. Although it is not the common path, several drugs have been approved with data from nonrandomized trials.[82,83] Randomization is not the only form of control available to drug sponsors. Randomization is adopted as a control mechanism when there is a lack of preexisting data on the condition and the treatment's effectiveness.[70,73,84] Randomization is often shorthand for the removal or mediation of known and unknown confounding variables and covariates, but it is an overstatement to claim that randomized trials are the only way to validate a treatment's safety and efficacy.

PUBLIC HEALTH IMPLICATIONS

Evidence from the use of GnRH analogs for both precocious puberty and gender dysphoria can be drawn together to satisfy some of the evidentiary requirements for approval as a supplemental indication for gender dysphoria. In 2019 and 2023, the FDA published draft guidance capturing its then-current thinking on the methods that might satisfy "substantial evidence of effectiveness."[74,85] This guidance continues the agency's growing inclination to embrace less rigid and prohibitive standards for evidence production. The agency recognizes inclusion of evidence drawn from a product's pharmacological class, a clinical investigation of efficacy for different but closely related approved indications, real-world evidence, and previous findings demonstrating the purported effects.[74,85]

Evidence from the use of these drugs among adolescents with precocious puberty easily conforms to the category of efficacy for different but closely related approved indications. According to the FDA, similarity can be constituted by the drug's mechanism of action and the similarity of the indications. Because the initial and supplementary indications involve the same mechanism of action (down regulation of sex hormone production) in the same population (adolescents), the same purpose (pubertal pause), and even the same products, it is appropriate to argue that precocious puberty qualifies as a "similar approved indication."

Additional evidence could be collected from the decades of research demonstrating the safety and efficacy of the drugs among transgender adolescents.[6,8,39,41–43,45,60,62,64,66,86] Analysis of the more than 3 decades of research accumulated regarding provision of GnRH analogs to transgender adolescents would produce substantive real-world evidence, albeit a different conceptualization of such evidence. These forms of evidence production may be novel but not prohibitively so, as the FDA previously boasted a "long-standing flexibility when considering the types of data and evidence that can meet the substantial evidence requirements."[85]

Should a "well-controlled" clinical investigation be required, there is no need to wait for a drug sponsor to conduct such a trial. The Best Pharmaceuticals for Children Act[87] may provide the Department of Health and Human Services a means to initiate this process. It is one of the express priorities of this law to address the prevalence of off-label use of drugs in pediatrics by sponsoring clinical trials of off-label products.[88] This legislation is therefore purpose built to address health disparities such as those described here. The Best Pharmaceuticals for Children Act enables the National Institutes of Health to identify off-label uses of drugs, sponsor clinical drug trials, and communicate data from those trials to the FDA for consideration of label modification.[88] Although such a path of approval for new drug indications is novel, it has been used for this exact purpose,[89] and the labeling of a number of pediatric drugs has been modified on the basis of this act.

Because the ability of GnRH analogs to pause puberty is well established, other means of control can be investigated. Alternative controls provide opportunities to better understand available forms of mediating interventions for bone health. Because bone health is dependent on genetic, dietary, physiological, environmental, and behavioral factors, a trial could specifically focus on bone health as its control basis. In both arms, patients would be given GnRH analogs, but controls would be in place to ensure that these patients remained relatively sedentary and were not provided with dietary or nutritional supplements. The experimental arm would then provide patients with standard exercise activities promoting mechanical loading and bone modeling as well as supplemental phosphorus, calcium, vitamin D, or low-dose estradiol. Such a trial, with proper management and diverse recruitment, could maintain the same level of scientific rigor as randomized trials while not risking the well-being of adolescents receiving placebo treatment.

SUMMARY

Although lawmakers have used off-label prescription of GnRH analogs to undermine the safety and efficacy of their use and justify restrictions, these attempts ring hollow for many reasons. Such claims are at odds with best practices in pediatric medicine, norms within drug development procedures, and an objective analysis of the evidence supporting this care. Such sentiments were recently expressed by the Utah Department of Health and Human Services in one of the most rigorous systematic reviews of pediatric transgender medicine.[90] This report, which echoes many of the perspectives presented here, similarly argues that the body of evidence supporting this field of medicine likely "exceeds the amount of evidence that often serves as the basis of FDA approval."

After more than 3 decades of clinical use and study, these drugs continue to be as safe as many other pediatric treatments. Yet, their use among transgender adolescents has been subjected to a degree of scrutiny that few treatments if any could be expected to withstand. Despite the safety profile of these medications' provision to transgender adolescents being equivalent to their on-label indication for precocious puberty, their use among transgender adolescents has been subject to ongoing and escalating legislative and administrative restrictions.

Why do drugs for 2 similar purposes, among the same population, face staggeringly unequal scrutiny, especially when transgender adolescents access these drugs at older ages than cisgender precocious puberty patients? Arguably, the more stringent standard is part of a broader ideologically motivated campaign against the rights of transgender people across all spheres of public life, from sports participation, use of public accommodations, and adolescent rights to education, identification documents, and attacks on gender transgression itself.

Withholding access to GnRH analogs places the well-being of all transgender adolescents at risk. Considering that nontreatment of gender dysphoria leads to a risk of depression and suicidality and to subsequent transition procedures becoming more invasive and costly, these restrictions on the use of GnRH analogs among transgender adolescents could endanger the health and well-being of tens of thousands of adolescents across the country. AJPH

ABOUT THE AUTHOR

At the time of the research, the author was unaffiliated.

CORRESPONDENCE

Correspondence should be sent to Sinéad Murano-Kinney, MFA, PO Box 7025, 940 Thayer Ave, Silver Spring, MD 20910 (e-mail: sinead.d.kinney@gmail.com). Reprints can be ordered at https://www.ajph.org by clicking the "Reprints" link.

PUBLICATION INFORMATION

Full Citation: Murano-Kinney S. Analogous analogs: considerations regarding off-label use of gonadotropin-releasing hormone analogs among transgender adolescents. *Am J Public Health*. 2025;115(10):1662–1670.

Acceptance Date: March 17, 2025.

DOI: https://doi.org/10.2105/AJPH.2025.308130

ORCID iD:

Sinéad Murano-Kinney https://orcid.org/0009-0001-0252-0072

ACKNOWLEDGMENTS

This article's creation was not funded in any part by any private or public entity.

I express my deepest gratitude to the editorial team and reviewers for their transformative insights. I would also like to express my deepest thanks to Florence Ashley for their notes on an early draft.

CONFLICTS OF INTEREST

The author reports no financial conflicts. The author discloses a belief in the rights of gender self-determination for all people.

HUMAN PARTICIPANT PROTECTION

No human participant trials were associated with the writing of this piece.

REFERENCES

1. Redfield C. The impact of 2024 anti-transgender legislation on youth. Available at: https://williamsinstitute.law.ucla.edu/publications/2024-anti-trans-legislation. Accessed September 12, 2024.
2. Twohey M, Jewett C. They paused puberty, but is there a cost? Available at: https://www.nytimes.com/2022/11/14/health/puberty-blockers-transgender.html. Accessed September 9, 2024.
3. Mireku A. Legal challenges put off label use of gender affirming care drugs in jeopardy. Available at: https://www.pharmaceutical-technology.com/features/legal-challenges-put-off-label-use-of-gender-affirming-care-drugs-in-jeopardy. Accessed January 18, 2025.
4. Grossman LA. Criminalizing transgender care. Available at: https://ilr.law.uiowa.edu/sites/ilr.law.uiowa.edu/files/2024-11/ILR-110-Grossman_1.pdf. Accessed January 18, 2025.
5. Chen M, Eugster EA. Central precocious puberty: update on diagnosis and treatment. *Paediatr Drugs*. 2015;17(4):273–281. https://doi.org/10.1007/s40272-015-0130-8
6. Finlayson C. *Pubertal Suppression in Transgender Youth*. Elsevier Inc; 2019.
7. Carswell JM, Lopez X, Rosenthal SM. The evolution of adolescent gender-affirming care: an historical perspective. *Horm Res Paediatr*. 2022;95(6):649–656. https://doi.org/10.1159/000526721
8. T'Sjoen G. Arcelus J, Gooren L, Klink DT, Tangpricha V. Endocrinology of transgender medicine. *Endocr Rev*. 2019;40(1):97–117. https://doi.org/10.1210/er.2018-00011
9. Rafferty J. Ensuring comprehensive care and support for transgender and gender-diverse children and adolescents. *Pediatrics*. 2018;142(4):e20182162. https://doi.org/10.1542/peds.2018-2162
10. Hembree WC, Cohen-Kettenis PT, Gooren L, et al. Endocrine treatment of gender-dysphoric/gender-incongruent persons: an Endocrine Society clinical practice guideline. *J Clin Endocrinol Metab*. 2017;102(11):3869–3903. https://doi.org/10.1210/jc.2017-01658
11. Day JK, Fish JN, Perez-Brumer A, Hatzenbuehler ML, Russell ST. Transgender youth substance use disparities: results from a population-based sample. *J Adolesc Health*. 2017;61(6):729–735. https://doi.org/10.1016/j.jadohealth.2017.06.024
12. Green AE, DeChants JP, Price MN, Davis CK. Association of gender-affirming hormone therapy with depression, thoughts of suicide, and attempted suicide among transgender and nonbinary youth. *J Adolesc Health*. 2022;70(4):643–649. https://doi.org/10.1016/j.jadohealth.2021.10.036
13. Marconi E, Monti L, Marfoli A, et al. A systematic review on gender dysphoria in adolescents and young adults: focus on suicidal and self-harming ideation and behaviours. *Child Adolesc Psychiatry Ment Health*. 2023;17(1):110. https://doi.org/10.1186/s13034-023-00654-3
14. Toomey RB, Syvertsen AK, Shramko M. Transgender adolescent suicide behavior. *Pediatrics*. 2018;142(4):e20174218. https://doi.org/10.1542/peds.2017-4218
15. Thoma BC, Salk RH, Choukas-Bradley S, Goldstein TR, Levine MD, Marshal MP. Suicidality disparities between transgender and cisgender adolescents. *Pediatrics*. 2019;144(5):e20191183. https://doi.org/10.1542/peds.2019-1183
16. de Vries ALC, McGuire JK, Steensma TD, Wagenaar ECF, Doreleijers TAH, Cohen-Kettenis PT. Young adult psychological outcome after puberty suppression and gender reassignment. *Pediatrics*. 2014;134(4):696–704. https://doi.org/10.1542/peds.2013-2958
17. Hughto JMW, Gunn HA, Rood BA, Pantalone DW. Social and medical gender affirmation experiences are inversely associated with mental health problems in a US non-probability sample of transgender adults. *Arch Sex Behav*. 2020;49(7):2635–2647. https://doi.org/10.1007/s10508-020-01655-5
18. Rowniak S, Bolt L, Sharifi C. Effect of cross-sex hormones on the quality of life, depression and anxiety of transgender individuals: a quantitative systematic review. *JBI Database System Rev Implement Rep*. 2019;17(9):1826–1854. https://doi.org/10.11124/JBISRIR-2017-003869
19. Turban JL, King D, Carswell JM, Keuroghlian AS. Pubertal suppression for transgender youth and risk of suicidal ideation. *Pediatrics*. 2020;145(2):e20191725. https://doi.org/10.1542/peds.2019-1725
20. Tordoff DM, Wanta JW, Collin A, Stepney C, Inwards-Breland DJ, Ahrens K. Mental health outcomes in transgender and nonbinary youths receiving gender-affirming care. *JAMA Netw Open*. 2022;5(2):e220978. https://doi.org/10.1001/jamanetworkopen.2022.0978
21. van der Miesen AIR, Steensma TD, de Vries ALC, Bos H, Popma A. Psychological functioning in transgender adolescents before and after gender-affirmative care compared with cisgender general population peers. *J Adolesc Health*. 2020;66(6):699–704. https://doi.org/10.1016/j.jadohealth.2019.12.018
22. Matouk K, Wald M. Gender-affirming care saves lives. Available at: https://www.columbiapsychiatry.org/news/gender-affirming-care-saves-lives. Accessed January 25, 2025.
23. Trump DJ. President Trump's plan to protect children from left-wing gender insanity. Available at: https://www.donaldjtrump.com/agenda47/president-trumps-plan-to-protect-children-from-left-wing-gender-insanity. Accessed December 19, 2024.
24. Trump DJ. Defending women from gender ideology extremism and restoring biological truth to the federal government. Available at: https://www.whitehouse.gov/presidential-actions/2025/01/defending-women-from-gender-ideology-extremism-and-restoring-biological-truth-to-the-federal-government. Accessed January 24, 2025.
25. Trump DJ. Protecting children from chemical and surgical mutilation. Available at: https://www.whitehouse.gov/presidential-actions/2025/01/protecting-children-from-chemical-and-surgical-mutilation. Accessed January 28, 2025.
26. Mervis J. Mass firings decimate US science agencies. Available at: https://www.science.org/content/article/mass-firings-decimate-u-s-science-agencies. Accessed February 19, 2025.
27. Neus N. The start of the national AIDS movement: Act Up's defining moment in queer protest history. Available at: https://www.theguardian.com/society/2023/oct/11/act-up-hiv-aids-1988-fda-protest. Accessed January 12, 2025.
28. King H. AIDS Coalition to Unleash Power (ACT-UP) demands access to drugs. Available at: https://nvdatabase.swarthmore.edu/content/us-aids-coalition-unleash-power-act-demands-access-drugs-1987-89. Accessed January 13, 2025.
29. Center for Drug Evaluation and Research. Frequently asked questions about the FDA drug approval process. Available at: https://www.fda.gov/drugs/special-features/frequently-asked-questions-about-fda-drug-approval-process. Accessed January 14, 2025.

30. Dwyer JB, Bloch MH. Antidepressants for pediatric patients. *Curr Psychiatr*. 2019;18(9):26–42F.

31. Furey K, Wilkins K. Prescribing "off-label": what should a physician disclose? *AMA J Ethics*. 2016;18(6):587–593. https://doi.org/10.1001/journalofethics.2016.18.6.ecas3-1606

32. Jenkins K. AAP policy clarifies acceptable off-label use of medical devices in children. Available at: https://publications.aap.org/aapnews/news/6950/AAP-policy-clarifies-acceptable-off-label-use-of. Accessed September 18, 2024.

33. Allen HC, Garbe MC, Lees J, et al. Off-label medication use in children, more common than we think: a systematic review of the literature. *J Okla State Med Assoc*. 2018;111(8):776–783.

34. Balan S, Hassali MAA, Mak VSL. Two decades of off-label prescribing in children: a literature review. *World J Pediatr*. 2018;14(6):528–540. https://doi.org/10.1007/s12519-018-0186-y

35. Sahragardjoonegani B, Beall RF, Kesselheim AS, Hollis A. Repurposing existing drugs for new uses: a cohort study of the frequency of FDA-granted new indication exclusivities since 1997. *J Pharm Policy Pract*. 2021;14(1):3. https://doi.org/10.1186/s40545-020-00282-8

36. Vokinger KN, Glaus CEG, Kesselheim AS, Serra-Burriel M, Ross JS, Hwang TJ. Therapeutic value of first versus supplemental indications of drugs in US and Europe (2011–20): retrospective cohort study. *BMJ*. 2023;382:e074166. https://doi.org/10.1136/bmj-2022-074166

37. Wouters OJ, McKee M, Luyten J. Estimated research and development investment needed to bring a new medicine to market, 2009–2018. *JAMA*. 2020;323(9):844–853. https://doi.org/10.1001/jama.2020.1166

38. Food and Drug Administration. FDA's drug review process: continued. Available at: https://www.fda.gov/drugs/information-consumers-and-patients-drugs/fdas-drug-review-process-continued. Accessed September 18, 2024.

39. Betsi G, Goulia P, Sandhu S, Xekouki P. Puberty suppression in adolescents with gender dysphoria: an emerging issue with multiple implications. *Front Endocrinol (Lausanne)*. 2024;15:1309904. https://doi.org/10.3389/fendo.2024.1309904

40. Magon N. Gonadotropin releasing hormone agonists: Expanding vistas. *Indian J Endocrinol Metab*. 2011;15(4):261. https://doi.org/10.4103/2230-8210.85575

41. Schagen SEE, Cohen-Kettenis PT, Delemarre-van de Waal HA, Hannema SE. Efficacy and safety of gonadotropin-releasing hormone agonist treatment to suppress puberty in gender dysphoric adolescents. *J Sex Med*. 2016;13(7):1125–1132. https://doi.org/10.1016/j.jsxm.2016.05.004

42. Mahfouda S, Moore JK, Siafarikas A, Zepf FD, Lin A. Puberty suppression in transgender children and adolescents. *Lancet Diabetes Endocrinol*. 2017;5(10):816–826. https://doi.org/10.1016/S2213-8587(17)30099-2

43. Ramos GGF, Mengai ACS, Daltro CAT, Cutrim PT, Zlotnik E, Beck APA. Systematic review: puberty suppression with GnRH analogues in adolescents with gender incongruity. *J Endocrinol Invest*. 2021;44(6):1151–1158. https://doi.org/10.1007/s40618-020-01449-5

44. Klink D, Caris M, Heijboer A, van Trotsenburg M, Rotteveel J. Bone mass in young adulthood following gonadotropin-releasing hormone analog treatment and cross-sex hormone treatment in adolescents with gender dysphoria. *J Clin Endocrinol Metab*. 2015;100(2):E270–E275. https://doi.org/10.1210/jc.2014-2439

45. Bragge N, Delafosse G, Temple-Smith S. Evidence for effective interventions for children and young people with gender dysphoria—update. Available at: https://www.saxinstitute.org.au/resource/evidence-for-effective-interventions-for-children-and-young-people-with-gender-dysphoria-update. Accessed September 11, 2024.

46. Boogers LS, Wiepjes CM, Klink DT, et al. Transgender girls grow tall: adult height is unaffected by GnRH analogue and estradiol treatment. *J Clin Endocrinol Metab*. 2022;107(9):e3805–e3815. https://doi.org/10.1210/clinem/dgac349

47. Ciancia S, Dubois V, Cools M. Impact of gender-affirming treatment on bone health in transgender and gender diverse youth. *Endocr Connect*. 2022;11(11):e220280. https://doi.org/10.1530/EC-22-0280

48. Giacomelli G, Meriggiola MC. Bone health in transgender people: a narrative review. *Ther Adv Endocrinol Metab*. 2022;13:20420188221099346. https://doi.org/10.1177/20420188221099346

49. Moustakli E, Tsonis O. Exploring hormone therapy effects on reproduction and health in transgender individuals. *Medicina (Kaunas)*. 2023;59(12):2094. https://doi.org/10.3390/medicina59122094

50. Schagen SEE, Wouters FM, Cohen-Kettenis PT, Gooren LJ, Hannema SE. Bone development in transgender adolescents treated with GnRH analogues and subsequent gender-affirming hormones. *J Clin Endocrinol Metab*. 2020;105(12):e4252–e4263. https://doi.org/10.1210/clinem/dgaa604

51. Willemsen LA, Boogers LS, Wiepjes CM, et al. Just as tall on testosterone; a neutral to positive effect on adult height of GnRHa and testosterone in trans boys. *J Clin Endocrinol Metab*. 2023;108(2):414–421. https://doi.org/10.1210/clinem/dgac571

52. Guaraldi F, Beccuti G, Gori D, Ghizzoni L. Management of endocrine disease: long-term outcomes of the treatment of central precocious puberty. *Eur J Endocrinol*. 2016;174(3):R79–R87. https://doi.org/10.1530/EJE-15-0590

53. Magiakou MA, Manousaki D, Papadaki M, et al. The efficacy and safety of gonadotropin-releasing hormone analog treatment in childhood and adolescence: a single center, long-term follow-up study. *J Clin Endocrinol Metab*. 2010;95(1):109–117. https://doi.org/10.1210/jc.2009-0793

54. Thornton P, Silverman LA, Geffner ME, Neely EK, Gould E, Danoff TM. Review of outcomes after cessation of gonadotropin-releasing hormone agonist treatment of girls with precocious puberty. *Pediatr Endocrinol Rev*. 2014;11(3):306–317.

55. Warton C, McDougall RJ. Fertility preservation for transgender children and young people in paediatric healthcare: a systematic review of ethical considerations. *J Med Ethics*. 2022;48(12):1076–1082. https://doi.org/10.1136/medethics-2021-107702

56. Brik T, Vrouenraets LJJJ, de Vries MC, Hannema SE. Trajectories of adolescents treated with gonadotropin-releasing hormone analogues for gender dysphoria. *Arch Sex Behav*. 2020;49(7):2611–2618. https://doi.org/10.1007/s10508-020-01660-8

57. Tornese G, Di Mase R, Munarin J, et al. Use of gonadotropin-releasing hormone agonists in transgender and gender diverse youth: a systematic review. *Front Endocrinol (Lausanne)*. 2025:16:1555186. https://doi.org/10.3389/fendo.2025.1555186

58. Fisher AD, Ristori J, Alessia Romani, et al. Back to the future: is GnRHa treatment in transgender and gender diverse adolescents only an extended evaluation phase? *J Clin Endocrinol Metab*. 2024;109(6):1565–1579. https://doi.org/10.1210/clinem/dgad729

59. Costa R, Dunsford M, Skagerberg E, Holt V, Carmichael P, Colizzi M. Psychological support, puberty suppression, and psychosocial functioning in adolescents with gender dysphoria. *J Sex Med*. 2015;12(11):2206–2214. https://doi.org/10.1111/jsm.13034

60. Cohen-Kettenis PT, van Goozen SH. Pubertal delay as an aid in diagnosis and treatment of a transsexual adolescent. *Eur Child Adolesc Psychiatry*. 1998;7(4):246–248. https://doi.org/10.1007/s007870050073

61. Kreukels BPC, Cohen-Kettenis PT. Puberty suppression in gender identity disorder: the Amsterdam experience. *Nat Rev Endocrinol*. 2011;7(8):466–472. https://doi.org/10.1038/nrendo.2011.78

62. Mejia-Otero JD, White P, Lopez X. Effectiveness of puberty suppression with gonadotropin-releasing hormone agonists in transgender youth. *Transgend Health*. 2021;6(1):31–35. https://doi.org/10.1089/trgh.2020.0007

63. Delemarre-van de Waal HA, Cohen-Kettenis PT. Clinical management of gender identity disorder in adolescents: a protocol on psychological and paediatric endocrinology aspects. Available at: https://academic.oup.com/ejendo/article-abstract/155/Supplement_1/S131/6695708?redirectedFrom=fulltext. Accessed September 9, 2024.

64. Rew L, Young CC, Monge M, Bogucka R. Review: Puberty blockers for transgender and gender diverse youth—a critical review of the literature. *Child Adolesc Ment Health*. 2021;26(1):3–14. https://doi.org/10.1111/camh.12437

65. Restar AJ. Gender-affirming care is preventative care. *Lancet Reg Health Am*. 2023;24:100544. https://doi.org/10.1016/j.lana.2023.100544

66. Cohen-Kettenis PT, Schagen SEE, Steensma TD, de Vries ALC, Delemarre-van de Waal HA. Puberty suppression in a gender-dysphoric adolescent: a 22-year follow-up. *Arch Sex Behav*. 2011;40(4):843–847. https://doi.org/10.1007/s10508-011-9758-9

67. Rothman MS, Ariel D, Kelley C, et al. The use of injectable estradiol in transgender and gender diverse adults: a scoping review of dose and serum estradiol levels. *Endocr Pract*. 2024;30(9):870–878. https://doi.org/10.1016/j.eprac.2024.05.008

68. Wang B, Kesselheim AS. Characteristics of efficacy evidence supporting approval of supplemental indications for prescription drugs in United States, 2005–14: systematic review. *BMJ*. 2015;351:h4679. https://doi.org/10.1136/bmj.h4679

69. Watson C, Davidson S, Bourke S, Bourchier L, Temple-Smith M, Sanci L. Evidence for effective interventions for children and young people with gender dysphoria. Available at: https://www.saxinstitute.org.au/wp-content/uploads/Evidence-for-effective-interventions-for-children-and-young-people-with-gender-dysphoria.pdf. Accessed September 9, 2024.

70. Frieden TR. Evidence for health decision making—beyond randomized, controlled trials.

N Engl J Med. 2017;377(5):465–475. https://doi.org/10.1056/NEJMra1614394

71. Oyelese Y. Randomized controlled trials: not always the "gold standard" for evidence in obstetrics and gynecology. *Am J Obstet Gynecol.* 2024;230(4):417–425. https://doi.org/10.1016/j.ajog.2023.10.015
72. Ashley F, Tordoff DM, Olson-Kennedy J, Restar AJ. Randomized-controlled trials are methodologically inappropriate in adolescent transgender healthcare. *Int J Transgend Health.* 2024;25(3):407–418. https://doi.org/10.1080/26895269.2023.2218357
73. Schall TE, Jaffe K, Moses JD. Roles of randomized controlled trials in establishing evidence-based gender-affirming care and advancing health equity. *AMA J Ethics.* 2024;26(9):E684–E689. https://doi.org/10.1001/amajethics.2024.684
74. Food and Drug Administration. Demonstrating substantial evidence of effectiveness for human drug and biological products. Available at: https://www.fda.gov/regulatory-information/search-fda-guidance-documents/demonstrating-substantial-evidence-effectiveness-human-drug-and-biological-products. Accessed September 16, 2024.
75. Brezin F, Busiah K, Leroy C, et al. Endocrine management of transgender adolescents: expert consensus of the French Society of Pediatric Endocrinology and Diabetology Working Group. *Arch Pediatr.* 2024;16:S0929-693X(24)00176-3. https://doi.org/10.1016/j.arcped.2024.08.003
76. Reed E. The myth of "low quality evidence" around transgender care. Available at: https://www.erininthemorning.com/p/the-myth-of-low-quality-evidence. Accessed September 18, 2024.
77. van der Zanden TM, Smeets NJL, de Hoop-Sommen M, et al. Off-label, but on-evidence? A review of the level of evidence for pediatric pharmacotherapy. *Clin Pharmacol Ther.* 2022;112(6):1243–1253. https://doi.org/10.1002/cpt.2736
78. Howick J, Koletsi D, Pandis N, et al. The quality of evidence for medical interventions does not improve or worsen: a metaepidemiological study of Cochrane reviews. *J Clin Epidemiol.* 2020;126:154–159. https://doi.org/10.1016/j.jclinepi.2020.08.005
79. UK National Archives. Cass Review final report. Available at: https://cass.independent-review.uk/home/publications/final-report. Accessed September 18, 2024.
80. Aaron DG, Konnoth C. The future of gender-affirming care—a law and policy perspective on the Cass Review. *N Engl J Med.* 2025;392(6):526–528. https://doi.org/10.1056/NEJMp2413747
81. Grijseels DM. Biological and psychosocial evidence in the Cass Review: a critical commentary. Available at: https://www.tandfonline.com/doi/full/10.1080/26895269.2024.2362304#d1e510. Accessed September 18, 2024.
82. Razavi M, Glasziou P, Klocksieben FA, Ioannidis JPA, Chalmers I, Djulbegovic B. US Food and Drug Administration approvals of drugs and devices based on nonrandomized clinical trials. *JAMA Netw Open.* 2019;2(9):e1911111. https://doi.org/10.1001/jamanetworkopen.2019.11111
83. Hatswell AJ, Baio G, Berlin JA, Irs A, Freemantle N. Regulatory approval of pharmaceuticals without a randomised controlled study: analysis of EMA and FDA approvals 1999–2014. *BMJ Open.* 2016;6(6):e011666. https://doi.org/10.1136/bmjopen-2016-011666
84. Grossman J, Mackenzie FJ. The randomized controlled trial: gold standard, or merely standard? *Perspect Biol Med.* 2005;48(4):516–534. https://doi.org/10.1353/pbm.2005.0092
85. Food and Drug Administration. Demonstrating substantial evidence of effectiveness based on one adequate and well-controlled clinical investigation and confirmatory evidence: draft guidance for industry. Available at: https://www.federalregister.gov/documents/2023/09/19/2023-20228/demonstrating-substantial-evidence-of-effectiveness-based-on-one-adequate-and-well-controlled. Accessed September 18, 2024.
86. Pine-Twaddell E, Newfield RS, Marinkovic M. Extended use of histrelin implant in pediatric patients. *Transgend Health.* 2023;8(3):264–272. https://doi.org/10.1089/trgh.2021.0130
87. US Congress. Best Pharmaceuticals for Children Act (2002). Available at: https://www.congress.gov/bill/107th-congress/senate-bill/1789. Accessed September 18, 2024.
88. Eunice Kennedy Shriver National Institute of Child Health and Human Development. About BPCA. Available at: https://www.nichd.nih.gov/research/supported/bpca/about. Accessed September 16, 2024.
89. Liu ITT, Kesselheim AS. Drug repurposing via the Best Pharmaceuticals for Children Act. *JAMA Pediatr.* 2024;178(9):855–856. https://doi.org/10.1001/jamapediatrics.2024.2287
90. US Department of Health and Human Services. Systematic medical evidence review of hormonal transgender treatment. Available at: https://le.utah.gov/AgencyRP/reportingDetail.jsp?rid=636. Accessed September 18, 2024.

Disaggregating Office of Management and Budget Race/Ethnicity Data to Examine Racial Disparities in Late-Stage HIV Diagnosis, Hawaii, 2010–2022

Fenfang Li, PhD, MPH, Breena K. Gaskov, MPH, Timothy J. McCormick, MA, Alan R. Katz, MD, MPH, and Diana J. Felton, MD

See also Kaholokula, p. 1551.

Objectives. To evaluate racial disparities when examining race at a more granular level than the broader 1997 Office of Management and Budget (OMB) categories.

Methods. We examined HIV diagnoses in Hawaii during 2010 to 2022 by OMB race/ethnicity categories and an 18-category granular race/ethnicity variable that included the 10 most frequent Asian and Native Hawaiian/other Pacific Islander groups. We used multivariable logistic regression, adjusting for potential confounders.

Results. During 2015 to 2022, using OMB race/ethnicity data and White people as the comparison group, we found that Asians were the only group at increased odds (adjusted odds ratio [AOR] = 3.69; 95% confidence interval [CI] = 1.86, 7.33) for late-stage HIV diagnosis. Using granular race/ethnicity and with White people as the comparison group, we found that Filipinos (AOR = 5.42; 95% CI = 2.27, 13.0), Asians with no ethnicity data (AOR = 8.21; 95% CI = 3.20, 21.06), and Pacific Islanders other than Native Hawaiians (AOR = 4.02; 95% CI = 1.10, 14.63) were at increased odds.

Conclusions. Disaggregating racial/ethnicity data revealed important disparities in late-stage HIV diagnosis that would otherwise be obscured.

Public Health Implications. Identification of racial disparities using granular data enables more targeted interventions to reduce late-stage HIV diagnoses and to improve health outcomes. (*Am J Public Health*. 2025;115(10):1671–1680. https://doi.org/10.2105/AJPH.2025.308192)

AJPH October 2025, Vol. 115, No. 10

The Centers for Disease Control and Prevention (CDC) reported that in 2016, among people in the United States living with HIV, 15% were undiagnosed and accounted for 38% of new HIV transmissions, emphasizing the importance of HIV testing and early diagnoses.[1] Delays in HIV diagnosis and timely treatment compromise the efficacy of therapeutic interventions, leading to poorer health outcomes, and amplify the risk of HIV transmission because of prolonged periods of undiagnosed infection.[1,2]

National data from the CDC revealed that the percentage of stage 3 HIV diagnoses (the stage at which a patient is considered to have AIDS) decreased significantly: from 28.4% in 2010 to 20.9% in 2022. The most significant decrease occurred in 2014 (22.6%), followed by a smaller but steady decrease during 2015 to 2022.[3,4] Despite these overall improvements, racial disparities were evident. For example, among Asians, the percentage of stage 3 HIV diagnoses increased from 24.9% in 2017 to 28.1% in 2022. Among Native Hawaiians/other Pacific Islanders (NHPIs), although the percentages decreased from 25.9% in 2017 to 24.1% in 2022, they were higher than those among White people, for whom the percentages decreased from 21.5% to 21.4% during this period.[3,4]

Hawaii has a unique racial and ethnic makeup. In 2020, among non-Hispanics/non-Latinos, Asians accounted for 36.5% of the state's population, followed by White people (21.6%), persons identifying as multiracial (20.1%), NHPIs (10.2%), and Black/African American people (1.5%). Hispanics/Latinos accounted for 9.5% of the total population.[5] In the general US population, among non-Hispanics/non-Latinos, White people accounted for 57.8%, followed by Black/African American people (12.1%), Asians (5.9%), persons identifying as multiracial (4.1%), and NHPIs (0.2%). Hispanics/Latinos accounted for 18.7% of the total population.[5] In Hawaii's Asian population, 41.2% identify as Filipino, 30.9% as Japanese, 10.0% as Chinese, and 4.3% as Korean. Among NHPIs in Hawaii, 59.7% identify as Native Hawaiian, 11.0% as Samoan, 5.5% as Marshallese, and 3.0% as Tongan.[6]

Geographically, Honolulu County (the island of Oahu) accounts for 69.9% of the state's population, whereas the neighboring islands, containing Hawaii County, Maui County, and Kauai County, account for about 30% of the population, with Kauai County having the smallest population at 5%. The neighboring islands, all rural, have long suffered from physician shortages, including HIV care providers.[7,8]

Hawaii's demographic distinctiveness extends into HIV diagnosis and care. Historically, Asians and NHPIs have been more likely than other racial groups to receive late-stage HIV diagnoses.[9–11] More recently, disparities in late-stage HIV diagnosis among Asians and NHPIs continued during 2010 to 2016, when the odds of being diagnosed at stage 3 (AIDS) were 3.7 times higher among NHPIs and more than twice as high among Asians compared to White people.[12]

Since the release of the 1997 Office of Management and Budget (OMB) standards for racial and ethnic data collection, the United States, including Hawaii, has seen growing racial diversity, especially among Asian and NHPI groups.[5,13,14] In Hawaii, from 2010 to 2020 the Asian population grew by 5.5%, and the population of NHPIs grew by 10.8%.[15] The newest census data reveal significant population growth among Pacific Islanders and Asians in the continental United States.[15–17] Broad categories such as "White," "Asian," and "NHPI" can mask important disparities in these groups.[12,13,17–19] In an earlier study of HIV characteristics among Asian and NHPI men who have sex with men in San Francisco, California, higher proportions of those who identified as multiethnic, Pacific Islander, Chinese, or Filipino had HIV than did those who identified as other Asian groups, such as Japanese and Korean.[20] A more recent study, in New York City, found lower HIV testing rates among Chinese adults than among other Asian subgroups.[21]

In March 2024, the OMB finalized revisions to the 1997 standards (Statistical Policy Directive No. 15), which require the use of a single combined question for race and ethnicity and encourage respondents to select as many ethnic categories as reflect their identity.[22] This enables collection of more granular data to better understand within-group disparities.[22] For example, under the Asian category, "Chinese," "Filipino," "Asian Indian," "Vietnamese," "Korean," and "Japanese" are new choices, together with an open space for additional details. Under the NHPI category, "Native Hawaiian," "Samoan," "Chamorro," "Tongan," "Fijian," "Marshallese," and an open space for additional detail are provided.[22] Federal agencies are required to make these changes to their surveys and other reports no later than March 2029.[23]

In Hawaii, the Department of Health's HIV surveillance program collected data on 12 Asian ethnic groups and 9 NHPI ethnic groups. Granular data have been collected in Hawaii since initiation of HIV/AIDS surveillance. The current categories have been in place since 2008. Using these data, we evaluated trends in racial/ethnic disparities in late-stage HIV diagnosis in Hawaii from 2010 through 2022. In addition, we aimed to examine how racial disparities differ when examined at a more granular level than the 1997 OMB categories.

METHODS

We used de-identified HIV surveillance information reported to the Hawaii Department of Health Enhanced HIV/AIDS Reporting System through July 1, 2024, which allowed an 18-month reporting delay and assessment of diagnoses for the year 2022. This statewide, population-based system collects, stores, and retrieves mandatory reports of confirmed HIV diagnoses among Hawaii residents.[3,4,12] Hawaii is 1 of 48 jurisdictions that require reporting of all levels of CD4 T-lymphocyte (CD4; a key measure of immune function used in HIV diagnosis and monitoring) test results to state or local health departments.[4] We included data from Hawaii residents who had their HIV infection diagnosed between 2010 and 2022. We did not include nonresidents, such as short-term visitors. The diagnosing medical provider determined residency status at the time of HIV diagnosis.

Stage 3 Classification at HIV Diagnosis

We used the 2008 CDC HIV case definition to classify cases diagnosed through 2013, and we used the 2014 case definition to classify cases diagnosed in 2014 and later.[24,25] We defined stage 3 (AIDS) as documentation of an AIDS-defining opportunistic illness or either a CD4 lymphocyte count of less than 200 cells per microliter or CD4 percentage of total lymphocytes of less than 14.[4,24,25] Documentation of an AIDS-defining opportunistic illness supersedes a CD4 lymphocyte count or percentage that would not, by itself, be the basis for a stage 3 (AIDS) classification. Stage 3 classification is based on opportunistic illness and CD4 test results within 3 months of the HIV diagnosis date.[4,24,25] Cases in which early HIV infection is documented by a previous negative test within 6 months of the first positive test are classified as stage 0 regardless of opportunistic illness or CD4.[25] We defined "stage 3 (AIDS)" at HIV diagnosis as late-stage HIV diagnosis, and we use this term interchangeably with "late-stage diagnosis."[12] Stage 3 at HIV diagnosis indicates that the individual has likely lived for years with undiagnosed HIV.

Race/Ethnicity

1997 OMB race/ethnicity. Race/ethnicity data based on the 1997 OMB classification reflect self-reported identification. We categorized ethnicity as either Hispanic/Latino or non-Hispanic/Latino. The Hispanic/Latino category included all races. The non-Hispanic group included 6 race categories: American Indians/Alaska Natives (AIAN), Asians, NHPIs, Black/African American people, White people, and individuals of multiple races.[14]

Granular race/ethnicity. In Hawaii, additional data on ethnicity are collected for non-Hispanic/non-Latino Asians and non-Hispanic/non-Latino NHPIs. For non-Hispanic/non-Latino Asians, data on 12 ethnic groups are collected—Japanese, Filipino, Chinese, Korean, Vietnamese, Laotian, Thai, Cambodian, Indonesian, Asian Indian, Pakistani, and Malaysian—and an additional category for all other Asians. For non-Hispanic/non-Latino NHPIs, data on 9 ethnic groups are collected—Hawaiian, Samoan, Guamanian, Tongan, Fijian, Marshallese, Tahitian, Northern Mariana, and Palauan—and 3 additional categories for other Micronesians, other Polynesians, and other Pacific Islanders. Race and ethnicity categories under the 1997 OMB, the 2024 OMB Statistical Policy Directive No. 15, and the Hawaii HIV surveillance program are summarized in Table A (available as a supplement to the online version of this article at http://www.ajph.org).

To protect patient confidentiality while attaining adequate statistical power for reliable estimates, we combined or "rolled up" categories of detailed race and ethnicity, except for the categories of "other" (e.g., "other Asian," "other Micronesian") or "unknown," to the next broader level, so that each category had a minimum of 10 persons for the specified period. As a result, we created a granular race/ethnicity variable with the following 11 categories: Hispanics (of any race), AIANs, Black/African American people, White people, more than 1 race, Filipinos, Japanese, other Asians not specified, other Asians specified, Native Hawaiians, and other NHPIs. The category "other Asians specified" included Asian Indian, Bangladeshi, Cambodian, Chinese, Indonesian, Korean, Laotian, Nepalese, Thai, and Vietnamese. The category, "other Asians not specified" included people with Asian as their race but with no additional data on ethnic groups under Asian. The category "other NHPIs" included Chamorro, Chuukese, Guamanian, Palauan, Samoan, Tongan, and all others with NHPI as their race but with no additional data on ethnic group.

Other Variables

We assessed additional variables for their associations with late-stage HIV diagnosis, including sex at birth (male or female), age at HIV diagnosis (< 45 or ≥ 45 years), county of residence at HIV diagnosis, birth country, and HIV transmission category. We further grouped birth countries as the United States, Asian countries, the Pacific region, and all other locations. The Pacific region included the US Affiliated Pacific Islands (American Samoa, Guam, the Commonwealth of the Northern Mariana Islands, and the Freely Associated States), the Kingdom of Tonga, and the Independent State of Samoa.

HIV transmission categories included male-to-male sexual contact, heterosexual contact, injection drug use, a dual-risk category for men who have sex with men and also inject drugs, and an "other" category. The men who have sex with men category included men who ever had sexual contact with both men and women. The heterosexual contact group included individuals who ever had heterosexual contact with a person known to have or to be at high risk for HIV infection (e.g., an injection drug user). The "other" category included those with hemophilia, blood transfusion recipients, and those with risk factors not reported or not identified.

Statistical Analysis

We used the χ^2 test for trend to evaluate the percentages of late-stage HIV diagnosis for the entire study period and intervals noted for trend difference in the national surveillance reports: 2010 to 2014 and 2015 to 2022.[3,4,11] We evaluated proportions of late-stage HIV diagnoses at the bivariate level by χ^2 test or Fisher exact test for small-sample comparisons. We used multivariable logistic regression to assess the relationship between late-stage HIV diagnosis and 1997 OMB race/ethnicity or the granular race/ethnicity separately after adjustment for sex at birth, age and county of residence at HIV diagnosis, birth location, and HIV transmission category. Adjusted odds ratios (AORs) and 95% confidence intervals (CIs) were the primary statistics reported from the multivariable models. We used SAS version 9.4 (SAS Institute Inc., Cary, NC) in conducting all statistical analyses.

RESULTS

Figure 1 presents the total number of HIV diagnoses and percentage of stage 3 (AIDS) classification at HIV diagnosis among Hawaii residents between 2010 and 2022. The total number of HIV diagnoses increased from 2011 to 2015 and then decreased through 2020. HIV diagnoses rebounded to pre–COVID-19 pandemic levels in 2021 and 2022. The percentage of stage 3 (AIDS) classification, or late-stage HIV diagnoses, decreased significantly from 32.0% in 2010 to 14.1% in 2016 but stalled around 20% from 2017 to 2022, except for 2020, when the percentage increased to 32.7%. The χ^2 test for trends showed a significant decrease for the entire 13-year study period of 2010 to 2022 ($P < .01$) but no significant change during 2010 to 2014 or 2015 to 2022.

Patient Characteristics and Late-Stage HIV Diagnosis

Of 1083 unique Hawaii residents with HIV infection diagnosed between 2010 and 2022, White people accounted for 30.1%, followed by Asians (22.5%), persons of multiple races (14.5%), NHPIs (13.3%), and Black/African American people (7.2%). When examined by granular race/ethnicity, White people continued to have the highest percentage (30.1%), followed by persons of multiple races (14.5%), Hispanics/Latinos (11.6%), Native Hawaiians (10.2%), Filipinos (8.9%), Black/African American people (7.2%), and other Asians specified (6.4%). The category "other Asians not specified" accounted for 3.8%. The category "other Pacific Islanders" accounted for 3.1% (Table 1).

During the study period, people with HIV infection diagnosed during 2010 to 2014 accounted for 42.8%, whereas those diagnosed during 2015 to 2022 accounted for 57.2% of the total. Males accounted for 88.8%. People younger

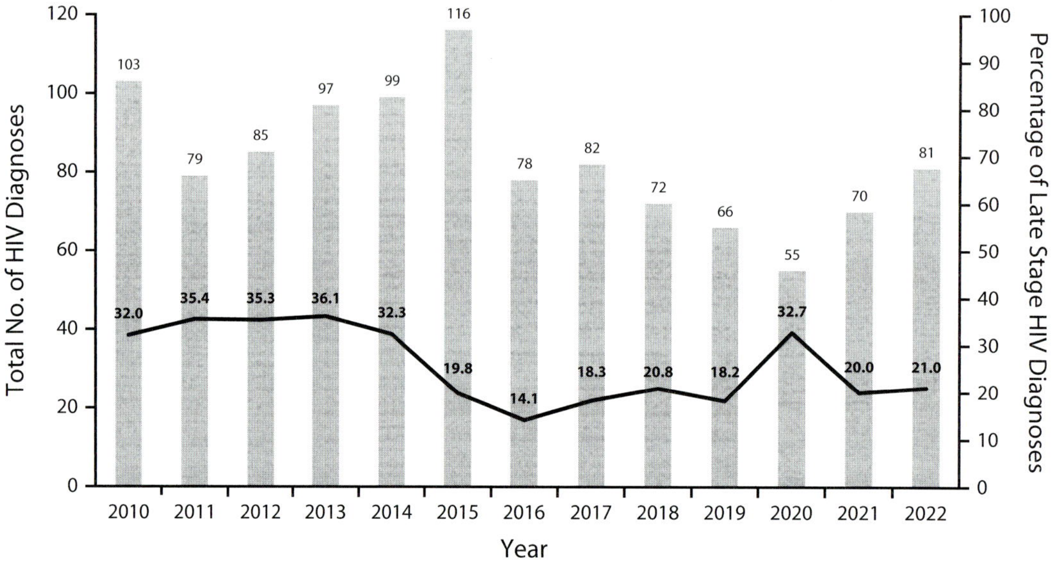

FIGURE 1— **Total Number of HIV Diagnoses and Percentage of Stage 3 AIDS Classification at HIV Diagnosis: Hawaii, 2010–2022**

TABLE 1— Distribution of HIV Diagnoses by the Office of Management and Budget (OMB) Race/Ethnicity and Granular Race/Ethnicity: Hawaii, 2010–2022

Race/Ethnicity	All Stages of HIV Diagnosis	Late-Stage of HIV Diagnosis		
	Total No. (% column)	"Yes," No. (% row)	"No," No. (% row)	P[a]
Total	1083 (100)	283 (26.1)	800 (73.9)	
1997 OMB race/ethnicity[b]				<.001
Hispanic, all races	126 (11.6)	24 (19.1)	102 (80.9)	
Asian	244 (22.5)	89 (36.5)	155 (63.5)	
Black	78 (7.2)	15 (19.2)	63 (80.8)	
Native Hawaiian/other Pacific Islander	144 (13.3)	50 (34.7)	94 (65.3)	
White	326 (30.1)	70 (21.5)	256 (78.5)	
Multiple races	157 (14.5)	34 (21.7)	123 (78.3)	
Other[c]	8 (0.7)	1 (12.5)	7 (87.5)	
Granular race/ethnicity				<.001
Hispanic, all races	126 (11.6)	24 (19.1)	102 (80.9)	
Filipino	96 (8.9)	40 (41.7)	56 (58.3)	
Japanese	38 (3.5)	13 (34.2)	25 (65.8)	
Other Asian specified[d]	69 (6.4)	19 (27.5)	50 (72.5)	
Other Asian unspecified[e]	41 (3.8)	17 (41.5)	24 (58.5)	
Black	78 (7.2)	15 (19.2)	63 (80.8)	
Native Hawaiian	110 (10.2)	35 (31.8)	75 (68.2)	
Other Pacific Islander[f]	34 (3.1)	15 (44.1)	19 (55.9)	
White	326 (30.1)	70 (21.5)	256 (78.5)	
Multiple races	157 (14.5)	34 (21.7)	123 (78.3)	
Other[c]	8 (0.7)	1 (12.5)	7 (87.5)	

[a]P value from the χ^2 test comparing proportions of late-stage HIV diagnosis. $P < .05$ represents statistically significant differences between the "yes" and "no" groups.
[b]Race/ethnicity categories follow the 1997 OMB standards: Hispanic (all races), White, Black, Asian, NHPI, and multiple races.
[c]The other category included American Indian/Alaska Native and people without data on race or ethnicity.
[d]Other Asian specified included Asian Indian, Bangladeshi, Cambodian, Chinese, Indonesian, Korean, Laotian, Nepalese, Thai, and Vietnamese.
[e]Other Asian not specified included people with Asian as their race but with no additional data on ethnic groups.
[f]Other Pacific Islander included Chamorro, Chuukese, Guamanian, Palauan, Samoan, Tongan, and all others with Native Hawaiian/other Pacific Islander as their race but with no additional data on ethnic groups.

than 45 years accounted for 68.7%. Almost three quarters (74.2%) of all HIV diagnoses were among residents of Honolulu County. Three quarters (74.8%) were born in the United States and 9.2% in Asian countries, with only 1.9% reporting being born in the Pacific region (Table B, available as a supplement to the online version of this article at http://www.ajph.org).

We found significant differences in the percentage of late-stage HIV diagnoses when classified by the OMB or the granular race/ethnicity method (Table 1). By OMB race/ethnicity, the highest percentages of late-stage HIV diagnosis were among Asians (36.5%) and NHPIs (34.7%). By granular race/ethnicity, other Pacific Islanders had the highest percentage (44.1%), followed by Filipinos (41.7%), other Asians unspecified (41.5%), Japanese (34.2%), and Native Hawaiians (31.8%). We also observed significant differences in the percentage of late-stage HIV diagnosis when classifying by HIV diagnosis period, age at HIV diagnosis, and HIV transmission category but not by sex at birth, county of residence, or birth country (Table B).

Logistic Regression Results

Table 2 presents the results of logistic regression models assessing late-stage HIV diagnosis by 1997 OMB race/ethnicity, while controlling for other selected patient characteristics across 2 time periods (those diagnosed during

TABLE 2— Logistic Regression Models of Late-Stage HIV Diagnosis by Office of Management and Budget (OMB) Race/Ethnicity, and Selected Patient Characteristics: Hawaii, 2010–2014 and 2015–2022

Variable	Late-Stage HIV Diagnosis, 2010–2014, OR (95% CI)	Late-Stage HIV Diagnosis, 2015–2022, OR (95% CI)
1997 OMB race/ethnicity[a]		
Hispanic vs White	1.41 (0.62, 3.21)	0.80 (0.34, 1.93)
Asian vs White	2.39 (1.10, 5.16)	3.69 (1.86, 7.33)
Black vs White	1.19 (0.40, 3.60)	0.92 (0.33, 2.53)
NHPI vs White	3.29 (1.65, 6.57)	1.66 (0.74, 3.72)
Multiple races vs White	1.48 (0.72, 3.02)	0.91 (0.39, 2.11)
Sex at birth, male vs female	2.05 (0.87, 4.81)	2.19 (0.95, 5.06)
Age at HIV diagnosis, ≥45 vs <45 y	2.32 (1.44, 3.75)	4.45 (2.75, 7.22)
Mode of transmission		
Heterosexual contact vs MSM	2.50 (0.94, 6.70)	1.63 (0.74, 3.55)
IDU vs MSM	2.64 (0.89, 7.89)	1.92 (0.84, 4.41)
MSM and IDU vs MSM	0.98 (0.28, 3.42)	0.90 (0.19, 4.25)
Other[b] vs MSM	1.53 (0.49, 4.82)	2.47 (1.11, 5.49)
County of residence at HIV diagnosis		
Hawaii County vs Honolulu County	0.82 (0.39, 1.70)	1.10 (0.56, 2.14)
Kauai County vs Honolulu County	4.30 (1.44, 12.83)	1.84 (0.55, 6.17)
Maui County vs Honolulu County	1.73 (0.86, 3.49)	0.45 (0.16, 1.29)
Birth country[c]		
Asia vs US	1.13 (0.45, 2.82)	0.70 (0.30, 1.60)
Pacific region vs US	4.53 (0.47, 43.36)	0.84 (0.16, 4.48)
Other vs US	0.22 (0.03, 1.88)	1.31 (0.49, 3.47)

Note. CI = confidence interval; IDU = injection drug use; MSM = male-to-male sexual contact; NHPI = Native Hawaiian/other Pacific Islander; OR = odds ratio. We ran 2 separate logistic regression models: one for 2010–2014 and the other for 2015–2022.
[a]Race/ethnicity categories follow the 1997 OMB standards: Hispanic (all races), White, Black, Asian, NHPI, and multiple races.
[b]The other category of mode of transmission refers to risk factors not reported or not identified.
[c]The Pacific region of birth country included the US Affiliated Pacific Islands (American Samoa, Guam, the Commonwealth of the Northern Mariana Islands, and the Freely Associated States), the Kingdom of Tonga, and the Independent State of Samoa. The other category of birth country refers to those whose birth country was unknown or any country or region other than Asia, the Pacific region, or the United States.

2010–2014 and those diagnosed during 2015–2022). During 2010 to 2014, both Asians (AOR = 2.39; 95% CI = 1.10, 5.16) and NHPIs (AOR = 3.29; 95% CI = 1.65, 6.57) were more likely to be diagnosed as late stage than were White people. During 2015 to 2022, only Asians (AOR = 3.69; 95% CI = 1.86, 7.33) were more likely to be diagnosed as late stage than White people.

Persons aged 45 years or older were also more likely to be diagnosed as late stage than were persons younger than 45 years for both periods. Residents from Kauai County were more likely to be diagnosed as late stage during 2010 to 2014 but not during 2015 to 2022. Neither birth sex, birth country, nor overall mode of HIV transmission was significantly associated with late-stage HIV diagnosis during either period.

Table 3 presents the results from logistic regression models of late-stage HIV diagnosis on the granular race/ethnicity, controlling for other selected patient characteristics by 2 periods (those diagnosed during 2010–2014 and those diagnosed during 2015–2022). During 2010 to 2014, Filipinos (AOR = 4.04; 95% CI = 1.58, 10.36), Native Hawaiians (AOR = 3.03; 95% CI = 1.48, 6.22), and Pacific Islanders other than Native Hawaiians (AOR = 6.27; 95% CI = 1.35, 29.08) were at increased odds of a late-stage HIV diagnosis compared to White people. During 2015 to 2022, the 3 groups with increased odds of a late-stage HIV diagnosis compared to White people were Filipinos (AOR = 5.42; 95% CI = 2.27, 13.0), Asians with no ethnicity data (AOR = 8.21; 95% CI = 3.20, 21.06), and Pacific Islanders other than Native Hawaiians (AOR = 4.02; 95% CI = 1.10, 14.63).

TABLE 3— Logistic Regression Models of Late-Stage HIV Diagnosis by Granular Race/Ethnicity and Selected Patient Characteristics: Hawaii, 2010–2014 and 2015–2022

Variable	Late-Stage HIV Diagnosis, 2010–2014, OR (95% CI)	Late-Stage HIV Diagnosis, 2015–2022, OR (95% CI)
Granular race/ethnicity		
Hispanic vs White	1.42 (0.62, 3.25)	0.81 (0.33, 1.98)
Filipino vs White	4.04 (1.58, 10.36)	5.42 (2.27, 13.0)
Japanese vs White	1.55 (0.46, 5.29)	0.85 (0.25, 2.85)
Other Asian specified[a] vs White	1.00 (0.28, 3.50)	1.46 (0.41, 5.17)
Other Asian not specified[b] vs White	1.98 (0.28, 13.81)	8.21 (3.20, 21.06)
Black vs White	1.22 (0.40, 3.70)	0.96 (0.34, 2.69)
Native Hawaiian vs White	3.03 (1.48, 6.22)	1.29 (0.50, 3.34)
Other Pacific Islander[c] vs White	6.27 (1.35, 29.08)	4.02 (1.10, 14.63)
Multiple races vs White	1.48 (0.72, 3.03)	0.95 (0.40, 2.24)
Sex at birth, male vs female	1.96 (0.83, 4.64)	2.55 (1.08, 6.03)
Age at HIV diagnosis, ≥45 y vs <45 y	2.48 (1.51, 4.07)	5.50 (3.28, 9.24)
Mode of transmission		
Heterosexual contact vs MSM[d]	2.51 (0.93, 6.79)	1.57 (0.71, 3.47)
IDU vs MSM	2.64 (0.88, 7.90)	2.16 (0.92, 5.06)
MSM and IDU vs MSM	1.05 (0.38, 2.87)	0.93 (0.19, 4.56)
Other[e] vs MSM	1.37 (0.54, 3.47)	2.79 (1.47, 5.29)
County of residence at HIV diagnosis		
Hawaii County vs Honolulu County	0.83 (0.40, 1.72)	1.04 (0.52, 2.08)
Kauai County vs Honolulu County	4.35 (1.45, 13.03)	2.14 (0.64, 7.13)
Maui County vs Honolulu County	1.71 (0.84, 3.48)	0.39 (0.13, 1.16)
Birth country[f]		
Asia vs US	1.77 (0.62, 5.09)	0.90 (0.37, 2.22)
Pacific region vs US	2.85 (0.24, 33.61)	0.54 (0.08, 3.51)
Other vs US	0.23 (0.03, 1.92)	1.33 (0.49, 3.59)

Note. CI = confidence interval; IDU = injection drug use; MSM = male-to-male sexual contact; OR = odds ratio. We ran 2 separate logistic regression models: one for period 2010–2014 and the other for 2015–2022.
[a]Other Asian specified included Asian Indian, Bangladeshi, Cambodian, Chinese, Indonesian, Korean, Laotian, Nepalese, Thai, and Vietnamese.
[b]Other Asian not specified included people with Asian as their race but with no additional data on ethnic groups under Asian.
[c]Other Pacific Islander included Chamorro, Chuukese, Guamanian, Palauan, Samoan, Tongan, and all others with Native Hawaiian/ Pacific Islander as their race but with no additional data on ethnic groups.
[d]Other category of HIV mode of transmission refers to risk factors not reported or not identified.
[e]The Pacific region included the US Affiliated Pacific Islands (American Samoa, Guam, the Commonwealth of the Northern Mariana Islands, and the Freely Associated States), the Kingdom of Tonga, and the Independent State of Samoa.
[f]The Other category of birth country refers to those whose birth country was unknown or any country/region other than Asia, Pacific region, or United States.

Persons aged 45 years or older were more likely to be diagnosed as late stage for both periods. Males were more likely to be diagnosed as late stage than were females during 2015 to 2022 but not during 2010 to 2014, as were persons whose HIV risk factors were not identified or reported. Residents from Kauai County were more likely to be diagnosed as late stage during 2010 to 2014 but not during 2015 to 2022. Birth country was not significantly associated with late-stage HIV diagnosis during either period.

DISCUSSION

By examining race/ethnicity at a more granular level, our study revealed racial disparities that would have been masked under the broader OMB categories. The disaggregated data allowed us to identify specific ethnic groups that are most affected by late-stage HIV diagnoses (e.g., Filipinos under Asians). By comparing data between recent and earlier periods, we also identified temporal shifts in disparities.

At the OMB level, Asians were at increased risk for late-stage HIV diagnosis during 2010 to 2014 and 2015 to 2022, consistent with previous research.[3,4,12] However, when we examined race/ethnicity at a more granular level, differences in specific subgroups emerged. Filipinos and Asians with unspecified ethnicity were particularly affected. This finding is consistent with previously reported health disparities in Asian subgroups[11,20,21] and can help better direct resources to increase testing and education. These findings can also help tailor appropriate interventions, such as HIV testing and education, to each subgroup's unique needs, for example, the creation of educational materials in common Filipino languages such as Tagalog and Ilocano.

NHPIs as a broad OMB category faced increased likelihood of late-stage HIV diagnosis during 2010 to 2014 (AOR = 3.29; 95% CI = 1.65, 6.57) but were no longer at significantly higher odds during 2015 to 2022 (AOR = 1.66; 95% CI = 0.74, 3.72). However, disaggregated data revealed that Pacific Islanders (e.g., Samoans, Tongans, Chamorros) other than Native Hawaiians were at significantly higher odds of late-stage HIV diagnosis than White people during 2010 to 2014 (AOR = 6.27; 95% CI = 1.35, 29.08) and during 2015 to 2022 (AOR = 4.02; 95% CI = 1.10, 14.63). Such findings highlight that Pacific Islanders other than Native Hawaiians have distinct health barriers and need targeted health interventions.

By comparing recent and earlier data, we identified groups consistently at higher odds of late-stage HIV diagnosis and demonstrated shifts in disparities over time. Filipinos and Pacific Islanders other than Native Hawaiians were consistently at increased odds of late-stage diagnosis, highlighting the need for targeted HIV testing and education.[10,11] Although Native Hawaiians experienced significantly higher odds than did White people during 2010 to 2014, they were no longer significantly different from White people during 2015 to 2022. By contrast, Asians of unspecified ethnicity were not significantly different from White people during 2010 to 2014 but faced significantly higher odds than did White people during 2015 to 2022. These trends suggest that interventions and services provided to Native Hawaiians may have been successful and could be replicated among other groups. Although there is limited literature on disparities specifically in HIV testing, certain Pacific Islanders were facing other barriers to health care, as demonstrated by research that found them less likely to be tested for COVID-19.[26,27]

In 2015, the CDC released a toolkit for expanding HIV partner services with the use of technology, possibly contributing to earlier diagnoses during subsequent years.[28] Data from Hawaii revealed the largest proportion of newly diagnosed HIV from HIV partner services during 2015 and 2016. However, whereas national trends showed a decline, Hawaii's late-stage HIV diagnoses stagnated from 2017 to 2022, potentially because of local disparities in health care access among marginalized communities.[4,26,27] Finally, the sharp decrease in late-stage HIV diagnoses observed nationally in 2014 and in Hawaii during 2015 to 2016 may partly reflect the updated 2014 case definition, which introduced stage 0 and reclassified some cases previously considered late stage.[3,4,25] Of note, the overall population of Hawaii increased from 2015 to 2016.[29]

Our finding that older adults are at increased odds of late-stage HIV diagnosis is consistent with the literature.[3,4,12] Although several studies have reported an association between late-stage HIV diagnosis and rural residence or foreign-born status,[30,31] our study did not find such associations, particularly during 2015 to 2022.

Limitations

Our study has several limitations. Surveillance data may not capture all relevant social determinants of health associated with late-stage diagnoses.[3,4,12,30] Self-reported race/ethnicity data also present challenges, as individuals may not consistently align with standard OMB categories, although new 2024 OMB categories may improve future representation.[3,4,12,22] Behavioral and demographic data may be incomplete or inconsistent because of reporting biases and misclassification.[3,4,10] As a cross-sectional study, the observed association between specific ethnic groups and late-stage HIV diagnosis cannot infer causation. Finally, unmeasured confounders such as HIV-related stigma and other factors affecting access to HIV testing are additional limitations of this study and warrant examination in future studies.

As one of the first studies to analyze HIV data by disaggregated race and ethnicity, this study highlights health disparities often hidden in broad racial/ethnic categories, emphasizing the need for granular data that reflect local population diversity. Future research should continue disaggregating broad OMB data to reveal subgroup-specific challenges in health care access and testing to enhance access to services and reduce health disparities.

In addition, studies investigating cultural strengths and barriers in HIV care, in particular HIV testing, would provide valuable insights for developing more tailored, effective interventions and preventive services to groups at consistently higher risk for late-stage HIV diagnosis.[32,33] Trends in Asian and NHPI populations during the COVID-19 pandemic indicated potential differences in health care access among specific subgroups, such as Filipinos compared to Japanese or Native Hawaiians compared to other Pacific Islanders.[26,27] It is possible that increased HIV testing and education were offered to and better received among Native Hawaiians but have not reached other Pacific Islanders. Future research examining HIV testing by granular race/ethnicity in parallel with HIV diagnosis data will shed light on disparities in HIV testing.

Public Health Implications

Identifying granular racial disparities allows more targeted, culturally responsive interventions that can effectively reduce late-stage HIV diagnoses among vulnerable populations. Specifically, the notable reduction in late-stage HIV diagnoses among Native Hawaiians suggests that certain policies or practices may have been impactful for this group. Understanding and replicating these strategies across other groups, such as Filipinos and other Pacific Islanders, may be beneficial in reducing disparities in late-stage HIV diagnosis. AJPH

ABOUT THE AUTHORS

Fenfang Li, Timothy J. McCormick, and Diana J. Felton are with the Communicable Disease and Public Health Nursing Division, Hawaii Department of Health, Honolulu, HI. Breena K. Gaskov and Alan R. Katz were with the Communicable Disease and Public Health Nursing Division, Hawaii Department of Health, Honolulu, at the time of the study. Alan R. Katz was also with the Thompson School of Social Work and Public Health, University of Hawaii at Manoa, Honolulu, at the time of the study.

CORRESPONDENCE

Correspondence should be sent to Fenfang Li, PhD, MPH, Communicable Disease and Public Health Nursing Division, Hawaii Department of Health, Room 423, 1250 Punchbowl St, Honolulu, HI 96813 (email: Fenfang.li@doh.hawaii.gov). Reprints can be ordered at http://www.ajph.org by clicking the "Reprints" link.

PUBLICATION INFORMATION

Full Citation: Li F, Gaskov BK, McCormick TJ, Katz AR, Felton DJ. Disaggregating Office of Management and Budget race/ethnicity data to examine racial disparities in late-stage HIV diagnosis, Hawaii, 2010–2022. *Am J Public Health*. 2025; 115(10):1671–1680.

Acceptance Date: May 7, 2025.

DOI: https://doi.org/10.2105/AJPH.2025.308192

ORCID iD:
Fenfang Li https://orcid.org/0000-0002-4617-6883

CONTRIBUTORS

F. Li led the study design and concept and completed the statistical analysis, the writing of the article, and the data interpretation. B. K. Gaskov contributed to article development. B. K. Gaskov, T. J. McCormick, A. R. Katz, and D. J. Felton participated in study design and concept, contributed to data interpretation, and critically reviewed the article for intellectual content. All authors have seen and approved the article.

ACKNOWLEDGMENTS

We thank all participating hospitals and medical providers for providing data and the best care to people living with HIV in Hawaii. Special thanks also go to the Hawaii HIV surveillance team, in particular Yuanshan (Sandy) Qiu, for collecting and managing HIV data at a high standard.

CONFLICTS OF INTEREST

The authors have no conflicts of interest to disclose.

HUMAN PARTICIPANT PROTECTION

The Hawaii Department of Health's institutional review board (IRB) determined that this study is public health surveillance and program improvement and therefore is not subject to IRB oversight (45 CFR 46.102 (1)(2)).

REFERENCES

1. Centers for Disease Control and Prevention. Vital signs: HIV transmission along the continuum of care—United States, 2016. *MMWR Morb Mortal Wkly Rep*. 2019;68(11):267–272. https://doi.org/10.15585/mmwr.mm6811e1
2. Spatz Friedman D, O'Byrne P, Roy M. Comparing those diagnosed early versus late in their HIV infection: implications for public health. *Int J STD AIDS*. 2017;28(7):693–701. https://doi.org/10.1177/0956462416664674
3. Centers for Disease Control and Prevention. HIV. Surveillance supplemental report: monitoring selected national HIV prevention and care objectives by using HIV surveillance data—United States and 6 dependent areas, 2017. July 2019. Available at: https://stacks.cdc.gov/view/cdc/149250. Accessed April 21, 2025.
4. Centers for Disease Control and Prevention. Monitoring selected national HIV prevention and care objectives by using HIV surveillance data—United States and 6 territories and freely associated states, 2022. May 21, 2024. Available at: https://stacks.cdc.gov/view/cdc/156511. Accessed April 21, 2025.
5. US Census Bureau. Profile of general population and housing characteristics, 2022. Available at: https://data.census.gov/table/ACSDP5Y2022.DP04?t=Homeownership+Rate&g=040XX00US41_050XX00US41013,41017,41031,41035&moe=false.+Accessed+on+January+19,+2024. Accessed April 17, 2025.
6. State of Hawaii, Department of Business, Economic Development & Tourism. Research & economic analysis. 2023 State of Hawaii data book (Table 1.32 and 1.33). Available at: https://dbedt.hawaii.gov/economic/databook/db2023. Accessed April 17, 2024.
7. Li F, McCormick TJ, Katz AR, Whiticar PM, Wasserman GM. Patient and provider characteristics associated with retention in HIV medical care and viral suppression among in care patients in Hawaii. *Int J STD AIDS*. 2021;32(10):919–926. https://doi.org/10.1177/09564624211002403
8. Hawaii State Department of Health. 2020 Hawaii HIV/AIDS integrated epidemiologic profile and impact of COVID-19 on HIV testing, diagnosis, and medical care. January 12, 2023. Available at: https://health.hawaii.gov/harmreduction/files/2023/01/Hawaii_2020-HIVAIDS-Epidemiologic-Profile_final-version_20230112.pdf. Accessed April 21, 2025.
9. Eckholdt HM, Chin JJ, Manzon-Santos JA, Kim DD. The needs of Asians and Pacific Islanders living with HIV in New York City. *AIDS Care*. 1997;9(6):493–504.
10. Wong FY, Campsmith ML, Nakamura GV, Crepaz N, Begley E. HIV testing and awareness of care-related services among a group of HIV-positive Asian Americans and Pacific Islanders in the United States: findings from a supplemental HIV/AIDS surveillance project. *AIDS Educ Prev*. 2004;16(5):440–447. https://doi.org/10.1521/aeap.16.5.440.48736
11. Shimizu SM, Chow DC, Katz AR, Richmond-Crum S, Miller D. Ethnic differences in HIV disease progression: a comparison of Asian/Pacific Islanders and White people living in Hawaii. *Ethn Dis*. 2006;16(1):262–267.
12. Li F, Juan BK, Wozniak M, et al. Trends and racial disparities of late-stage HIV diagnosis: Hawaii, 2010–2016. *Am J Public Health*. 2018;108(suppl 4):S292–S298. https://doi.org/10.2105/AJPH.2018.304506
13. Quint J, Matagi C, Kaholokula JK. The Hawai'i NHPI data disaggregation imperative: preventing

data genocide through statewide race and ethnicity standards. *Hawaii J Health Soc Welf.* 2023; 82(10 suppl 1):67–72.

14. White House, Office of Management and Budget. Revisions to the standards for the classification of federal data on race and ethnicity. Available at: https://obamawhitehouse.archives.gov/node/15626. Accessed April 21, 2025.
15. US Census Bureau. Hawaii added more than 94,000 people since 2010. August 25, 2021. Available at: https://www.census.gov/library/stories/state-by-state/hawaii.html. Accessed April 21, 2025.
16. Budiman A, Ruiz NG. Key facts about Asian Americans, a diverse and growing population. April 29, 2021. Available at: https://coilink.org/20.500.12592/w73v65. Accessed April 21, 2025.
17. Rico B, Hahn JK, and Jacobs P. Detailed look at Native Hawaiian and other Pacific Islander groups. September 21, 2023. Available at: https://www.census.gov/library/stories/2023/09/2020-census-dhc-a-nhpi-population.html. Accessed April 21, 2025.
18. Becker T, Babey SH, Dorsey R, Ponce NA. Data disaggregation with American Indian/Alaska Native population data. *Popul Res Policy Rev.* 2021;40:103–125. https://doi.org/10.1007/s11113-020-09635-2
19. Zhang X, Kaholokula JK, Kahn-John M, et al. Elevating voice and visibility: health research for American Indian and Alaska Native, Asian American, and Native Hawaiian and Pacific Islander populations in the United States. *Am J Public Health.* 2024;114(suppl 1):S25–S28. https://doi.org/10.2105/AJPH.2023.307494
20. Choi KH, McFarland W, Neilands TB, et al. An opportunity for prevention: prevalence, incidence, and sexual risk for HIV among young Asian and Pacific Islander men who have sex with men, San Francisco. *Sex Transm Dis.* 2004;31(8):475–480. https://doi.org/10.1097/01.olq.0000135988.19969.62
21. King L, Deng WQ. Health disparities among Asian New Yorkers. March 2018. Available at: https://www.nyc.gov/assets/doh/downloads/pdf/epi/databrief100.pdf. Accessed April 21, 2025.
22. Office of Management and Budget. Revisions to OMB's statistical policy directive No. 15: standards for maintaining, collecting, and presenting federal data on race and ethnicity. *Fed Regist.* 2024;89(62):22182–22196. Available at: https://www.govinfo.gov/content/pkg/FR-2024-03-29/pdf/2024-06469.pdf. Accessed April 7, 2025.
23. Orvis K. OMB's 2024 revisions to SPD No. 15 are final. What's happening now? October 16, 2024. Available at: https://spd15revision.gov/content/spd15revision/en/news/2024-10-16-omb-blog.html. Accessed April 21, 2025.
24. Centers for Disease Control and Prevention. Revised surveillance case definitions for HIV infection among adults, adolescents, and children aged <18 months and for HIV infection and AIDS among children aged 18 months to <13 years—United States, 2008. *MMWR Recomm Rep.* 2008; 57(RR-10):1–12.
25. Centers for Disease Control and Prevention. Revised surveillance case definition for HIV infection—United States, 2014. *MMWR Recomm Rep.* 2014;63(RR-03):1–10.
26. Penaia CS, Morey BN, Thomas KB, et al. Disparities in Native Hawaiian and Pacific Islander COVID-19 mortality: a community-driven data response. *Am J Public Health.* 2021;111(suppl 2):S49–S52. https://doi.org/10.2105/AJPH.2021.306370
27. Cha L, Le T, Ve'e T, Ah Soon NT, Tseng W. Pacific Islanders in the era of COVID-19: an overlooked community in need. *J Racial Ethn Health Disparities.* 2022;9(4):1347–1356. https://doi.org/10.1007/s40615-021-01075-8
28. Centers for Disease Control and Prevention. Introducing technology into partner services: a toolkit for programs. December 2015. Available at: https://stacks.cdc.gov/view/cdc/44484. Accessed April 21, 2025.
29. US Census Bureau. Intercensal estimates of the resident population for the United States, regions, states, District of Columbia, and Puerto Rico: April 1, 2010 to April 1, 2020 (NST-EST2020INT-POP). Available at: https://www.census.gov/data/tables/time-series/demo/popest/intercensal-2010-2020-national.html. Accessed April 7, 2025.
30. Centers for Disease Control and Prevention. Social determinants of health and selected HIV care outcomes among adults with diagnosed HIV infection in 37 states and the District of Columbia, 2015. Available at: https://stacks.cdc.gov/view/cdc/49710. Accessed April 7, 2025.
31. Trepka MJ, Fennie KP, Sheehan DM, Lutfi K, Maddox L, Lieb S. Late HIV diagnosis: differences by rural/urban residence, Florida, 2007–2011. *AIDS Patient Care STDS.* 2014;28(4):188–197. https://doi.org/10.1089/apc.2013.0362
32. Sabato TM. Deconstructing the model minority myth: exploring health risk behaviors of American Asian and Pacific Islander young adults. *J Health Dispar Res Pract.* 2017;10(3):136–149. Available at: https://oasis.library.unlv.edu/cgi/viewcontent.cgi?article=1653&context=jhdrp. Accessed August 11, 2025.
33. Sen S, Nguyen HD, Kim SY, Aguilar J. HIV knowledge, risk behavior, stigma, and their impact on HIV testing among Asian Americans and Pacific Islanders: a review of literature. *Soc Work Public Health.* 2017;32(1):11–29. https://doi.org/10.1080/19371918.2016.1173612

Inequities in Excess Pandemic Mortality Among Documented and Undocumented Immigrants in California, 2020–2023

Alicia R. Riley, PhD, MPH, MA, Ye Ji Kim, PhD, MPH, Josefina Flores Morales, PhD, Marie-Laure Charpignon, PhD, MSc, Michelle A. DeVost, MPH, and Yea-Hung Chen, PhD, MS

See also Guadamuz, p. 1554.

Objectives. To examine how excess mortality during the COVID-19 pandemic differed by legal status and its intersections with sociodemographic factors, overall and among working-age Latinos.

Methods. Using death records from Californian adults (aged ≥ 25 years) with a natural cause of death, we estimated excess mortality between March 2020 and May 2023, using ARIMA (autoregressive integrated moving average) models fit to prepandemic data spanning January 2016 through February 2020. We used country of birth and social security number (SSN) to classify decedents as US-born, foreign-born with a valid SSN ("documented"), or foreign-born without a valid SSN ("undocumented"). We assessed intersectional disparities with 5 sociodemographic factors.

Results. Pandemic period relative excess mortality was twice as high among undocumented as documented immigrants. Across subgroups, undocumented Latino essential workers experienced the highest relative excess mortality (91% increase; 95% prediction interval [PI] = 60%, 138%); US-born White adults experienced the lowest relative excess mortality (8% increase; 95% PI = 3%, 14%).

Conclusions. Undocumented legal status increased the risk of death during the pandemic among immigrants in California.

Public Health Implications. Our findings urge attention to the exclusion of immigrants from health care and social services in the aftermath of the COVID-19 pandemic. (*Am J Public Health*. 2025;115(10):1681–1690. https://doi.org/10.2105/AJPH.2025.308150)

AJPH October 2025, Vol. 115, No. 10

Studies of excess mortality during the COVID-19 pandemic revealed alarmingly high death rates among Latino people across the United States.[1–3] Language, nativity, health insurance, multigenerational housing, and occupation have been posited as contributing factors.[3–5] However, because of the absence of information about immigrant legal status in death-reporting systems, 2 major questions have remained unanswered: How did legal status differentiate risk of death during the pandemic? And to what extent did the high burden of pandemic mortality among Latino people reflect legal status inequities?

Legal status, also known as immigration status, results from racialized policies that restrict citizenship and lawful statuses and distinguish groups of people based on how and when they arrived in the United States.[6] Racist ideologies, such as colorblind racism and White supremacy, are used to justify the entitlement of certain immigrants, particularly European immigrants and immigrants racialized as White, to the privileges of US citizenship or legal residency. By contrast, these same racial logics are used to exclude other immigrants from lawfully obtaining employment opportunities and safety net benefits.[6,7] The resulting legal status gradient, in which birthright citizens are the most included and undocumented immigrants without a social security number (SSN) are the most excluded, has health consequences.[8]

Legal status, as captured by nativity and possession of a valid SSN, likely differentiated risk of severe illness and death during the COVID-19 pandemic through multiple pathways, both direct and indirect, including heightened exposure in the workplace, lack of paid time off, and limited access to health care. Directly, lacking an SSN is the basis for exclusion from public medical insurance, labor rights, and economic security programs such as unemployment insurance—all critical determinants of health during the pandemic.[9,10] Although recent state policy changes are expanding Medicaid access to undocumented immigrants,[11] working-age undocumented adults in California were ineligible for Medicaid and many safety net benefits during the pandemic. Indirectly, the pandemic coincided with an era of criminalization and racialized targeting of Latino undocumented immigrants by Immigration and Customs Enforcement.[12–14]

Living under the threat of arrest, detention, and deportation is traumatic for immigrants and their family members.[15,16] This stress adversely affects the immune system, putting people at greater risk for developing severe COVID-19.[9,14] In times of crisis, the threat of punishment can also dissuade people from seeking emergency medical care or from reporting safety violations in the workplace.[14] We hypothesized that a combination of these direct and indirect mechanisms put immigrants lacking SSNs at greater risk for death during the pandemic.

Although both theory and previous research suggest that legal status is a key driver of COVID-19 inequities,[17–20] COVID-19 surveillance data do not include any direct measure of legal status. Therefore, the influence of legal status on pandemic inequities remains unknown. Predominant explanations of observed COVID-19 inequities affecting Latino people have emphasized the role of individual behavior and comorbidities.[21–23] Fewer studies have gone further and examined the intersections of race/ethnicity with education, occupation, language, or geography.[3,24–26] These studies have highlighted heterogeneity in the risk of COVID-19 illness and death among Latino people. For instance, a study of excess mortality in California found that the pandemic resulted in a 58% increase in mortality among foreign-born Latinos in essential occupations (e.g., agriculture, manufacturing) with less than a high school education but only a 30% increase among foreign-born Latinos in nonessential occupations with a high school education or more.[3] This finding raises concerns that legal status may have contributed to differences in COVID-19 mortality risk.

California is home to 10.6 million immigrants and has the highest share of foreign-born residents and the largest undocumented immigrant population of any US state, making it an appropriate setting to analyze inequities in pandemic mortality across the legal status gradient. Our study extends previous research on pandemic disparities by combining information available on death certificates to classify decedents into 3 groups that broadly capture the legal status gradient: US-born ("birthright citizens"), foreign-born with a valid SSN ("documented immigrants"), and foreign-born with an invalid or missing SSN ("undocumented immigrants"). We conceptualized legal status as an axis of social inclusion or exclusion that intersects with other social determinants of health associated with pandemic-related excess mortality. Latino ethnicity, male sex, lower educational attainment, and essential worker status have each been independently associated with a greater risk of death during the pandemic.[3,27] Our examination of intersectional disparities in pandemic period mortality, by legal status and race/ethnicity, sex, educational attainment, and occupation, has the potential to implicate racialized immigration policy as a form of structural exclusion that put Latinos at greater risk for COVID-19 death.

METHODS

We drew on restricted death certificates of California residents aged 25 years and older who died from a natural cause between 2016 and 2023 in California (n = 936 132). Our focus on natural cause deaths means that we excluded deaths from intentional and unintentional injuries (e.g., suicide, car accident, fatal overdose), which are unlikely to be misclassified as COVID-19 deaths. Natural cause deaths include any cause of death from acute or chronic disease of any organ system (e.g., COVID-19, cancer, stroke). An advantage of estimating excess mortality for all natural cause deaths is that we minimize bias because of socioeconomic disparities in the classification of COVID-19 deaths.

We used the information available on death certificates to generate a logical proxy for legal status. Specifically, we classified decedents into 3 categories based on their country of birth (US-born or foreign-born) and the presence or absence of a valid SSN on their death certificate: US-born (birthright citizens), foreign-born with a reported valid SSN (including naturalized citizens and legal permanent residents and any immigrant with a valid SSN), or foreign-born without a reported valid SSN (including unauthorized immigrants, asylum seekers, and nonimmigrant visa

AJPH October 2025, Vol. 115, No. 10

holders). Previous studies have employed a similar SSN proxy approach.[28–30] We classified a decedent's SSN as invalid when it was missing or unknown or when the provided sequence of numbers was implausible. We classified sex as male or female and did not measure it separately from gender. We used a dichotomous measure of educational attainment that distinguished having less than a high school diploma from completing high school or more education. To capture differences in occupation, we first converted the free text for "usual occupation" provided on each death certificate into a census occupation code. Then, we categorized the occupation codes as either "essential" or "nonessential," according to California's essential sectors designations.[31]

In our analytic approach, we estimated natural cause excess mortality during the pandemic period (March 2020–May 2023) using seasonal ARIMA (autoregressive integrated moving average) models fit to death counts from the prepandemic period (January 2016–February 2020) and modeling up to 4 seasonal parameters. We estimated the models using the Hyndman and Khandakar automatic forecasting algorithm implemented in the corresponding forecast package in R version 4.2.1 (RStudio, Boston, MA). Model selection employed a stepwise algorithm that prioritized models according to Akaike information criterion value. In further model fit assessments, the mean absolute percentage error ranged from 1.9% for the model pertaining to documented foreign-born individuals to 4.7% for the undocumented foreign-born model—values that were appropriately low and indicated satisfactory model fit without overfitting.[32] Using each subgroup-specific model, we projected the number of deaths per month that would have been expected had the pandemic not occurred, along with corresponding 95% prediction intervals (PIs) generated through bootstrapping.

We report results for both absolute and relative excess mortality. Absolute excess mortality is defined as the difference between the observed number of deaths during the pandemic period and the expected number of deaths based on prepandemic trends. Relative excess mortality is defined as the ratio of the observed number of deaths during the pandemic period to the expected number of deaths based on prepandemic trends, which we refer to as the observed/expected ratio ("O/E ratio"). We estimated monthly excess mortality during the pandemic period among all adults aged 25 years and older and by categories of race/ethnicity (non-Hispanic Asian, non-Hispanic Black, Latino/x, non-Hispanic White, and other non-Hispanic), age (25–64 years, ≥ 65 years), sex (female, male), education (high school diploma, no high school diploma), and occupation (essential sector, nonessential sector). We then examined pandemic period excess mortality among working-age (aged 18–64 years) Latino adults by legal status and the intersections of legal status with sex, education, and occupation.

RESULTS

Excess mortality during the COVID-19 pandemic differed by inferred legal status. We estimated that 7430 (95% PI = 6911, 7957) excess natural cause deaths occurred between March 2020 and May 2023 among California residents who were foreign-born adults aged 25 years and older and did not have a reported valid SSN (subsequently referred to as "undocumented immigrants"). Such a toll equates to a 55% (95% PI = 49%, 61%) increase in mortality above prepandemic levels among undocumented immigrants. By contrast, over the same period, we estimated a 22% (95% PI = 19%, 25%) increase in mortality among foreign-born adults with a reported valid SSN (subsequently referred to as "documented immigrants") and a 12% (95% PI = 8%, 17%) increase in mortality among US-born citizens. As visualized in Figure A (available as a supplement to the online version of this article at http://www.ajph.org), these legal status inequities in relative excess mortality accumulated over the pandemic period, with the largest inequities experienced during summer 2020 and the 2021 winter surge.

As shown in Table 1 and Figure 1, legal status inequities in pandemic period excess mortality were further stratified by the sociodemographic factors we considered: race/ethnicity, age, sex, educational attainment, and occupation. At the lower extreme, US-born White people had the lowest relative excess mortality of any sociodemographic subgroup (O/E ratio = 1.08; 95% PI = 1.03, 1.14). At the upper extreme, we observed the highest relative excess mortality among undocumented essential workers (O/E ratio = 1.76; 95% PI = 1.51, 2.10).

Within most sociodemographic subgroups, our results demonstrated the hypothesized legal status gradient: excess mortality was highest among undocumented foreign-born adults, followed by documented foreign-born adults, and it was lowest among US-born adults. The male–female gap in relative excess mortality was more extreme among undocumented immigrants (male = 68%; 95% PI = 61%, 77%; female = 30%; 95% PI = 7%, 66%) than among documented immigrants

TABLE 1— Absolute and Relative Excess Mortality Among Californian Adults Aged 25 Years and Older by Inferred Legal Status: March 2020–May 2023

	Undocumented Foreign-Born		Documented Foreign-Born		US-Born	
	Excess Mortality (95% PI)	O/E Ratio (95% PI)	Excess Mortality (95% PI)	O/E Ratio (95% PI)	Excess Mortality (95% PI)	O/E Ratio (95% PI)
Overall	7430 (6911, 7957)	1.55 (1.49, 1.61)	48 495 (43 428, 53 604)	1.22 (1.19, 1.25)	69 394 (48 322, 90 792)	1.12 (1.08, 1.17)
Race/ethnicity						
Latino/x	6556 (6087, 7030)	1.57 (1.51, 1.63)	28 006 (26 903, 29 109)	1.34 (1.32, 1.36)	16 172 (14 875, 17 483)	1.23 (1.21, 1.26)
Black	30 (5, 54)	1.23 (1.03, 1.53)	794 (684, 903)	1.41 (1.34, 1.50)	9195 (7965, 10 438)	1.16 (1.14, 1.19)
Asian	168 (−230, 571)	1.13 (0.87, 1.61)	11 286 (8797, 13 793)	1.14 (1.11, 1.18)	2477 (1691, 3274)	1.19 (1.12, 1.27)
Other race	37 (26, 48)	1.66 (1.39, 2.05)	561 (167, 959)	1.30 (1.07, 1.64)	2295 (1923, 2672)	1.22 (1.18, 1.27)
White	151 (96, 204)	1.18 (1.11, 1.25)	6989 (6082, 7881)	1.13 (1.11, 1.15)	33 236 (12 011, 54 895)	1.08 (1.03, 1.14)
Age, y						
25–64	4956 (3842, 6080)	1.62 (1.42, 1.89)	12 582 (11 563, 13 602)	1.34 (1.30, 1.38)	22 482 (20 085, 24 909)	1.22 (1.19, 1.25)
≥65	730 (−3179, 4720)	1.10 (0.72, 2.42)	36 600 (31 904, 41 342)	1.20 (1.17, 1.23)	51 163 (27 720, 75 064)	1.11 (1.06, 1.18)
Sex						
Female	1861 (510, 3232)	1.30 (1.07, 1.66)	22 057 (19 508, 24 638)	1.20 (1.17, 1.23)	28 424 (13 937, 43 196)	1.10 (1.05, 1.16)
Male	5227 (4878, 5580)	1.68 (1.61, 1.77)	26 631 (23 550, 29 746)	1.24 (1.21, 1.28)	40 854 (34 000, 47 794)	1.14 (1.12, 1.17)
Education						
No HS diploma	4626 (4200, 5057)	1.52 (1.45, 1.60)	22 908 (21 003, 24 837)	1.30 (1.27, 1.33)	9951 (7536, 12 373)	1.18 (1.13, 1.24)
HS diploma	2520 (2120, 2913)	1.66 (1.50, 1.85)	23 636 (19 704, 27 611)	1.17 (1.14, 1.21)	65 776 (48 330, 83 506)	1.13 (1.10, 1.18)
Occupation[a]						
Essential sector	4207 (3295, 5130)	1.76 (1.51, 2.10)	8407 (7583, 9240)	1.33 (1.29, 1.37)	14 239 (12 810, 15 687)	1.23 (1.20, 1.25)
Nonessential sector	871 (781, 960)	1.47 (1.40, 1.55)	2548 (1980, 3117)	1.22 (1.16, 1.28)	7653 (6535, 8786)	1.22 (1.18, 1.26)

Note. HS = high school; O/E = observed/expected; PI = prediction interval. We inferred legal status based on the presence of a valid Social Security number on the death certificate and foreign birth.
Source. California Department of Public Health.
[a]We restricted estimates for categories of occupation to working-age decedents (aged 25–64 y at the time of death).

(male = 24%; 95% PI = 21%, 28%; female = 20%; 95% PI = 17%, 23%) and US-born citizens (male = 14%; 95% PI = 12%, 17%; female = 10%; 95% PI = 5%, 16%). We found higher relative excess mortality (O/E ratio = 1.66; 95% PI = 1.50, 1.85) among undocumented immigrants with a high school diploma or more education than among those with less education (O/E ratio = 1.52; 95% PI = 1.45, 1.60). However, prepandemic mortality was also higher among undocumented people without a high school diploma.

Figure 2 provides a closer look at the dynamics between the absolute counts of observed and expected natural cause deaths and the relative increase in excess death among undocumented adults. Although there was a male–female disparity in natural cause deaths among undocumented decedents before the pandemic, it worsened during the pandemic. Similarly, the absolute number of excess deaths was higher among undocumented adults with less than a high school diploma than among their more educated counterparts, reflecting mortality inequities that preceded the pandemic.

We found that 88% of excess natural cause deaths occurred among Latino people. Figure 3 displays the results of our intersectional analysis focused on working-age Latino adults in California. Pandemic period mortality among working-age undocumented Latinos was 57% (95% PI = 51%, 63%) higher than expected. By contrast, mortality was 34% (95% PI = 32%, 36%) higher than expected for documented foreign-born Latinos and 23% (95% PI = 21%, 26%) higher than expected for US-born Latinos. We found an interaction between legal status, essential worker status, and race/ethnicity, which resulted in an exacerbated risk of premature death during the pandemic for

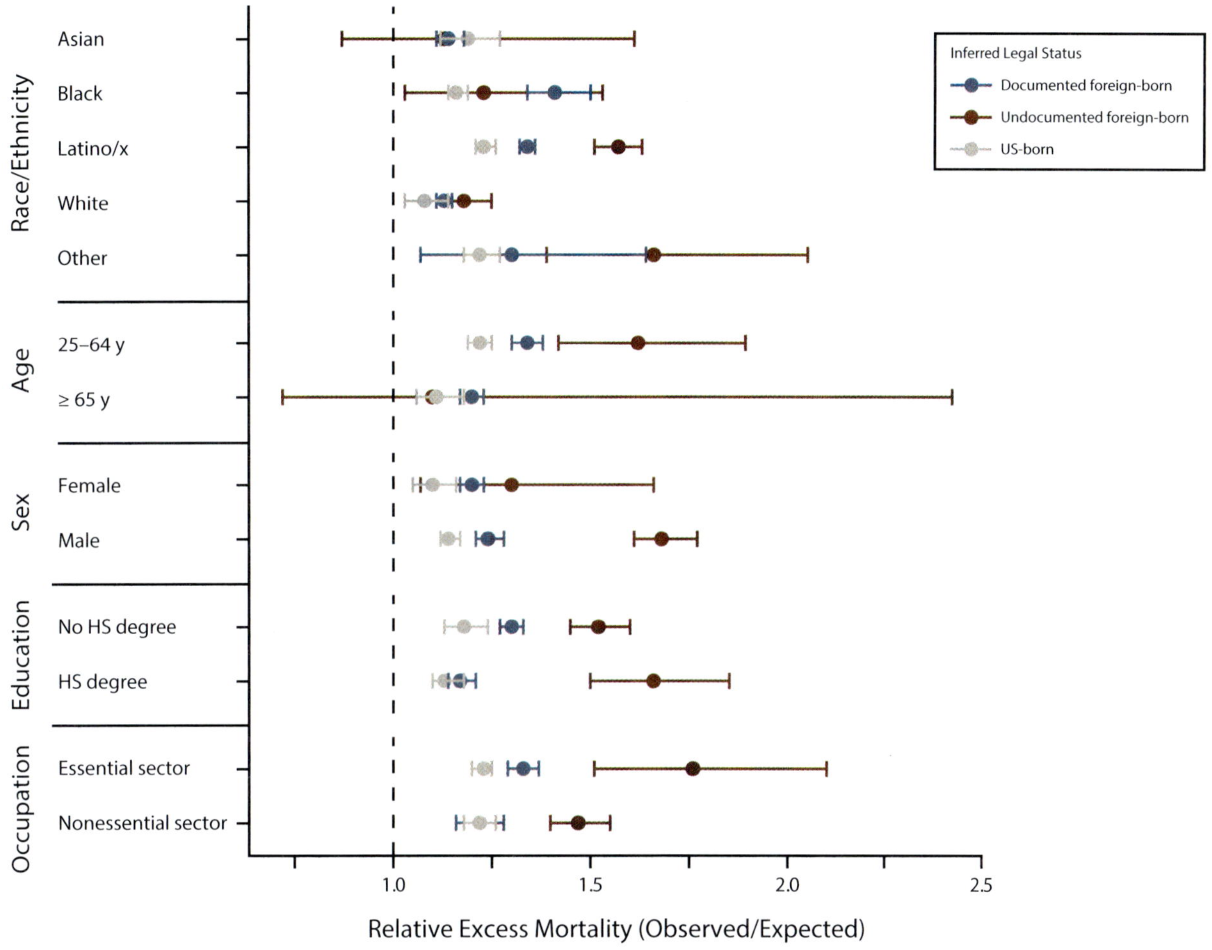

	O/E Ratio (95% PI)		
	DFB	UFB	USB
Asian	1.14 (1.11, 1.18)	1.13 (0.87, 1.61)	1.19 (1.12, 1.27)
Black	1.41 (1.34, 1.50)	1.23 (1.03, 1.53)	1.16 (1.14, 1.19)
Latino/x	1.34 (1.32, 1.36)	1.57 (1.51, 1.63)	1.23 (1.21, 1.26)
Other	1.30 (1.07, 1.64)	1.66 (1.39, 2.05)	1.22 (1.18, 1.27)
White	1.13 (1.11, 1.15)	1.18 (1.11, 1.25)	1.08 (1.03, 1.14)
Age: 25–64 y	1.34 (1.30, 1.38)	1.62 (1.42, 1.89)	1.22 (1.19, 1.25)
Age: ≥ 65 y	1.20 (1.17, 1.23)	1.10 (0.72, 2.42)	1.11 (1.06, 1.18)
Sex: female	1.20 (1.17, 1.23)	1.30 (1.07, 1.66)	1.10 (1.05, 1.16)
Sex: male	1.24 (1.21, 1.28)	1.68 (1.61, 1.77)	1.14 (1.12, 1.17)
Education: no HS	1.30 (1.27, 1.33)	1.52 (1.45, 1.60)	1.18 (1.13, 1.24)
Education: HS	1.17 (1.14, 1.21)	1.66 (1.50, 1.85)	1.13 (1.10, 1.18)
Occupation: essential	1.33 (1.29, 1.37)	1.76 (1.51, 2.10)	1.23 (1.20, 1.25)
Occupation: nonessential	1.22 (1.16, 1.28)	1.47 (1.40, 1.55)	1.22 (1.18, 1.26)

FIGURE 1— Excess Natural Cause Mortality by Legal Status and Social Factors: California, 2020–2023

Note. DFB = documented foreign-born; HS = high school; O/E = observed/expected; PI = prediction interval; UFB = undocumented foreign-born; USB = US-born. We restricted our analyses to individuals aged 25 y and older at the time of death, except for occupation categories, which we restricted to individuals aged 25–64 y at the time of death. For all subgroups, we compared natural cause deaths during the pandemic (March 2020–May 2023) to natural cause deaths before the pandemic (January 2016–February 2020) to estimate excess mortality. We inferred legal status based on the presence of a valid Social Security number on the death certificate and foreign birth.
Source. California Department of Public Health.

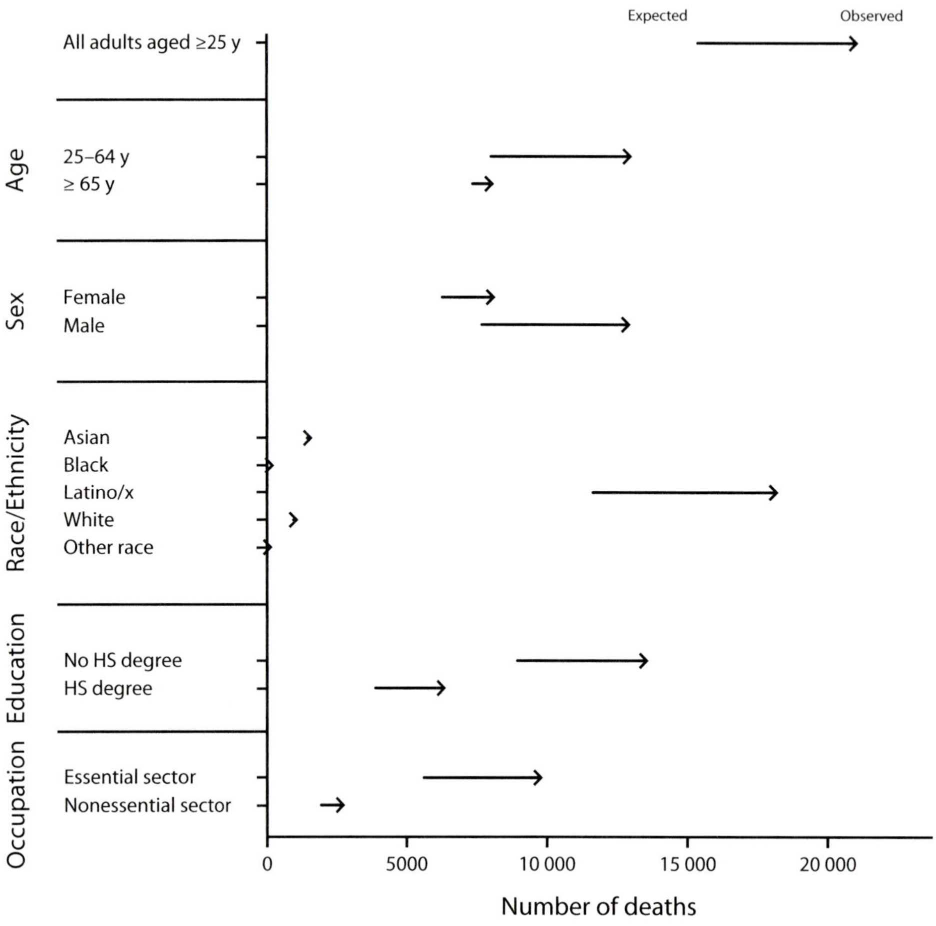

FIGURE 2— Absolute Increases in Natural Cause Deaths Among Undocumented Californians During the COVID-19 Pandemic, by Subgroup: 2020–2023

Note. HS = high school. Arrows show the difference between the number of natural cause deaths expected based on prepandemic trends and the number of deaths observed during the pandemic period (March 2020–May 2023) among undocumented Californians. We estimated undocumented status based on the absence of a valid Social Security number on the death certificate and foreign birth. We restricted results for occupation subgroups to decedents aged 25–64 y.
Source. Mortality data are from the California Department of Public Health.

undocumented Latinos in essential occupations. Working-age undocumented Latinos with an essential sector occupation experienced a 91% increase in natural cause mortality, relative to prepandemic levels. Although all Latino essential workers experienced excess mortality because of the pandemic, increases among documented immigrants and US-born citizens were less pronounced, at 46% and 36%, respectively. The association between sex and excess mortality was also moderated by legal status and race/ethnicity, so that relative excess mortality was the highest for undocumented Latino men (O/E ratio = 1.89; 95% PI = 1.58, 2.36).

Finally, although population denominators were not available for any of the social factor subgroups, we drew on multiple estimates of the California undocumented population to calculate crude estimates of absolute excess mortality for the 3 legal status subgroups in Figure B (available as a supplement to the online version of this article at http://www.ajph.org). The estimated absolute excess mortality for undocumented immigrants ranged from 271 to 369 deaths per 100 000 population. The estimated absolute excess mortality for documented immigrants ranged from 568 to 621 deaths per 100 000 population. These crude rates did not adjust for differences in age structure between subgroups.

DISCUSSION

Legal status is a fundamental cause of health inequity.[6] However, research on mortality inequities during the COVID-19 pandemic has left legal status relatively unexamined because of its absence from available data.[1,3,5] This is the first

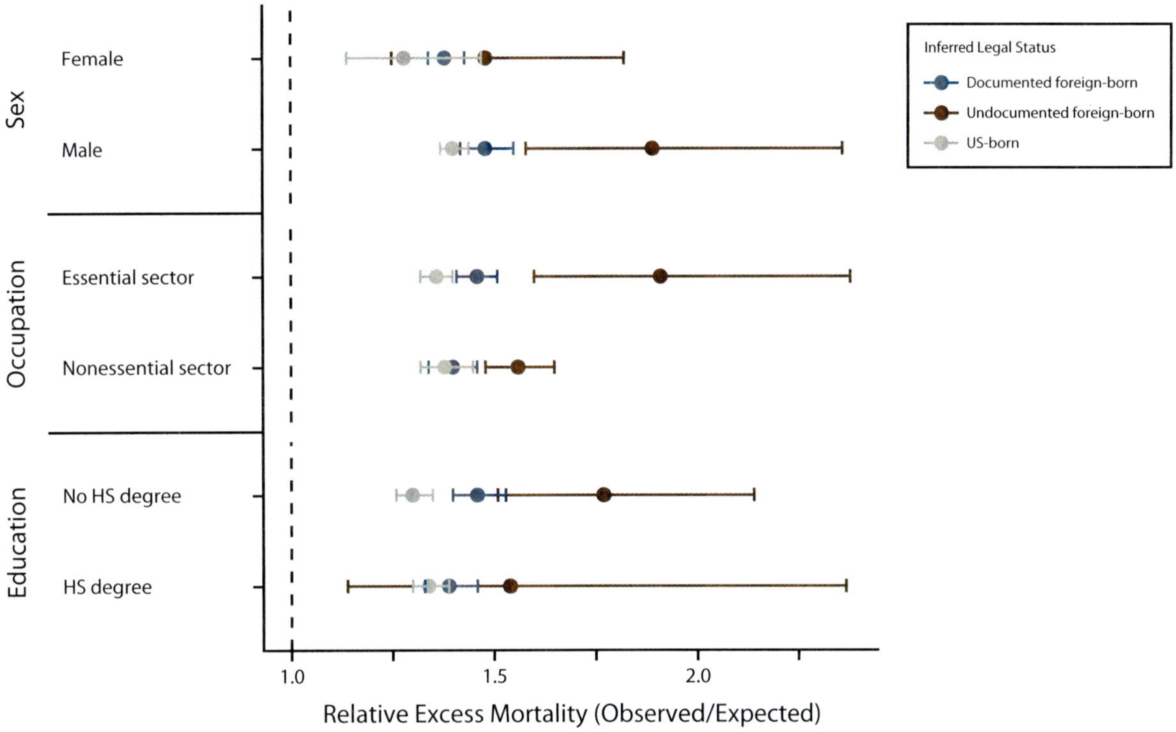

	O/E Ratio (95% PI)		
	DFB	UFB	USB
Sex: female	1.38 (1.34, 1.43)	1.48 (1.25, 1.82)	1.28 (1.14, 1.47)
Sex: male	1.48 (1.42, 1.55)	1.89 (1.58, 2.36)	1.40 (1.37, 1.44)
Occupation: essential	1.46 (1.41, 1.51)	1.91 (1.60, 2.38)	1.36 (1.32, 1.40)
Occupation: nonessential	1.40 (1.34, 1.46)	1.56 (1.48, 1.65)	1.38 (1.32, 1.45)
Education: no HS	1.46 (1.40, 1.53)	1.77 (1.51, 2.14)	1.30 (1.26, 1.35)
Education: HS	1.39 (1.33, 1.46)	1.54 (1.14, 2.37)	1.34 (1.30, 1.39)

FIGURE 3— Excess Natural Cause Mortality During the COVID-19 Pandemic Among Working-Age Latino Californians by Legal Status and Social Factors: 2020–2023

Note. DFB = documented foreign-born; HS = high school; O/E = observed/expected; PI = prediction interval; UFB = undocumented foreign-born; USB = US-born. We restricted our analyses to Latino/a/x individuals aged 25–64 y at the time of death. For each subgroup, we compared natural cause deaths during the pandemic (March 2020–May 2023) to natural cause deaths before the pandemic (January 2016–February 2020) to estimate excess mortality. We inferred legal status based on the presence of a valid Social Security number on the death certificate and foreign birth.
Source. Mortality data are from the California Department of Public Health.

study to the best of our knowledge to use death records to provide evidence linking legal status to inequities in excess mortality during the pandemic. To overcome the absence of direct measures of legal status in surveillance or vital statistics data, we introduced a proxy approach for classifying legal status that used country of birth and the presence of a valid SSN on the death certificate. Applying this SSN proxy approach to death certificates from California between March 2016 and May 2023, we found that lacking a valid SSN was consistently associated with higher pandemic period relative excess natural cause mortality among adults overall and in subgroups of intersecting sociodemographic factors. These results suggest that the legal status gradient was a fundamental cause of mortality during the pandemic.

Our results have several implications for understanding the expansion of health inequities during the COVID-19 pandemic and for advocacy to protect the health of all Californians, regardless of legal status. First, our study reveals that people without a reported valid SSN faced a dramatic increase in natural cause mortality risk during the COVID-19 pandemic relative to prepandemic levels. Indeed, relative excess mortality was 2 times higher among undocumented immigrants than among documented immigrants. Further, the disparity in excess mortality between documented immigrants and US-born citizens was smaller than the disparity between undocumented and documented immigrants. Immigrants without valid SSNs were likely at greater risk for COVID-19 death from lack of paid time off when sick, overrepresentation in jobs with few workplace protections, lack of health insurance, stress associated with immigration enforcement, and more. It is important to consider that our study focused on individuals in California, a state that has adopted policies to extend health care, drivers licenses, and emergency pandemic relief to undocumented immigrants. Consequently, our results may underestimate the extent to which legal status contributed to inequities in pandemic period excess mortality at the national level.

Second, we did not see evidence of an immigrant health advantage in our results. Legal status inequity may restrict immigrant health advantages to certain groups, such as those with a valid SSN. However, it also appears that legal status–related marginalization may have offset any protective effects of nativity on mortality risk even among immigrants with a valid SSN.

Third, we demonstrated that this increased risk of death was unevenly distributed across race/ethnicity subgroups. In doing so, our study challenges previous attempts to explain racialized inequities in COVID-19 mortality that relied on behavioral or biological stereotypes and omitted any discussion of immigrant legal status.[33] Although the legal status gradient appeared less pronounced among working-age Latino people, pandemic period increases in mortality were much higher in relative terms among Latino people, particularly Latino men, than among other race/ethnicity subgroups. We see this as evidence that legal status is an intersectional driver of previously documented racialized inequities in COVID-19 mortality, reflecting the racist ways that undocumented legal status is assigned and enforced.[10]

Fourth, our study introduces a novel approach to studying legal status disparities during the COVID-19 pandemic and beyond by inferring legal status using only information available on the death certificate. The SSN proxy approach we applied built on work by Ka-Yuet Liu[34] and is similar to other SSN proxy approaches to classifying legal status.[30] Our SSN proxy approach reduced self-report bias and, unlike probabilistic methods, allowed a rough assessment of the legal status gradient in a large population-based data set with restricted covariates. But it has important limitations. First, it may misclassify decedents because of SSN reporting errors or challenges in defining true legal status. Sensitivity analyses suggest that the impacts of plausible levels of misclassification because of SSN reporting errors (which we estimated could be as high as 1.96%) are small for documented immigrants but more influential for undocumented immigrants because of their lower numbers. Second, our proxy approach classifies any immigrant without a reported valid SSN as "undocumented," which is sure to misclassify some documented individuals. Again, we expect that this kind of misclassification would attenuate our excess mortality estimates for undocumented immigrants because individuals with less-marginalized statuses, such as nonimmigrant visa holders, are included in the undocumented subgroup. Third, our approach relies on access to restricted mortality data because of the sensitive nature of SSN identifiers. Therefore, our approach cannot be readily used by community organizations. Given these complexities, we have interpreted our results to reflect how SSN serves as a marker of immigrant marginalization or inclusion, which likely contributes to mortality disparities.

Limitations

The results of this study should be considered in light of several additional limitations. First, we focused on relative measures of excess mortality, as opposed to per capita measures, because of the lack of reliable estimates of the population size of undocumented immigrants necessary to construct mortality rates. Because we defined excess mortality in relative terms, the increases in mortality we report may appear more severe for subgroups with low mortality before the COVID-19 pandemic than for those with high prepandemic mortality. For reference, selected estimates of absolute excess mortality can be found in Table A (available as a supplement to the online version of this article at http://www.ajph.org). Second, the race/ethnicity, occupation, and SSN fields on death certificates are completed by next of kin or medical providers and are known to have inaccuracies that can introduce biases into a study like ours.

Third, our SSN proxy approach categorizes immigrant legal status using only 3 static categories and is, thus, an explicitly imperfect proxy. In reality, legal status is fluid and includes a broad range of noncitizen statuses that do not map consistently onto the possession of a valid SSN.[30] Because the likelihood of misclassification is highest for the undocumented group, our findings provide a conservative estimate of the mortality disadvantage associated with undocumented legal status during the COVID-19 pandemic. Further, our study design does not distinguish between naturalized citizens and documented noncitizens. However, previous work suggests that naturalized citizens enjoy a better health profile than do documented noncitizens.[35] It follows that classifying naturalized citizens as documented immigrants may make the documented death toll seem less severe than it would if naturalized citizens were analyzed separately. Fourth, although our intersectional analyses show that legal status inequities influence previously documented social disparities in COVID-19 deaths, some intersectional subgroups are very small, resulting in wide PIs that should be interpreted with caution.

Fifth, our results should not be extrapolated into the future because of the unprecedented nature of the COVID-19 pandemic and the limits of excess death projections. Our ARIMA models, trained with data from January 2016 through February 2020, are sensitive to the mortality patterns of this prepandemic period. Finally, our approach assumes that the population composition of immigrants in California was stable over the study period. However, changes to immigration policy and enforcement during the pandemic may have altered this composition. For instance, Title 42, which used public health emergency powers to expel migrants who reached US borders, was imposed in March 2020 and ended in May 2023. Although Title 42 overlapped with our study period, reports suggest it shifted border crossing away from ports of entry, rather than deterring overall immigration. Recent immigration trends indicate that the decline in new arrivals (both authorized and unauthorized) in 2020 to 2021 was followed by a rebound in 2022 to 2023.[36] Our excess mortality estimates effectively average over this period of fluctuation, but if declines in the immigrant population were greater than we assumed, our estimates would underestimate excess mortality. Notwithstanding these limitations, our study demonstrates how the SSN proxy approach can be applied to death certificate data to investigate the impacts of inferred legal status on mortality.

Public Health Implications

With this evidence of the striking legal status gradient in excess death during the pandemic, it becomes clear that many policies that were intended to provide universal protections, such as lockdowns and free testing campaigns, played out in ways that were stratified by legal status. Our results raise an alarm about the increased risk of death faced by undocumented immigrants during the COVID-19 pandemic and its implications for long COVID, mental health, and the physical health of survivors. However, our study also challenges the obfuscation of legal status inequities in mortality that preceded the pandemic and the ongoing normalization of mortality inequities.

We join others in calling to eliminate immigration status as a determinant of eligibility for publicly funded health insurance and safety net programs, including disaster relief payments. Our analysis also highlights the need for expanded worker protections, paid leave, and enforcement of workplace safety for undocumented workers. Until changes are enacted at the federal level, state and local efforts to include immigrants in health insurance and public benefits, such as unemployment insurance, are urgently needed.[10] Inclusive access to health care and social services requires policies that block the encroachment of racist immigration enforcement into local policing so that all people can access life-saving care without the threat of detention, deportation, and family separation. AJPH

ABOUT THE AUTHORS

Alicia R. Riley is with the Department of Sociology, University of California, Santa Cruz. Ye Ji Kim is with the Department of Epidemiology, Boston University School of Public Health, Boston, MA. Josefina Flores Morales is with the Department of Epidemiology and Population Health, Stanford University, Stanford, CA. Marie-Laure Charpignon is with the Institute for Data, Systems, and Society, Massachusetts Institute of Technology, Cambridge, MA. Michelle A. Devost is with the Department of Epidemiology and Biostatistics, University of California, San Francisco. Yea-Hung Chen is with the Department of Epidemiology and Biostatistics, University of California, San Francisco.

CORRESPONDENCE

Correspondence should be sent to Alicia R. Riley, Assistant Professor, University of California Santa Cruz, Department of Sociology, 1156 High St, Santa Cruz, CA 95060 (e-mail: alicia.riley@ucsc.edu). Reprints can be ordered at https://www.ajph.org by clicking the "Reprints" link.

PUBLICATION INFORMATION

Full Citation: Riley AR, Kim YJ, Flores Morales J, Charpignon M-L, DeVost MA, Chen Y-H. Inequities in excess pandemic mortality among documented and undocumented immigrants in California, 2020–2023. *Am J Public Health*. 2025;115(10): 1681–1690.

Acceptance Date: April 1, 2025.

DOI: https://doi.org/10.2105/AJPH.2025.308150

ORCID iDs:

Alicia R. Riley https://orcid.org/0000-0002-3341-6892

Ye Ji Kim https://orcid.org/0000-0003-1583-1408

CONTRIBUTORS

A. R. Riley created the figures and tables and wrote the first draft of the article. A. R. Riley and Y-H. Chen conceptualized the study. Y. J. Kim and Y-H. Chen analyzed the data. Y-H. Chen obtained the data. All authors interpreted the data and contributed to and revised the article.

ACKNOWLEDGMENTS

We thank the several anonymous reviewers for their constructive feedback and the Pandemic Equity and Analytics Research Lab members for supporting the development of this study.

CONFLICTS OF INTEREST

The authors have no conflicts of interest to disclose.

HUMAN PARTICIPANT PROTECTION

The study protocol was approved by the State of California Committee for the Protection of Human Subjects (project no. 2020-109).

REFERENCES

1. De Ramos IP, Lazo M, Schnake-Mahl A, et al. COVID-19 outcomes among the Hispanic population of 27 large US cities, 2020–2021. *Am J Public Health*. 2022;112(7):1034–1044. https://doi.org/10.2105/AJPH.2022.306809
2. Chen YH, Glymour MM, Catalano R, et al. Excess mortality in California during the Coronavirus disease 2019 pandemic, March to August 2020. *JAMA Intern Med*. 2021;181(5):705–707. https://doi.org/jamainternmed.2020.7578
3. Riley AR, Chen YH, Matthay EC, et al. Excess mortality among Latino people in California during the COVID-19 pandemic. *SSM Popul Health*. 2021;15:100860. https://doi.org/10.1016/j.ssmph.2021.100860
4. Page KR, Venkataramani M, Beyrer C, Polk S. Undocumented US immigrants and COVID-19. *N Engl J Med*. 2020;382(21):e62. https://doi.org/10.1056/NEJMp2005953
5. Lee H, Andrasfay T, Riley A, Wu Q, Crimmins E. Do social determinants of health explain racial/ethnic disparities in COVID-19 infection? *Soc Sci Med*. 2022;306:115098. https://doi.org/10.1016/j.socscimed.2022.115098
6. Asad AL, Clair M. Racialized legal status as a social determinant of health. *Soc Sci Med*. 2018;199:19–28. https://doi.org/10.1016/j.socscimed.2017.03.010
7. Bonilla-Silva E. *Racism Without Racists: Color-Blind Racism and the Persistence of Racial Inequality in the United States*. Lanham, MD: Rowman & Littlefield; 2006.
8. Menjívar C, Abrego LJ. Legal violence: immigration law and the lives of Central American immigrants. *Am J Sociol*. 2012;117(5):1380–1421. https://doi.org/10.1086/663575
9. Castañeda H, Holmes SM, Madrigal DS, Young MED, Beyeler N, Quesada J. Immigration as a social determinant of health. *Annu Rev Public Health*. 2015;36:375–392. https://doi.org/10.1146/annurev-publhealth-032013-182419
10. Lebrón AMW, Torres IR, Kline N, Lopez WD, Trinidad Young MEDE, Novak N. Immigration and immigrant policies, health, and health equity in the United States. *Milbank Q*. 2023;101(suppl 1):119–152. https://doi.org/10.1111/1468-0009.12636
11. Department of Health Care Services. Ages 26 through 49 adult full scope Medi-Cal expansion. Available at: https://www.dhcs.ca.gov/services/medi-cal/eligibility/Pages/Adult-Expansion.aspx. Accessed April 12, 2024.
12. Natta MV. *Medical Legal Violence: Health Care and Immigration Enforcement Against Latinx Noncitizens*. New York, NY: New York University Press; 2023. https://doi.org/10.18574/nyu/9781479807444.001.0001
13. Marfo EA, Fernandez-Sanchez H, Annor BOH. Challenges of undocumented immigrants in Canada and the USA during the COVID-19 pandemic: a review. *IJMHSC*. 2022;18(4):332–340. https://doi.org/10.1108/IJMHSC-07-2020-0072
14. Lopez MM, Holmes SM. Raids on immigrant communities during the pandemic threaten the country's public health. *Am J Public Health*. 2020;110(7):958–959. https://doi.org/10.2105/AJPH.2020.305704
15. Novak NL, Geronimus AT, Martinez-Cardoso AM. Change in birth outcomes among infants born to Latina mothers after a major immigration raid. *Int J Epidemiol*. 2017;46(3):839–849. https://doi.org/10.1093/ije/dyw346
16. Lopez WD, Gudino J, Shull T, Godinez G, Novak NL. Large-scale immigration worksite raids: community disaster, community response. *J Community Pract*. 2024;32(1):86–106. https://doi.org/10.1080/10705422.2024.2311246
17. Franco K, Patler C, Pirtle WL. COVID-19's unequal toll: differences in health-related quality of life by gendered and racialized groups. *J Health Soc Behav*. 2024;65(1):60–74. https://doi.org/10.1177/00221465231199734
18. Riley AR. Advancing the study of health inequality: fundamental causes as systems of exposure. *SSM Popul Health*. 2020;10:100555. https://doi.org/10.1016/j.ssmph.2020.100555
19. García SJ, Trummel T, Cornejo M, et al. Immigrant health inequities: exposing diversions and White supremacy. *Soc Sci*. 2021;10(9):341. https://doi.org/10.3390/socsci10090341
20. Schut RA, Boen C. State immigration policy contexts and racialized legal status disparities in health care utilization among US agricultural workers. *Demography*. 2022;59(6):2079–2107. https://doi.org/10.1215/00703370-10342687
21. Kricorian K, Turner K. COVID-19 vaccine acceptance and beliefs among Black and Hispanic Americans. *PLoS One*. 2021;16(8):e0256122. https://doi.org/10.1371/journal.pone.0256122
22. Webb Hooper M, Nápoles AM, Pérez-Stable EJ. COVID-19 and racial/ethnic disparities. *JAMA*. 2020;323(24):2466–2467. https://doi.org/10.1001/jama.2020.8598
23. Garcini LM, Pham TT, Ambriz AM, Lill S, Tsevat J. COVID-19 diagnostic testing among underserved Latino communities: barriers and facilitators. *Health Soc Care Community*. 2022;30(5):e1907–e1916. https://doi.org/10.1111/hsc.13621
24. Rodriguez-Diaz CE, Guilamo-Ramos V, Mena L, et al. Risk for COVID-19 infection and death among Latinos in the United States: examining heterogeneity in transmission dynamics. *Ann Epidemiol*. 2020;52:46–53.e2. https://doi.org/10.1016/j.annepidem.2020.07.007
25. Reitsma MB, Claypool AL, Vargo J, et al. Racial/Ethnic disparities in COVID-19 exposure risk, testing, and cases at the subcounty level in California. *Health Aff (Millwood)*. 2021;40(6):870–878. https://doi.org/10.1377/hlthaff.2021.00098
26. Macias Gil R, Marcelin JR, Zuniga-Blanco B, Marquez C, Mathew T, Piggott DA. COVID-19 pandemic: disparate health impact on the Hispanic/Latinx population in the United States. *J Infect Dis*. 2020;222(10):1592–1595. https://doi.org/10.1093/infdis/jiaa474
27. Chen YH, Matthay EC, Chen R, et al. Excess mortality in California by education during the COVID-19 pandemic. *Am J Prev Med*. 2022;63(5):827–836. https://doi.org/10.1016/j.amepre.2022.06.020
28. Lowry SJ, Blecker H, Camp J, et al. Possibilities and challenges in occupational injury surveillance of day laborers. *Am J Ind Med*. 2010;53(2):126–134. https://doi.org/10.1002/ajim.20741
29. Hotchkiss JL, Quispe-Agnoli M, Rios-Avila F. The wage impact of undocumented workers: evidence from administrative data. *South Econ J*. 2015;81(4):874–906. https://doi.org/10.1002/soej.12020
30. Trinidad Young MEDE, Madrigal DS. Documenting legal status: a systematic review of measurement of undocumented status in health research. *Public Health Rev*. 2017;38:26. https://doi.org/10.1186/s40985-017-0073-4
31. California Department of Public Health. Essential critical infrastructure workers list. Available at: https://broadbandcouncil.ca.gov/wp-content/uploads/sites/68/2020/05/EssentialCriticalInfrastructureWorkers.pdf. Accessed July 1, 2025.
32. Gill B, Kehler T, Schneider M. Meaning and prediction of "excess mortality": a comparison of COVID-19 and pre-COVID-19 mortality data in 31 Eurostat countries from 1965 to 2021. *Biol Methods Protoc*. 2024;9(1):bpae031. https://doi.org/10.1093/biomethods/bpae031
33. Warth G, Cook M. Increased outbreaks near trigger point to reassess openings. *San Diego Union Tribune*. June 18, 2020. Available at: https://www.sandiegouniontribune.com/news/health/story/2020-06-17/county-gives-update-on-coronavirus. Accessed May 28, 2024.
34. Liu KY. Are undocumented immigrants more likely to die unnaturally? A population-wide study of 1.7 million death records. Paper presented at: Population Association of American Annual Meeting. Denver, CO; April 26–28, 2018. Available at: https://paa.confex.com/paa/2018/meetingapp.cgi/Paper/21938. Accessed July 1, 2025.
35. Guadamuz JS, Durazo-Arvizu RA, Morales JF, Qato DM. Citizenship status and mortality among young Latino adults in the US, 1998–2015. *Am J Prev Med*. 2022;62(5):777–781. https://doi.org/10.1016/j.amepre.2021.11.005
36. Penn Wharton. The Impact of COVID-19 on immigration to the United States. October 15, 2024. Available at: https://budgetmodel.wharton.upenn.edu/issues/2024/10/15/the-impact-of-covid-19-on-immigration-to-the-united-states. Accessed March 24, 2025.

Health Hazards of Migration in People Seeking Asylum in New York City, 2023

Christian Olivo-Freites, MD, Patricia Miguez-Arosemena, MD, Andrés Henao-Martínez, MD, PhD, Jose Antonio Suarez, MD, Carlos Franco-Paredes, MD, MPH, Deborah Edelman, MD, Cristina Olivo-Freites, MD, Jennifer Marquez, MPH, Carlos Plazola, MD, Kayla Leschly, BA, Jayme Leschly, BA, Nathan Gundacker, MD, and Amir M. Mohareb, MD

See also Payton, p. 1557.

Objectives. To identify hazardous migration experiences among asylum seekers and associations with psychiatric illness.

Methods. We conducted a cross-sectional study of asylum seekers in a federally qualified health center in New York City from January 1 to November 30, 2023, to determine the frequency of and factors associated with hazardous migration events: physical or sexual assault, kidnapping, extortion, illnesses, and incarceration.

Results. Of 530 people (median age = 28 years, 55.5% female), most were from Venezuela (38.5%), Ecuador (20.0%), and other countries in South America (27.0%). They reported physical assault (24.9%), sexual assault (1.9%), kidnapping (4.7%), extortion (48.3%), and illness (19.4%) during migration. Crossing the Darien Gap was independently associated with experiencing physical or sexual violence (as a composite outcome, adjusted odds ratio [AOR] = 2.71; 95% confidence interval [CI] = 1.47, 5.10), illness (AOR = 3.71; 95% CI = 1.70, 8.58), and extortion (AOR = 1.94; 95% CI = 1.12, 3.34). Among adults, 10.7% (95% CI = 7.7%, 14.3%) were diagnosed with psychiatric illness during their initial evaluation, and this was more common in those who were incarcerated in immigration detention centers (OR = 2.02; 95% CI = 1.13, 3.66).

Conclusions. Asylum seekers journeying through the Darien Gap frequently encounter hazardous traumatic events. Detention by immigration authorities is associated with psychiatric illnesses. (*Am J Public Health*. 2025;115(10):1691–1699. https://doi.org/10.2105/AJPH.2025.308065)

AJPH October 2025, Vol. 115, No. 10

The number of people seeking asylum in the United States has been rising, with over 2 million asylum applications currently awaiting processing.[1] People seeking asylum enter the United States independently after migrating from their countries of origin and subsequently apply for asylum. Asylum seekers may leave their countries of origin through fear of persecution based on race, religion, nationality, membership in a particular social group, or political opinion.[2] Many people seeking asylum in the United States traverse the Mexico–US border after taking irregular migration routes through South and Central America, which may take months or years.[1,3] US Customs and Border Protection reports increased encounters or apprehensions with migrating people seeking entry through the Mexico–US border, with 1.7 million encounters in 2021 and 2.4 million in 2023.[4] The total number of people granted asylum in 2023 was 54 350. Given the lengthy backlogs in immigration court, asylum seekers frequently wait years for a decision on their applications; more than 1.1 million people filed for asylum in the United States in 2023.[1]

HEALTH HAZARDS DURING MIGRATION

For people seeking asylum in the United States, the migration process is frequently hazardous and can compound preexisting physical and psychological conditions in people who are forcibly displaced from their countries of origin.[3] Traveling through South America, Central America, and Mexico can expose people to hostile natural elements, vector-borne infections, and traumatic injury.[5–7] Migration also puts people at risk for suffering violence, extortion, and detention at the hands of political authorities, gangs, and traffickers who control various routes of the journey.[8,9] Migrating families report limited access to nutrition and health care during their journey, which can complicate acute and chronic illnesses.[10] Detention in carceral facilities, both outside of and within the United States, can introduce risks of infectious diseases and mental health disorders.[11–13] Such hazardous events encountered during migration can greatly affect the health and well-being of people resettling in the United States.

One site of unique hazards in this journey is in the Darien Gap, an area of dense rainforest between Colombia and Panama with no secure land connection.[5,7] People who migrate through the Darien Gap travel on foot or in boats.[9] Travel through the Darien Gap is hazardous because of the risk of violence, drowning, attack by wild animals, and injuries along the uncharted terrain.[5] Hazardous migration experiences such as physical and sexual assault, kidnappings, and financial extortion are believed to be pervasive among people who traverse the Darien Gap.[14]

STUDY OBJECTIVES

The hazards encountered by people completing this journey have not been formally studied in a population following resettlement in the United States, even though their clinical and public health implications may be substantial. Additionally, the association between hazardous migration experiences and psychiatric illness has been understudied in the current population of US asylum seekers. This study aimed to determine the frequency of hazardous migration experiences, such as physical and sexual assault, acute illness, and financial extortion, and their association with demographic characteristics, migration through the Darien Gap, and mental health illness in people seeking asylum in New York City in 2023.

METHODS

We conducted a cross-sectional study of recently arrived people seeking asylum who were unstably housed in New York City and who sought primary care in a federally qualified health center between January 1, 2023, and November 30, 2023. People from the shelter sites operated by the New York City Humanitarian Emergency Response and Relief Center presented to care in this clinic through self-referral, referral through a case manager or social worker, or referral from emergency departments and hospitals in the city following discharge. We created a note template for clinicians to use for the first evaluation of asylum-seeking patients. Clinicians screened patients for hazardous migration experiences and referred patients to behavioral health services when appropriate. Our primary analysis aimed to determine the frequency and associations with hazardous migration experiences. Our secondary analysis aimed to determine the association between hazardous experiences and psychiatric diagnoses made during the medical screening visit. We used the STROBE guidelines for reporting of cross-sectional observational studies.[15]

Study Population

We identified eligible participants by searching medical records for patients who had a medical encounter that matched a diagnostic code for a refugee health examination (*International Classification of Diseases, Tenth Revision* [*ICD-10*] code Z02.89; Geneva, Switzerland: World Health Organization; 1992). Clinicians in our clinic used this *ICD* code as a matter of internal practice when seeing patients who identified as asylum seekers being sheltered through the city's emergency assistance shelter system and who had not been previously evaluated by other clinicians in the primary care practice. This was verified by medical record review. Asylum status was identified in clinic patients as it influenced the social services offered. Participants were those seeking asylum in the United States within 1 year of their initial medical visit. Status as asylum seekers was verified in the clinic through documentation from the US Citizenship and Immigration Services. We did not restrict participation based on age, and we included reporting from parents or guardians for participants aged younger than 18 years. We excluded people who had altered mental status or who required immediate hospitalization at the time of evaluation. No unaccompanied minors were evaluated in our clinic during the study period. We limited the analysis to participants who reported details of their migration history.

Data Collection: Demographic Variables

We collected demographic information from the clinical record, including age, biological sex, preferred language, and country of origin. We report countries (or regions) of origin, such as Mexico,

Central America, the Caribbean, Venezuela, Ecuador, Colombia, Peru, other South American countries, and other regions, including African and Asian countries.

Data Collection: Migration History

Using methods in trauma-informed care,[16,17] we collected a detailed history from patients regarding their migration. This history included the reasons for forced displacement, the route and mode of migration, and the estimated cost per individual for migration (in present-day US dollars). For people reporting travel through the Darien Gap, we asked about the duration of travel through the rainforest, the illnesses encountered during this part of their journey (regardless of the receipt of medical care), and whether they witnessed a death or human remains along their travel route. We also recorded whether people underwent secondary migration, which we defined as migration following a minimum of 1 year in an intermediate country prior to arriving in the United States. Given the time required to complete this detailed history-taking, most patients presenting for urgent care visits in our clinical site could not complete the assessment of their migration history. However, all people were screened for mental health conditions and were referred to behavioral health for more in-depth psychiatric screening and longitudinal care when appropriate. Primary care providers in this clinic have extensive experience in screening, diagnosing, and treating mental health disorders in people experiencing homelessness and in patients newly arrived in the United States.

Outcome Measures

For the primary analysis, outcome measures were the hazardous events encountered during their journey to the United States. We defined a hazardous migration event as physical assault, sexual assault or rape, kidnapping, financial extortion, and developing an illness during migration. Clinicians used a shared definition for these experiences based on a template intake questionnaire used during their evaluation (Appendix, available as a supplement to the online version of this article at http://www.ajph.org). We defined financial extortion as the appropriation of money under the threat of violence by a political or nonstate authority; this definition did not include voluntary payment to traffickers or smugglers for transportation services under financial extortion. We also recorded and separately report whether police or border authorities incarcerated participants during their travel before or after crossing into the United States. We could not distinguish between US Customs and Border Protection detention or US Immigration and Customs Enforcement (online Appendix). We excluded from the analysis any hazardous events that preceded their migration. For our secondary analysis, our outcome measure was any psychiatric diagnosis made by the clinician during the screening visit. To measure this outcome, we reviewed the clinical diagnosis codes of each screening visit. Clinicians screened for depression, most often with Patient Health Questionnaire-9, and made other psychiatric diagnoses based on their individual clinical evaluation.

Statistical Analysis

We report categorical variables as frequencies (percentages) and continuous variables as medians (interquartile ranges [IQRs]). We used z scores to compute the 95% confidence interval (CI) of the proportion of participants who experienced hazardous migration events. We used multivariable logistic regression to determine factors associated with hazardous migration experiences. In this analysis, we separately analyzed 3 different regression models. Model 1 analyzed a composite outcome of physical or sexual assault. Model 2 analyzed the need for medical care during the journey. Model 3 analyzed financial extortion under the threat of violence. We report an adjusted odds ratio (AOR) for metrics controlling for age group (child, adolescent, and adult), sex assigned at birth, country (or region) of origin, secondary migration, and travel across the Darien Gap. We incorporated region of origin into the multivariable models because we hypothesized an independent association between the region of origin and travel through the Darien Gap. Therefore, we categorized regions of origin in geographic relation to the Darien Gap: Mexico, Central America, and the Caribbean; Venezuela; Ecuador; other South America; and other (Africa, Asia). For the secondary analysis, we used χ^2 analysis and univariable logistic regression to determine the association between hazardous migration experiences and a psychiatric illness diagnosed at the medical screening visit. We restricted this secondary analysis to adults (≥ 18 years) given the challenges of diagnosing psychiatric illness in children within 1 medical visit. We chose $P < .05$ as our threshold of significance. We used R version 4.0.3 for all statistical analyses.

RESULTS

Our clinic cared for 1486 sheltered people seeking asylum during the study period (online Appendix). The final study population that completed a detailed migration history included 530 people with median (IQR) age of 28 (12–35) years and 294 (55.5%) identifying as female (Table 1). The countries and regions of origin included Venezuela (204; 38.5%), Ecuador (106; 20.0%), Colombia (90; 17.0%), Peru (36; 6.8%), other countries of South America (17; 3.2%), Mexico and Central America (29; 5.5%), the Caribbean (23; 4.3%), and other parts of the world, including Africa and Asia (25; 4.7%). Secondary migration was reported by 127 participants (24.0%), of whom 90 (70.9%) were from Venezuela. The most common intermediate countries for secondary migrants were Colombia and Ecuador. Commonly reported reasons for displacement were fear of violence (291; 54.9%) and political persecution (115; 21.7%). Most people exclusively used ground transportation during their journey, whereas 85 people (16.0%) used air travel (Figure 1). The reported costs of migration ranged up to $20 000 per person.

TABLE 1— Characteristics of Unhoused Asylum Seekers Screened at a Federally Qualified Health Center: New York, NY, 2023

Characteristic	Value (n = 530), Median (IQR) or No. (%)
Age, y	28 (12–35)
Sex assigned at birth	
Female	294 (55.5)
Male	236 (44.5)
Country/region of origin	
Venezuela	204 (38.5)
Ecuador	106 (20.0)
Colombia	90 (17.0)
Peru	36 (6.8)
Mexico and Central America	29 (5.5)
Caribbean	23 (4.3)
Other (Africa, Asia)	25 (4.7)
Other (South America)	17 (3.2)
Secondary migration[a]	
Yes	127 (24.0)
No or unknown	403 (76.0)
Crossed Darien Gap	
Yes	312 (58.9)
No	213 (40.2)
Unknown	5 (1.0)
Detained or incarcerated during journey	
Yes	95 (17.9)
No	435 (82.1)
Detained or incarcerated after arrival in United States	
Yes	301 (57.7)
No	221 (42.3)
Hazardous migration experiences[b]	
Physical assault	132 (24.9)
Sexual assault	10 (1.9)
Kidnapping	25 (4.7)
Financial extortion	255 (48.3)
Illness requiring medical care	103 (19.4)
Multiple hazardous experiences	143 (27.0)
None or unknown	198 (37.4)

Note. IQR = interquartile range.
[a]Secondary migration was defined as migration to the United States following a minimum of 1 year in an intermediate country (i.e., not their country of origin).
[b]The experiences listed are not mutually exclusive and do not sum to 100%.

Hazardous Migration Experiences

We found that 62.6% (95% CI = 58.4%, 66.8%) of people reported at least 1 hazardous migration experience while traveling to the United States. Participants reported physical and sexual assault during migration (24.9% and 1.9%, respectively). Twenty-five people (4.7%) were kidnapped during their journey, most commonly in Mexico (19 of 25; 76%). Roughly half (255; 48.3%) experienced financial extortion under the threat of violence, many of whom reported extortion at multiple points during the journey. The most common sites of extortion were Mexico (174; 68.2%) and Guatemala (124; 48.6%). Approximately one quarter (143; 27.0%) reported multiple hazardous experiences during their journey. Most participants (301; 57.7%) reported experiencing detention or incarceration by immigration authorities in the United States, whereas 95 (17.9%) reported detention or incarceration in other countries during their journey.

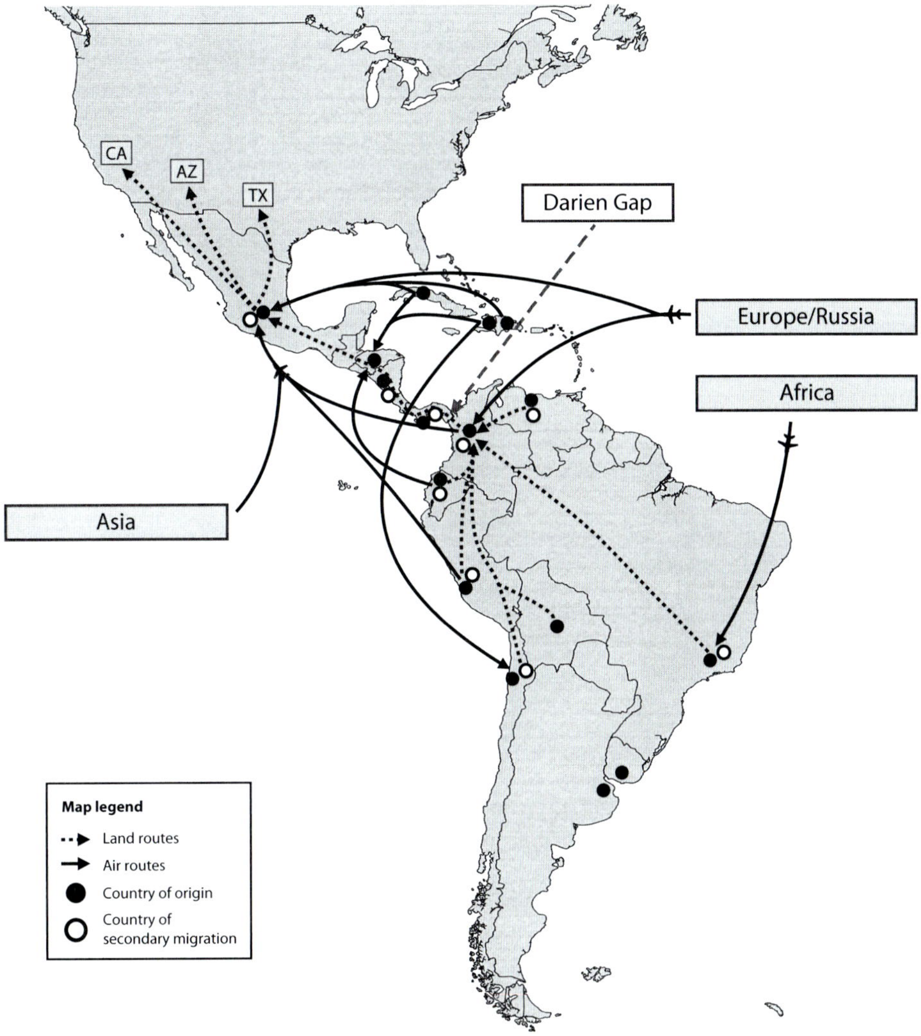

FIGURE 1— Map of Reported Routes of Migration of People Seeking Asylum and Experiencing Unstable Housing: New York, NY, 2023

Note. Land routes of migration are depicted in dashes; air travel is depicted in solid lines. Secondary migration is defined as residence in a second country outside one's country of origin for at least 1 year before resettlement in the United States. Some individuals (e.g., those from Argentina and Uruguay) did not provide details of their migration routes.

Exposure to the Darien Gap

The majority of participants (312; 58.9%) crossed the Darien Gap (Table 2), 213 (40.2%) did not cross the Darien Gap, and 5 (1.0%) did not have information recorded. The median (IQR) duration in the Darien Gap was 5 (4–7) days, although 1 participant was there for nearly 4 weeks. A total of 107 people (34.3%) experienced illnesses in the Darien Gap, of whom 62 (57.9%) reported gastrointestinal illness and 15 (14.0%) reported dermatological diseases, including cutaneous leishmaniasis and trench foot. Fewer people reported respiratory tract illness (10; 9.3%), genitourinary tract disease (4; 3.7%), multiple overlapping conditions, nonspecific febrile illnesses, and pregnancy-related complications. Many people who crossed the Darien Gap (161; 51.6%) reported witnessing deaths or finding human remains during their journey.

After adjusting for age group, sex, country or region of origin, and secondary migration, travel through the Darien Gap was independently associated with physical or sexual violence (AOR = 2.71; 95% CI = 1.47, 5.10; Table 3). People who traveled through the Darien Gap were also more likely to require medical care during their journey (AOR = 3.71; 95% CI = 1.70, 8.58) and to experience financial extortion with the threat of violence (AOR = 1.94; 95% CI = 1.12, 3.34). Secondary migration was associated with lower odds of physical or sexual violence (AOR = 0.54; 95%

TABLE 2— Migration Experiences in the Darien Gap, Panama, Among Asylum Seekers Evaluated in a Federally Qualified Health Center: New York, NY, 2023

Characteristic	Value (n = 312), Median (IQR) or No. (%)
Days in Darien Gap	5 (4–7)
Experienced illness in Darien Gap	
Yes	107 (34.3)
No	160 (51.3)
Unknown	45 (14.4)
Types of illnesses (n = 107)	
Gastrointestinal disease	62 (57.9)
Dermatological disease	15 (14.0)
Respiratory tract disease	10 (9.3)
Genitourinary tract disease	4 (3.7)
Other conditions[a]	9 (8.4)
Multiple conditions	7 (6.5)
Witnessed deaths or human remains in Darien Gap	
Yes	161 (51.6)
No	131 (42.0)
Unknown	20 (6.4)

Note. IQR = interquartile range.
[a]Other conditions included malaria, acute febrile illness not otherwise specified, and pregnancy-related complications.

CI = 0.31, 0.91) and higher odds of financial extortion (AOR = 2.68; 95% CI = 1.64, 4.43) after adjustment for other factors.

Secondary Analysis: Psychiatric Diagnosis

Among the 365 adults (≥ 18 years) in the sample, 39 (10.7%; 95% CI = 7.7%, 14.3%) were diagnosed with a psychiatric illness at their initial medical evaluation. These diagnoses were most commonly depression, generalized anxiety, and posttraumatic stress disorder. Psychiatric illness was not more common in adults who had experienced physical or sexual violence (*P* = 1.0), acute illness (*P* = .70), or financial extortion (*P* = 1.0) during migration. Psychiatric illness was associated with incarceration after arrival into the United States by immigration authorities (χ^2 = 6.067; *P* = .014) with an odds ratio of 2.02 (95% CI = 1.13, 3.66).

DISCUSSION

In this study of unhoused asylum seekers in New York City, we found that 62.6% experienced hazardous events during their migration, including physical and sexual assault, kidnappings, financial extortion, and illnesses or injuries requiring medical attention. Our clinic was uniquely positioned to interview and treat recently migrated people experiencing unstable housing in New York City, whose migrant population has surpassed 200 000 people since 2022.[18] The demographic composition of our study population reflects the population of asylum seekers who enter the United States through the Mexico–US border, with a relatively young age and a high percentage of people from South and Central America.[1] Given the high number of people embarking on this journey, our study suggests that hundreds of thousands of people traveling to the United States annually are affected by numerous underappreciated health hazards of migration.

Hazardous Migration and the Darien Gap

A critical finding of this study is the association of hazardous migration experiences with traversing the Darien Gap. Although there has been much press and news reporting on the migration through the Darien Gap, there are few epidemiological studies on the health hazards of this migration route. We found that travel through the Darien Gap was independently associated with experiencing physical or sexual violence, a need for acute medical care, and financial extortion. The Darien region has a widespread gang and cartel presence in addition to human traffickers, which increases the risk of violence for people who are migrating.[9] We found that 51.6% of people who crossed the Darien Gap reported witnessing a death or finding human remains along their journey in the jungle, which reflects the high lethality associated with this journey. A recent study of postmortem evaluations of human remains in the Darien Gap demonstrated a high prevalence of deaths caused by interpersonal violence and drowning, with over 12.3% of deaths among children and young adults.[5] It is not known how many people die or disappear through this route of migration each year, but based on the findings

TABLE 3— Factors Associated With Hazardous Migration Experiences Among Asylum Seekers Evaluated in a Federally Qualified Health Center: New York, NY, 2023

	OR (95% CI)		
Characteristic	**Model 1, Outcome: Physical/Sexual Violence[a]**	**Model 2, Outcome: Need for Medical Care**	**Model 3, Outcome: Financial Extortion**
Age group			
Adult (> 25 y) (Ref)	1	1	1
Child (< 13 y)	0.75 (0.46, 1.22)	0.91 (0.51, 1.60)	0.89 (0.56, 1.40)
Adolescent (13–25 y)	0.69 (0.37, 1.23)	1.10 (0.59, 2.00)	0.68 (0.40, 1.16)
Sex assigned at birth			
Female (Ref)	1	1	1
Male	1.40 (0.93, 2.11)	1.09 (0.66, 1.68)	1.12 (0.77, 1.65)
Country/region of origin			
Venezuela (Ref)	1	1	1
Mexico, Central America, or the Caribbean	2.65 (1.14, 6.13)	1.22 (0.43, 3.36)	0.73 (0.33, 1.61)
Ecuador	0.97 (0.55, 1.72)	1.06 (0.57, 1.94)	1.98 (0.58, 1.67)
Other (South America)	1.01 (0.49, 2.07)	0.38 (0.13, 0.97)	0.43 (0.22, 0.81)
Other (Africa, Asia)	1.19 (0.38, 3.31)	0.45 (0.07, 1.77)	0.17 (0.05, 0.50)
Secondary migration			
No/unknown (Ref)	1	1	1
Yes	0.54 (0.31, 0.91)	1.56 (0.91, 2.66)	2.68 (1.64, 4.43)
Crossed Darien Gap			
No/unknown (Ref)	1	1	1
Yes	2.71 (1.47, 5.10)	3.71 (1.70, 8.58)	1.94 (1.12, 3.34)

Note. CI = confidence interval; OR = odds ratio. Multivariable logistic regression was used.
[a]Physical/sexual violence included physical assault, sexual assault, and kidnapping. For definitions, see Appendix (available as a supplement to the online version of this article at http://www.ajph.org).

from this study, enhancing the quality of medical care and the safety of people migrating through the Darien Gap should be made an urgent public health priority.

The hazards reported in this study complicate the already difficult migration process for people displaced from their countries of origin, particularly in an era of increasing restrictions on refugee resettlement and asylum worldwide. The lifetime prevalence of physical and sexual violence among asylum seekers is likely higher than what is reported here, as this study is limited to events encountered during the course of migration and not in countries of origin or the United States since resettlement.[19,20] Our study population's predominant mode of transportation was overland, likely attributed to the changing visa requirements in the region.[21,22] Paradoxically, these visa requirements and other forms of migration restriction do not appear to decrease migration volume. Instead, they compel individuals seeking asylum to use irregular land pathways, possibly exposing them to more migration hazards.[7]

Clinical and Public Health Implications

The findings of this study have important clinical and policy implications. To our knowledge, this study is the first to provide detailed accounts of specific migration experiences for the current unstably housed asylum-seeking population in the United States, many of whom traveled through the Darien Gap. Clinicians should identify these events as they represent risk factors for physical and mental health conditions for asylum seekers following resettlement. However, these experiences may be underreported in general clinical settings, given their associated stigma and the sensitive and potentially retraumatizing nature of recounting past events. State and municipal public health authorities should invest resources, particularly through community-based organizations, to help identify asylum seekers with traumatic experiences and link them to appropriate social and mental health supports.

Although the Centers for Disease Control and Prevention provides guidelines for the medical screening and care of patients who have arrived in the United States through the formal refugee resettlement program,[23] there are no evidence-based guidelines available for clinicians who care for the hundreds of thousands of migrants and asylum seekers who are not formally resettled as refugees. This represents a major public health gap, given the higher volume of displaced people who resettle in the United States seeking asylum compared with the refugee resettlement program. For example, in 2023 alone, more than 1.1 million individuals were included in asylum filings in the United States, compared with 60 050 admitted refugees that same year.[1] Clinicians who care for this population should use methods of trauma-informed care to screen for hazards during the migration process and provide medical care for this growing patient population. Clinical and public health experts should develop the evidence base to help inform guidelines for screening and care for forcibly displaced persons outside the refugee resettlement program.

Hazardous Migration and Psychiatric Illness

Past studies have demonstrated that major depression and posttraumatic stress disorder are present in 45% to 48% of the refugees and asylum seekers who have experienced violence, kidnappings, and torture.[24] Our study found that 10.7% of adult asylum seekers received a psychiatric diagnosis at their initial medical visit. Still, this study likely underestimates the true prevalence of mental illness in this population as our analysis relied on clinical diagnoses made in the initial screening visit, and diagnoses may occur after their initial visit. As in past studies, we found higher odds of experiencing psychiatric illness among those who were incarcerated in US immigration detention centers.[12] Past studies have also shown that hypertension, dyslipidemia, and physical disabilities are prevalent in asylum seekers who report physical and sexual violence prior to resettlement.[25] There are also risks of infectious diseases associated with detention and incarceration, particularly in overcrowded facilities.[26,27] Policymakers should aim to minimize the carceral detention of asylum seekers given the deleterious individual and societal effects of incarceration.

Study Limitations

Several limitations should be considered when interpreting these study results. First, as this was a single-center study, generalizability has limitations. The findings reported here are most reflective of asylum seekers experiencing unstable housing after traveling across the Mexico–US border to enter the United States. Second, as this was a cross-sectional study, we cannot use these findings to determine causation, and unmeasured variables may confound some findings in the regression analyses. For example, unmeasured variables may be associated with the exposure of crossing the Darien Gap and the outcomes of interest. Not all individuals evaluated in our clinic during the study were asked detailed migration histories because of time constraints and discomfort with trauma-informed questioning. Given that the referral process to our clinic included post–emergency department and hospitalization visits, our sample may overestimate the prevalence of some outcomes. However, because of stigma, retraumatization risks, and underreporting, sexual violence likely remains underestimated. For the reasons stated, we believe the prevalence of psychiatric illness is higher than what is reported here. We did not analyze the prevalence of psychiatric conditions in children, given the challenges of making accurate diagnoses in a single medical screening visit.

Conclusions

This study demonstrates that 62.6% of unhoused asylum seekers presenting for care at a federally qualified health center in New York City reported a hazardous event during their migration. We found that 24.9% reported an instance of physical violence and 1.9% reported sexual violence. Approximately half reported financial extortion, and one fifth required medical care during their journey. Travel through the Darien Gap was associated with these hazardous experiences, and detention by US immigration authorities was associated with psychiatric illness after arrival. Many of the traumatic experiences that asylum seekers experience during their migration may leave long-term sequelae that can influence their resettlement and health. Public health authorities should formulate policies that address the substantial risk of traumatic events among the growing asylum-seeking population. AJPH

ABOUT THE AUTHORS

At the time this work was conducted, Christian Olivo-Freites, Jennifer Marquez, Kayla Leschly, and Jayme Leschly were with Ryan Health, New York, NY. Patricia Miguez-Arosemena was with the Department of Internal Medicine, Mount Sinai Health System, New York, NY. Andrés Henao-Martínez was with the Division of Infectious Diseases, University of Colorado, Anschutz

Medical Campus, Aurora. Jose Antonio Suarez was with Senacyt, Panama City, Panama. Carlos Franco-Paredes was with Hospital Infantil de Mexico, Federico Gomez, Mexico City, Mexico. Deborah Edelman was with the Department of Internal Medicine, Mount Sinai Health System and Icahn School of Medicine at Mount Sinai, New York, NY. Cristina Olivo-Freites was with the Division of Hematology and Oncology, University of Texas Health Science Center, Houston. Carlos Plazola was with the Division of Infectious Diseases, University of Miami Miller School of Medicine, Miami, FL. Nathan Gundacker was with the Medical College of Wisconsin and Zablocki VA Medical Center, Milwaukee. Amir M. Mohareb was with the Massachusetts General Hospital Center for Global Health and Division of Infectious Diseases and Harvard Medical School, Boston, MA.

CORRESPONDENCE

Correspondence should be sent to Amir M. Mohareb, MD, Center for Global Health, Massachusetts General Hospital, 125 Nashua St, #7222, Boston, MA 02114 (e-mail: amohareb@mgh.harvard.edu). Reprints can be ordered at https://www.ajph.org by clicking the "Reprints" link.

PUBLICATION INFORMATION

Full Citation: Olivo-Freites C, Miguez-Arosemena P, Henao-Martínez A, et al. Health hazards of migration in people seeking asylum in New York City, 2023. *Am J Public Health*. 2025;115(10):1691–1699.

Acceptance Date: February 5, 2025.

DOI: https://doi.org/10.2105/AJPH.2025.308065

ORCID iDs:

Christian Olivo-Freites https://orcid.org/0000-0002-0779-921X

Carlos Franco-Paredes https://orcid.org/0000-0001-8757-643X

Deborah Edelman https://orcid.org/0000-0002-7198-2879

Amir M. Mohareb https://orcid.org/0000-0002-3761-6154

CONTRIBUTORS

Christian Olivo-Freites and A. M. Mohareb conceptualized the study. Christian Olivo-Freites, J. Marquez, J. A. Suarez, N. Gundacker, C. Franco-Paredes, and A. Henao-Martínez designed the questionnaire. Christian Olivo-Freites, C. Plazola, J. Marquez, J. Leschly, and K. Leschly undertook data collection. Christian Olivo-Freites and A. M. Mohareb conducted statistical analysis. Christian Olivo-Freites, A. M. Mohareb, C. Franco-Paredes, and D. Edelman interpreted the results. Christian Olivo-Freites and A. M. Mohareb primarily drafted the manuscript. All authors reviewed the manuscript and critically revised its contents for intellectual content.

CONFLICTS OF INTEREST

None of the authors report any financial disclosures or conflicts of interest related to this article.

HUMAN PARTICIPANT PROTECTION

This study was approved by the Ryan Health board of directors and the MassGeneral Brigham institutional review board.

REFERENCES

1. US Dept of Homeland Security, Office of Homeland Security Statistics. Annual flow report: refugees and asylees: 2023. November 2024. Available at: https://ohss.dhs.gov/topics/immigration/refugees-and-asylees/refugees-and-asylees-annual-flow-report. Accessed June 20, 2025.
2. UN High Commissioner for Refugees. Global trends. Available at: https://www.unhcr.org/media/40152. Accessed June 20, 2025.
3. Ward N, Batalova J. Refugees and asylees in the United States. June 15, 2023. Available at: https://www.migrationpolicy.org/article/refugees-and-asylees-united-states. Accessed June 20, 2025.
4. US Customs and Border Patrol. Nationwide encounters. Available at: https://www.cbp.gov/newsroom/stats/nationwide-encounters. Accessed April 20, 2023.
5. Lucio JVP, Congram D, Franco-Paredes C, et al. Mortality during migration through the Darién Gap in Panama in 2018–22. *Lancet*. 2023;402(10410):1321–1322. https://doi.org/10.1016/S0140-6736(23)01635-5
6. Reynolds CW, Cheung AW, Draugelis S, et al. Epidemiology of asylum seekers and refugees at the Mexico–US border: a cross-sectional analysis from the migrant settlement camp in Matamoros, Mexico. *BMC Public Health*. 2024;24(1):489. https://doi.org/10.1186/s12889-024-17947-7
7. Higuita NA, Suarez JA, Millender E, et al. US bound journey of migrant peoples InTransit across Dante's Inferno and Purgatory in the Americas. *Travel Med Infect Dis*. 2022;47:102317. https://doi.org/10.1016/j.tmaid.2022.102317
8. Abaya M, Lesley B, Williams C, Chaves-Gnecco D, Flores G. Forcible displacement, migration, and violence against children and families in Latin America. *Pediatr Clin North Am*. 2021;68(2):371–387. https://doi.org/10.1016/j.pcl.2020.12.003
9. Naranjo L, Williams Y, Levy J, et al. The endless vulnerability of migrant children in-transit across the Darién Gap. *Am J Trop Med Hyg*. 2023;109(3):515–519. https://doi.org/10.4269/ajtmh.22-0765
10. Ahmed D, Benavente P, Diaz E. Food insecurity among international migrants during the COVID-19 pandemic: a scoping review. *Int J Environ Res Public Health*. 2023;20(7):5273. https://doi.org/10.3390/ijerph20075273
11. Tellez D, Tejkl L, McLaughlin D, Vallet M, Abrahim O, Spiegel PB. The United States detention system for migrants: patterns of negligence and inconsistency. *J Migr Health*. 2022;6:100141. https://doi.org/10.1016/j.jmh.2022.100141
12. von Werthern M, Robjant K, Chui Z, et al. The impact of immigration detention on mental health: a systematic review. *BMC Psychiatry*. 2018;18(1):382. https://doi.org/10.1186/s12888-018-1945-y
13. Robjant K, Hassan R, Katona C. Mental health implications of detaining asylum seekers: systematic review. *Br J Psychiatry*. 2009;194(4):306–312. https://doi.org/10.1192/bjp.bp.108.053223
14. Taylor L. Health crisis for migrants crossing the Darién Gap is intensifying, MSF warns. *BMJ*. 2022;377:o1323. https://doi.org/10.1136/bmj.o1323
15. von Elm E, Altman DG, Egger M, et al. The strengthening the reporting of observational studies in epidemiology (STROBE) statement: guidelines for reporting observational studies. *Ann Intern Med*. 2007;147(8):573–577. https://doi.org/10.1136/bmj.39335.541782.AD
16. Forkey H, Szilagyi M, Kelly ET, et al. Trauma-informed care. *Pediatrics*. 2021;148(2):e2021052580. https://doi.org/10.1542/peds.2021-052580
17. Im H, Swan LET. Capacity building for refugee mental health in resettlement: implementation and evaluation of cross-cultural trauma-informed care training. *J Immigr Minor Health*. 2020;22(5):923–934. https://doi.org/10.1007/s10903-020-00992-w
18. City of New York Website. Mayor Adams announces New York City has cared for more than 100,000 asylum seekers since last Spring. August 16, 2023. Available at: https://www.nyc.gov/office-of-the-mayor/news/600-23/mayor-adams-new-york-city-has-cared-more-100-000-asylum-seekers-since-last-spring. Accessed June 20, 2025.
19. Aguirre NG, Milewski AR, Shin J, Ottenheimer D. Gender-based violence experienced by women seeking asylum in the United State: a lifetime of multiple traumas inflicted by multiple perpetrators. *J Forensic Leg Med*. 2020;72:101959. https://doi.org/10.1016/j.jflm.2020.101959
20. Khouani J, Landrin M, Boulakia RC, et al. Incidence of sexual violence among recently arrived asylum-seeking women in France: a retrospective cohort study. *Lancet Reg Health Eur*. 2023;34:100731. https://doi.org/10.1016/j.lanepe.2023.100731
21. Jokisch B. Ecuador juggles rising emigration and challenges accommodating Venezuelan arrivals. October 18, 2023. Available at: https://www.migrationpolicy.org/article/ecuador-migration-trends-emigration-venezuelans. Accessed June 20, 2025.
22. Human Rights Watch. Mexico/Central America: new visa restrictions harm Venezuelans. July 5, 2022. Available at: https://www.hrw.org/news/2022/07/05/mexico/central-america-new-visa-restrictions-harm-venezuelans. Accessed June 20, 2025.
23. Centers for Disease Control and Prevention. Refugee health guidance. Available at: https://www.cdc.gov/immigrant-refugee-health/hcp/domestic-guidance/index.html. Accessed June 20, 2025.
24. Tamblyn JM, Calderon AJ, Combs S, O'Brien MM. Patients from abroad becoming patients in everyday practice: torture survivors in primary care. *J Immigr Minor Health*. 2011;13(4):798–801. https://doi.org/10.1007/s10903-010-9429-2
25. Al-Rousan T, AlHeresh R, Saadi A, et al. Epidemiology of cardiovascular disease and its risk factors among refugees and asylum seekers: systematic review and meta-analysis. *Int J Cardiol Cardiovasc Risk Prev*. 2022;12:200126. https://doi.org/10.1016/j.ijcrp.2022.200126
26. Lo NC, Nyathi S, Chapman LAC, et al. Influenza, varicella, and mumps outbreaks in US migrant detention centers. *JAMA*. 202112;325(2):180–182. https://doi.org/10.1001/jama.2020.20539
27. Leibowitz AI, Siedner MJ, Tsai AC, Mohareb AM. Association between prison crowding and COVID-19 incidence rates in Massachusetts prisons, April 2020–January 2021. *JAMA Intern Med*. 2021;181(10):1315–1321. https://doi.org/10.1001/jamainternmed.2021.4392

Impacts of a Healthy Checkout Ordinance on Added Sugars, Sodium, and Other Nutrients at Checkout 1 Year After Implementation: Berkeley, California, 2021–2022

Alexandria E. Reimold, PhD, Ethan C. Wolf, MPH, Kris Jayme G. Matas, MLIS, Samantha Marinello, PhD, Lisa M. Powell, PhD, Rebecca M. Schermbeck, MPH, MS, RD, and Jennifer Falbe, ScD, MPH

See also Pomeranz, p. 1561.

Objectives. To assess the impact of the world's first mandatory healthy checkout policy on added sugars, sodium, and other nutrients available at retail checkouts in Berkeley, California.

Methods. We collected data on food and beverage facings before (2021) and after (2022) policy implementation in 23 Berkeley (8786 facings) and 75 California comparison stores (40 617 facings). Our analysis used difference-in-differences models.

Results. Between 2021 and 2022, there was a 70% reduction in added sugars per serving of food and beverage facings (b = 0.30; 95% confidence interval [CI] = 0.15, 0.59) and a 53% reduction in sodium per serving of beverage facings (b = 0.47; 95% CI = 0.28, 0.81) at Berkeley checkouts relative to comparison city checkouts. There was a 41% reduction in saturated fat and a 47% increase in fiber per serving of food and beverage facings (b = 0.59; 95% CI = 0.44, 0.79 and b = 1.47; 95% CI = 1.05, 2.06, respectively).

Conclusions. One year after implementation, the policy reduced added sugars and saturated fat per serving of food and beverage facings, reduced sodium per serving of beverage facings, and increased fiber per serving of food and beverage facings.

Public Health Implications. Healthy checkout policies have potential to increase the healthfulness of checkout food environments. (*Am J Public Health*. 2025;115(10):1700–1712. https://doi.org/10.2105/AJPH.2025.308159)

AJPH October 2025, Vol. 115, No. 10

Retail food environments influence food purchasing behaviors and, thus, diet quality of populations, partially through the placement of products in prominent store locations.[1–3] Checkout areas hold particular significance. All customers must walk through a checkout to complete their purchases, and roughly 1 in 3 customers purchase foods or beverages displayed at checkout.[4] Because of marketing contracts between retailers and manufacturers, checkout areas encourage sales of items like candy, sugar-sweetened beverages (SSBs), and salty snacks[5] by capitalizing on consumers' last-minute, impulse purchasing decisions.[6–8] These items are often high in nutrients of concern like added sugars and sodium, which can increase the risk of type 2 diabetes, high blood pressure, heart disease, and stroke when consumed in excess.[9–11] Checkout areas may also contribute to nutrition and health disparities,[4,12] as stores in neighborhoods with higher poverty and higher Black and Hispanic residential compositions are more likely to stock unhealthy foods and beverages at checkout.[5,13,14]

To ensure that large food retailers offer healthy options rather than unhealthy foods at checkout, Berkeley, California, implemented a healthy checkout ordinance (HCO) in 2021,[15] the world's first mandatory healthy checkout policy, to our knowledge.[16–19] This ordinance (i.e., city-level law) requires that stores display only the following at checkout: nonfood and nonbeverage products, unsweetened beverages, sugar-free gum and mints, fruits, vegetables, nuts, seeds, legumes, yogurt, cheese, and whole grains with no more than 5 grams of added sugars and no more than 200 milligrams of sodium per serving.[15] The Berkeley HCO was championed by a grass-roots community coalition.[19] Before implementation, only 29% of food and beverage products at checkout met the HCO requirements.[5] One year after implementation, candy, SSBs, and other sweets were replaced with a combination of nonfood products and compliant food and beverage products.[20] However, no study has examined the impact of the HCO on the nutrient content of food and beverage products remaining at checkout.

To evaluate the HCO's impact on the nutrients it limits, we assessed changes in added sugars and sodium in the food and beverage products available in store checkouts in Berkeley before and 1 year after implementation compared with other Northern California cities. We also examined the HCO's impacts on nutrients related to the HCO food group restrictions, including saturated fat and fiber, as well as calories.

METHODS

The Berkeley HCO implementation in March 2021[15] created a natural experiment in which we conducted a cohort study of products available at retail checkouts in Berkeley and comparison cities before (February 2021; ≤ 1 month before implementation) and 1 year after (February 2022) implementation.[15] This study included a census of Berkeley stores initially identified as subject to the HCO (n = 23) and comparison stores, matched by store type and chain, from 3 California cities matched to Berkeley by sociodemographic characteristics: Davis, Oakland, and Sacramento (n = 75). The sampling strategy is described elsewhere.[20] Table A (available as a supplement to the online version of this article at https://ajph.org) shows the store sample.

All product facings[5] in up to 3 randomly selected checkouts (i.e., designated waiting area including endcaps and any space within 3 feet of the register) were assessed in each store. A product facing refers to each product visible to customers, not including products stacked behind it. Each facing was counted separately, including side-by-side facings for identical products. Using the highly reliable Store Check-OUt Tool (SCOUT),[21] trained data collectors photographed and assessed characteristics (e.g., brand, flavor, and size) of each facing. Using methods reported previously,[5] nutrient and ingredient data from manufacturer and retailer websites were linked for each food and beverage facing. Of the resulting 50 061 food and beverage facings, 658 (1%) did not have nutrient information for at least 1 outcome (e.g., imported or discontinued products with no manufacturer website), leaving an analytic sample of 49 403 (8786 in Berkeley and 40 617 in comparison cities).

Of the 49 403 food and beverage facings evaluated, 8258 (17%) did not have retrievable nutrient data for the exact product or package size. These facings were linked with nutrient information using similar products with a different flavor (e.g., strawberry instead of watermelon) or size (> 1 unit [e.g., ounce, milliliter] difference in size). We conducted a sensitivity analysis without these 8258 facings, restricting to the 41 145 facings with nutrient data from the same product or package size.

Outcomes and Measures

Based on the HCO nutrient limits, the 2 primary outcomes are average grams of added sugars and milligrams of sodium per serving of food and beverage facings. Based on HCO food category limits, 3 secondary outcomes include average grams of saturated fat and fiber, and calories per serving of food and beverage facings. To assess changes in the whole product shoppers take home, we also report outcomes per package of food and beverage facings (amount per serving multiplied by servings per package).

To understand variation in HCO implementation, we report the primary outcomes stratified by store type (chain supermarket, independent supermarket, chain mass merchandiser, chain specialty food, chain dollar, independent grocery, and chain drug), defined by the North American Industry Classification System, store observations, and name recognition.

Statistical Analysis

We report summary statistics for all outcomes before and after policy implementation in Berkeley and comparison cities. We then report changes in each outcome from before to after implementation using difference-in-differences generalized linear models with cluster-robust standard errors clustered at the store level, log link, and γ distribution to account for the right skew of nutrient distributions.

Specifically, we estimated the following model:

$$(1)\quad Nutrient_{ist} = \exp(\beta_0 + \beta_1 Post_t + \beta_2 Berkeley_s + \beta_3 (Post_t \times Berkeley_s) + \varepsilon_{ist})$$

where $Nutrient_{ist}$ is the nutrient outcome for product facing *i*, in site *s*, at time *t*. Two indicator variables, *Post* and *Berkeley*, indicate if the product facing was at checkout before or after implementation and in Berkeley or a comparison city, respectively. With this modeling approach, exponentiated coefficients (i.e., [b−1]×100 for b < 1.0 and [1-b]×100 for b ≥ 1.0) are interpreted as the percent change in Berkeley relative to comparison cities. We ran models for all food and beverage facings (including gum and mints) and for food facings and beverage facings separately. We also report percent change in nutrient outcomes attributable to changes in product type (e.g., SSBs, fruits) offered at checkout. We then stratified the analyses for primary outcomes by store type.

We conducted analyses in August to October 2024 with Stata/SE version 18.0 (StataCorp LLC, College Station, TX). We followed Strengthening the Reporting of Observational Studies in Epidemiology (STROBE) reporting guidelines.

RESULTS

The number of food and beverage facings in the analytic sample decreased by 42% (5572–3214 facings) after implementation in Berkeley, whereas there was little change (4%) in the number of food and beverage facings in comparison cities (19 914–20 703 facings; Table 1).

Primary Outcomes

One year after Berkeley HCO implementation, there was a 70% reduction (95% confidence interval [CI] = −85%, −41%) in grams of added sugars per serving of food and beverage facings remaining at checkouts in Berkeley relative to comparison cities (b = 0.30; 95% CI = 0.15, 0.59). When we examined beverage facings and food facings separately, there were 72% (95% CI = −89%, −27%) and 73% (95% CI = −84%, −55%) relative reductions in added sugars per serving, respectively (b = 0.28; 95% CI = 0.11, 0.73 and b = 0.27; 95% CI = 0.16, 0.45). This pattern was consistent in sensitivity analyses using added sugars per package of food and beverage facings (Figure 1; Table 1).

There was not a statistically significant change in milligrams of sodium per serving of food and beverage facings (b = 0.81; 95% CI = 0.57, 1.14) or per serving of food facing alone (b = 0.94; 95% CI = 0.64, 1.37), likely because before implementation, only 9% of food facings at Berkeley checkouts were high in sodium (i.e., > 200 milligrams per serving). However, there was a 53% reduction (95% CI = −72%, −19%) in sodium per serving of beverage facings at checkout in Berkeley relative to comparison cities (b = 0.47; 95% CI = 0.28, 0.81). There was no statistically significant relative reduction in sodium content per package of food and beverage facings in Berkeley (Figure 1; Table 1).

Secondary Outcomes

There were changes in saturated fat, fiber, and calorie content of food and beverage facings at Berkeley checkouts. There was a 41% reduction (95% CI = −56%, −21%) in saturated fat content per serving of food and beverage facings displayed at checkout in Berkeley relative to comparison cities (b = 0.59; 95% CI = 0.44, 0.79), with a 38% reduction (95% CI = −54%, −17%) in saturated fat content per serving of food facings (b = 0.62; 95% CI = 0.46, 0.83). There was also a 47% increase (95% CI = 5%, 106%) in fiber content per serving of food and beverage facings displayed at checkout in Berkeley relative to comparison cities (b = 1.47; 95% CI = 1.05, 2.06), again, driven by a 56% increase (95% CI = 13%, 115%) in fiber content per serving of food (b = 1.56; 95% CI = 1.13, 2.15) in Berkeley relative to comparison cities. Beverage facings contained negligible saturated fat and fiber content per serving; thus, there were no significant changes for these nutrients from these products. Finally, there was a 27% reduction (95% CI = −40%, −12%) in calories per serving of food and beverage facings displayed at checkout in Berkeley relative to comparison cities (b = 0.73; 95% CI = 0.60, 0.88), an 18% reduction (95% CI = −31%, −1%) for food and a 58% reduction (95% CI = −77%, −22%) for beverage facings (b = 0.82; 95% CI = 0.69, 0.99 and b = 0.42; 95% CI = 0.23, 0.78, respectively; Figure A [available as a supplement to the online version of this article at https://ajph.org]; Table 1).

Nutrient and calorie reductions in food and beverage facings were largely driven by the removal of candy and SSBs (e.g., soda, energy drinks) from checkouts, which accounted for 50% and 39% of the reduction in added sugars, 88% and 2% of the reduction in saturated fat, and 72% and 8% of the reduction in calories, respectively. The increase in fiber was largely driven by the addition of bars (granola and protein) and nuts, which accounted for

TABLE 1— Nutrient Composition of Food and Beverage Products per Serving and per Package Facing at Retail Checkouts Before and After Implementation of the Berkeley Healthy Checkout Ordinance: Berkeley, California, and Comparison Cities, 2021–2022

	Berkeley, CA		Comparison Cities		b (95% CI)	% Change,[a] Berkeley vs Comparison
	Preimplementation	Postimplementation	Preimplementation	Postimplementation		
Added sugars (grams)						
Per serving food and beverage					0.30 (0.15, 0.59)	−70
Mean (SD)	11.1 (15.6)	3.4 (10.7)	11.4 (15.8)	11.7 (16.3)		
No.	5 498	3 135	19 594	20 114		
Per serving beverage					0.28 (0.11, 0.73)	−72
Mean (SD)	23.0 (26.0)	6.7 (17.9)	22.8 (26.7)	24.1 (26.6)		
No.	1 110	864	3 741	4 134		
Per serving food					0.27 (0.16, 0.45)	−73
Mean (SD)	8.0 (9.4)	2.1 (5.4)	8.6 (10.2)	8.5 (10.1)		
No.	4 388	2 271	15 853	15 980		
Per package food and beverage					0.29 (0.16, 0.53)	−71
Mean (SD)	29.6 (63.5)	7.6 (29.1)	28.0 (67.4)	24.7 (50.3)		
No.	5 394	3 009	19 099	19 743		
Per package beverage					0.27 (0.10, 0.72)	−73
Mean (SD)	24.9 (28.7)	7.3 (18.5)	24.7 (28.0)	26.9 (33.0)		
No.	1 105	803	3 580	3 986		
Per package food					0.30 (0.17, 0.51)	−70
Mean (SD)	30.8 (69.7)	7.7 (32.1)	28.8 (73.5)	24.1 (53.8)		
No.	4 289	2 206	15 519	15 757		
Sodium (milligrams)						
Per serving food and beverage					0.81 (0.57, 1.14)	NS
Mean (SD)	78.6 (119.6)	66.1 (109.0)	85.1 (170.6)	88.9 (163.7)		
No.	5 543	3 142	19 608	20 506		
Per serving beverage					0.47 (0.28, 0.81)	−53
Mean (SD)	97.3 (99.8)	45.0 (76.1)	90.6 (99.6)	88.9 (99.5)		
No.	1 115	812	3 667	4 081		
Per serving food					0.94 (0.64, 1.37)	NS
Mean (SD)	73.9 (123.7)	73.4 (117.5)	83.9 (183.0)	88.9 (176.0)		
No.	4 428	2 330	15 941	16 425		
Per package food and beverage					0.60 (0.35, 1.04)	NS
Mean (SD)	271.0 (1202.1)	194.5 (447.6)	243.2 (892.9)	290.7 (1391.8)		
No.	5 435	3 062	19 178	20 142		

Continued

TABLE 1— Continued

	Berkeley, CA		Comparison Cities			
	Preimplementation	Postimplementation	Preimplementation	Postimplementation	b (95% CI)	% Change,[a] Berkeley vs Comparison
Per package beverage					0.95 (0.41, 2.21)	NS
Mean (SD)	110.1 (109.5)	108.7 (277.3)	103.6 (136.2)	107.3 (237.4)		
No.	1 110	801	3 576	3 994		
Per package food					0.59 (0.33, 1.05)	NS
Mean (SD)	312.3 (1343.3)	224.8 (490.6)	275.2 (985.0)	336.0 (1546.6)		
No.	4 325	2 261	15 602	16 148		
Saturated fat (grams)						
Per serving food and beverage					0.59 (0.44, 0.79)	−41
Mean (SD)	2.0 (2.7)	1.2 (2.0)	2.0 (2.8)	2.0 (2.8)		
No.	5 536	3 148	19 589	20 486		
Per serving beverage					1.85 (0.28, 12.00)	NS
Mean (SD)	0.2 (0.7)	0.1 (0.4)	0.2 (0.7)	< 0.1 (0.3)		
No.	1 115	819	3 684	4 087		
Per serving food					0.62 (0.46, 0.83)	−38
Mean (SD)	2.4 (2.8)	1.5 (2.2)	2.4 (2.9)	2.4 (2.9)		
No.	4 421	2 329	15 905	16 399		
Per package food and beverage					0.65 (0.43, 0.96)	−35
Mean (SD)	6.8 (16.5)	4.3 (10.0)	5.2 (12.1)	5.0 (12.4)		
No.	5 427	3 061	19 155	20 128		
Per package beverage					3.72 (0.33, 42.02)	NS
Mean (SD)	0.4 (3.4)	0.4 (3.2)	0.3 (2.8)	0.1 (1.7)		
No.	1 110	801	3 589	4 006		
Per package food					0.67 (0.45, 1.00)	NS
Mean (SD)	8.5 (18.1)	5.6 (11.1)	6.3 (13.1)	6.2 (13.6)		
No.	4 317	2 260	15 566	16 122		
Fiber (grams)						
Per serving food and beverage					1.47 (1.05, 2.06)	47
Mean (SD)	0.8 (1.4)	1.3 (2.4)	0.7 (1.4)	0.8 (1.5)		
No.	5 568	3 149	19 840	20 623		
Per serving beverage					1.91 (0.38, 9.56)	NS
Mean (SD)	< 0.1 (0.2)	< 0.1 (0.3)	< 0.1 (0.4)	< 0.1 (0.3)		
No.	1 115	815	3 684	4 093		

Continued

TABLE 1— Continued

	Berkeley, CA		Comparison Cities			
	Preimplementation	Postimplementation	Preimplementation	Postimplementation	b (95% CI)	% Change,[a] Berkeley vs Comparison
Per serving food					1.56 (1.13, 2.15)	56
Mean (SD)	1.0 (1.5)	1.7 (2.6)	0.9 (1.5)	0.9 (1.6)		
No.	4 453	2 334	16 156	16 530		
Per package food and beverage					1.28 (0.88, 1.87)	NS
Mean (SD)	3.0 (7.3)	4.4 (9.2)	2.0 (5.7)	2.2 (6.3)		
No.	5 441	3 064	19 242	20 170		
Per package beverage					1.20 (0.28, 5.11)	NS
Mean (SD)	0.1 (0.8)	0.2 (1.0)	0.1 (0.8)	0.1 (1.1)		
No.	1 110	803	3 590	4 012		
Per package food					1.36 (0.95, 1.95)	NS
Mean (SD)	3.8 (8.0)	5.9 (10.3)	2.4 (6.2)	2.8 (6.9)		
No.	4 331	2 261	15 652	16 158		
Calories (kilocalories)						
Per serving food and beverage					0.73 (0.60, 0.88)	−27
Mean (SD)	115.7 (94.9)	85.9 (87.9)	113.4 (96.4)	115.8 (95.0)		
No.	5 550	3 135	19 657	20 525		
Per serving beverage					0.42 (0.23, 0.78)	−58
Mean (SD)	101.8 (103.1)	42.7 (72.8)	103.7 (103.5)	102.6 (100.4)		
No.	1 115	813	3 684	4 089		
Per serving food					0.82 (0.69, 0.99)	−18
Mean (SD)	119.1 (92.4)	101.1 (87.7)	115.6 (94.6)	119.1 (93.4)		
No.	4 435	2 322	15 973	16 436		
Per package food and beverage					0.88 (0.65, 1.19)	NS
Mean (SD)	413.7 (622.1)	355.4 (561.1)	334.9 (537.5)	328.0 (508.7)		
No.	5 441	3 063	19 227	20 161		
Per package beverage					0.71 (0.34, 1.49)	NS
Mean (SD)	122.3 (147.1)	86.3 (196.8)	119.7 (136.4)	118.1 (143.2)		
No.	1 110	802	3 593	4 002		
Per package food					0.93 (0.69, 1.26)	NS
Mean (SD)	488.4 (673.3)	450.8 (614.8)	384.3 (581.3)	380.0 (551.5)		
No.	4 331	2 261	15 634	16 159		

Note. CI = confidence interval; NS = not significant. The sample size was n = 49 403. Variation in cell sizes between nutrients is attributable to missing data for some nutrients. Variation in cell sizes between the main outcome (per serving) and sensitivity analyses (per package of food-and-beverage facings) is attributable to missing data in the servings per package variable.

[a]% change calculated as (b−1)×100 for b < 1.0 and (1−b)×100 for b ≥ 1.0.

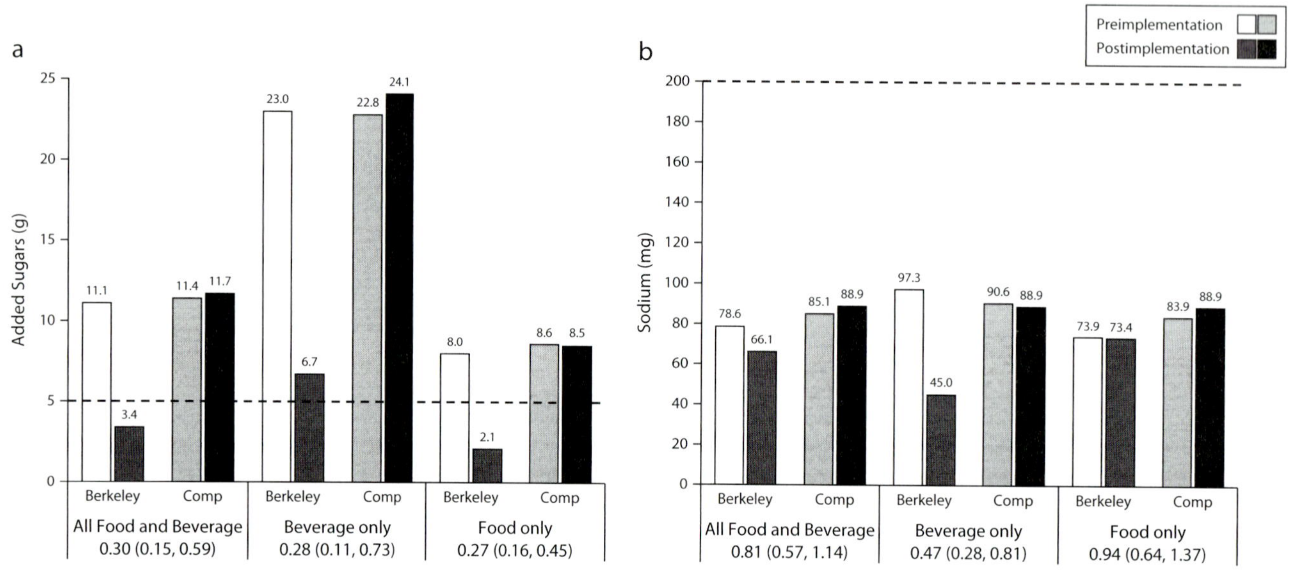

FIGURE 1— Mean (a) Added Sugars and (b) Sodium Content of Food and Beverage Products at Retail Checkouts Before and After Implementation of the Healthy Checkout Ordinance in Berkeley, California, and Comparison Cities (Comp): 2021–2022

Note. Difference-in-differences models were used to determine the significance of nutrient changes compared to comparison cities, reported as b (95% confidence interval). Dotted lines indicate the maximum content of added sugars (5 grams) and sodium (200 mg) per serving of food products permitted at checkout by the Berkeley Healthy Checkout Ordinance.

47% and 25% of the increase in fiber, respectively. The sodium reduction in beverage facings was driven by the removal of regular and diet energy drinks, which accounted for 44% and 26% of the reduction, respectively.

The pattern of results for saturated fat, but not fiber or calories, was similar in sensitivity analyses examining changes per package of food and beverage facings (Table 1). There was a 35% reduction (95% CI = −57%, −4%) in saturated fat content per package of food and beverage facings displayed at checkout in Berkeley relative to comparison cities (b = 0.65; 95% CI = 0.43, 0.96). However, there were no statistically significant changes in fiber or calories per package of food and beverage facings at checkout in Berkeley relative to comparison cities. For fiber, the lack of significant increase per package was attributable to the large proportion of products that were gum and mints. After excluding these products, there was a significant 57% increase (95% CI = 9%, 124%) in fiber per package in Berkeley relative to comparison cities (b = 1.57; 95% CI = 1.09, 2.24). For calories, the lack of significant reduction per package was attributable to the larger package sizes (i.e., more servings per package) of healthier compliant products, including nuts, seeds, and whole grains. In a sensitivity analysis excluding these products, there was a significant 41% reduction (95% CI = −55%, −22%) in calories per package in Berkeley relative to comparison cities (b = 0.59; 95% CI = 0.45, 0.78).

Results did not vary substantially when we restricted the sample to the 41 145 food and beverage facings with exact nutrient data (Table B, available as a supplement to the online version of this article at https://ajph.org). However, there were 2 differences for secondary outcomes: saturated fat per package and calories per serving. The reductions in saturated fat per package of food and beverage facings and calories per serving of food displayed at checkout in Berkeley relative to comparison cities were no longer statistically significant, but the magnitude of change was similar to when including the full sample. Thus, these differences may be attributable to a loss in power from restricting the sample.

Primary Outcomes by Store Type

One-year changes in added sugars and sodium per serving of food and beverage facings at checkouts varied by store type (Figure 2, Table 2). Relative to comparison checkouts, in Berkeley checkouts, there were reductions in added sugars content per serving of food and beverage facings by 97% (95% CI = −98%, −94%) in chain

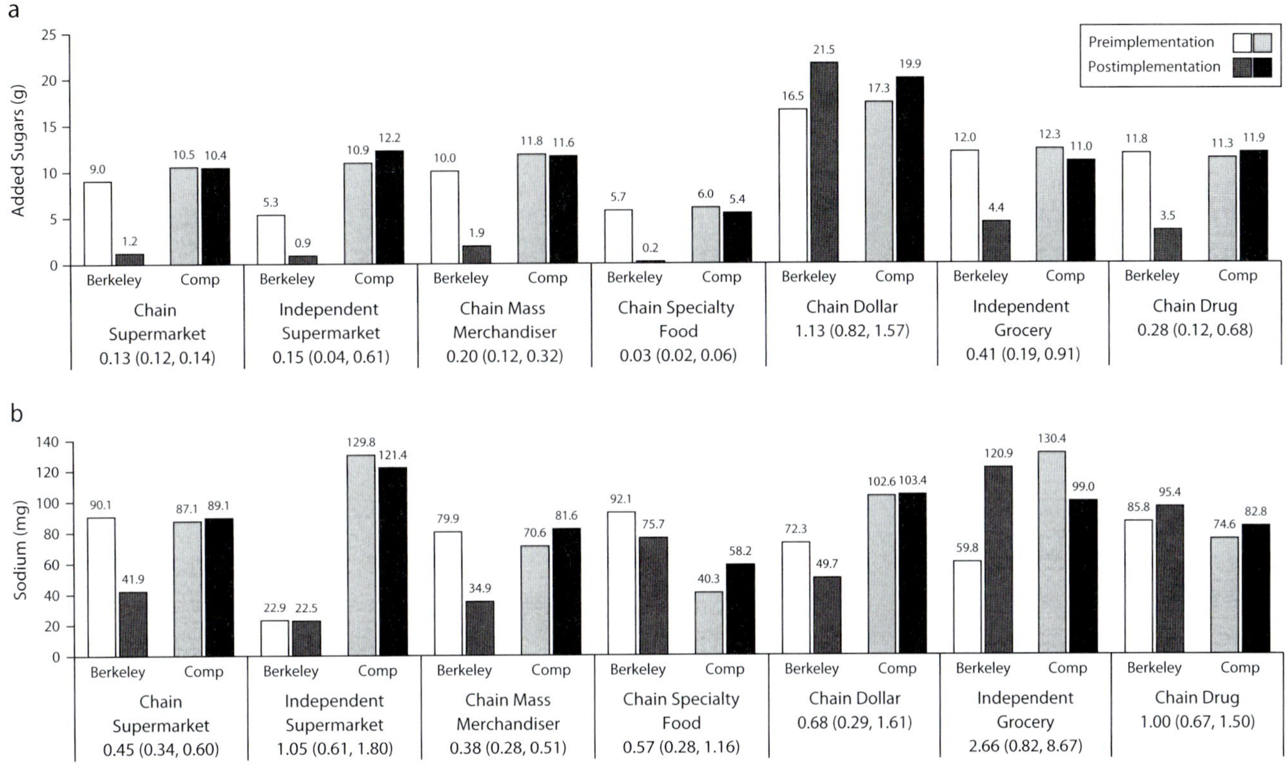

FIGURE 2— Mean (a) Added Sugars and (b) Sodium Content of Food and Beverage Products at Retail Checkouts by Store Type Before and After Implementation of the Healthy Checkout Ordinance in Berkeley, California, and Comparison Cities (Comp): 2021–2022

Note. Difference-in-differences models were used to determine the significance of nutrient changes compared to comparison cities, reported as b (95% confidence interval).

specialty food stores (b = 0.03; 95% CI = 0.02, 0.06), 87% (95% CI = −88%, −86%) in chain supermarkets (b = 0.13; 95% CI = 0.12, 0.14), 85% (95% CI = −96%, −39%) in independent supermarkets (b = 0.15; 95% CI = 0.04, 0.61), 80% (95% CI = −88%, −68%) in chain mass merchandisers (b = 0.20; 95% CI = 0.12, 0.32), 72% (95% CI = −88%, −32%) in chain drug stores (b = 0.28; 95% CI = 0.12, 0.68), and 59% (95% CI = −81%, −9%) in independent grocery stores (b = 0.41; 95% CI = 0.19, 0.91). There was no statistically significant change in added sugars content per serving of food and beverage facings displayed in chain dollar store checkouts in Berkeley relative to comparison cities. This was driven by 1 of 2 dollar stores in Berkeley, which reduced the number of food and beverage facings at sampled checkouts (275–148 facings) but did not reduce the added sugars content of the foods and beverage facings at checkout (24.4–27.9 grams per serving).

Relative to comparison checkouts, in Berkeley checkouts, there were reductions in sodium content per serving of food and beverage facings by 62% (95% CI = −72%, −49%) in chain mass merchandisers (b = =0.38; 95% CI = 0.28, 0.51) and 55% (95% CI = −66%, −40%) in chain supermarkets (b = 0.45; 95% CI = 0.34, 0.60). There were no statistically significant changes in sodium content per serving of food and beverage facings in other store types.

DISCUSSION

To our knowledge, this study is the first to quantify changes in the nutrient content of food and beverage facings available at retail checkouts before and after a healthy checkout policy. Roughly 1 year after the Berkeley HCO was implemented, there was a 42% reduction in the number of food and beverage facings available at sampled checkouts. Among the remaining food and beverage facings that were available at Berkeley checkouts, there were significant reductions in the added sugars and saturated fat content per serving of food and beverage facings, a significant reduction in sodium per serving of beverage facings, and a significant increase in fiber per serving of

TABLE 2— Added Sugar and Sodium per Serving of Food and Beverage Products at Retail Checkouts Before and After Implementation of the Berkeley Healthy Checkout Ordinance by Store Type: Berkeley, California, and Comparison Cities, 2021–2022

	Berkeley, CA		Comparison Cities		b (95% CI)	% Change,[a] Berkeley vs Comparison
	Preimplementation	Postimplementation	Preimplementation	Postimplementation		
Added sugars (grams)						
Chain supermarket					0.13 (0.12, 0.14)	−87
Mean (SD)	9.0 (15.6)	1.2 (4.6)	10.5 (15.9)	10.4 (15.8)		
No.	538	602	6131	6360		
Independent supermarket					0.15 (0.04, 0.61)	−85
Mean (SD)	5.3 (8.3)	0.9 (1.6)	10.9 (14.3)	12.2 (14.5)		
No.	319	295	1597	1602		
Chain mass merchandiser					0.20 (0.12, 0.32)	−80
Mean (SD)	10.0 (16.3)	1.9 (5.4)	11.8 (18.1)	11.6 (19.4)		
No.	895	464	2503	2330		
Chain specialty food					0.02 (0.02, 0.06)	−97
Mean (SD)	5.7 (6.3)	0.2 (0.7)	6.0 (7.8)	5.4 (7.2)		
No.	461	317	1027	1277		
Chain dollar					1.13 (0.82, 1.57)	NS
Mean (SD)	16.5 (19.9)	21.5 (27.4)	17.3 (21.2)	19.9 (22.8)		
No.	857	191	1702	1755		
Independent grocery					0.41 (0.19, 0.91)	−59
Mean (SD)	12.0 (10.5)	4.4 (9.8)	12.3 (10.9)	11.0 (10.4)		
No.	280	185	647	805		
Chain drug					0.28 (0.12, 0.68)	−72
Mean (SD)	11.8 (15.3)	3.5 (9.6)	11.3 (14.2)	11.9 (14.7)		
No.	2148	1081	5987	5985		
Sodium (milligrams)						
Chain supermarket					0.45 (0.34, 0.60)	−55
Mean (SD)	90.1 (128.9)	41.9 (90.4)	87.1 (144.9)	89.1 (138.5)		
No.	543	603	6137	6491		
Independent supermarket					1.05 (0.61, 1.80)	NS
Mean (SD)	22.9 (42.7)	22.5 (50.7)	129.8 (278.3)	121.4 (246.1)		
No.	327	307	1650	1728		

Continued

TABLE 2— Continued

	Berkeley, CA		Comparison Cities		b (95% CI)	% Change,[a] Berkeley vs Comparison
	Preimplementation	Postimplementation	Preimplementation	Postimplementation		
Chain mass merchandiser					0.38 (0.28, 0.51)	−62
Mean (SD)	79.9 (101.6)	34.9 (64.3)	70.6 (109.5)	81.6 (126.5)		
No.	897	464	2467	2314		
Chain specialty food					0.57 (0.28, 1.16)	NS
Mean (SD)	92.1 (119.3)	75.7 (119.6)	40.3 (76.7)	58.2 (94.0)		
No.	477	296	1026	1283		
Chain dollar					0.68 (0.29, 1.61)	NS
Mean (SD)	72.3 (102.9)	49.7 (100.6)	102.6 (267.5)	103.4 (267.1)		
No.	854	188	1660	1801		
Independent grocery					2.66 (0.82, 8.67)	NS
Mean (SD)	59.8 (76.0)	120.9 (172.6)	130.4 (255.3)	99.0 (215.0)		
No.	294	200	672	872		
Chain drug					1.00 (0.67, 1.50)	NS
Mean (SD)	85.8 (139.0)	95.4 (116.5)	74.6 (133.8)	82.8 (128.6)		
No.	2151	1084	5996	6017		

Note. CI = confidence interval; NS = not significant. The sample size was n = 49 403.
[a]% change calculated as (b−1)×100 for b < 1.0 and (1−b)×100 for b ≥ 1.0.

food and beverage facings. There was also a significant reduction in calorie content per serving. These findings are consistent with a previous evaluation of Berkeley HCO compliance, which found decreased presence of noncompliant products like SSBs, candy, and other sweets, along with increased presence of both nonfood and nonbeverage products and compliant food and beverage facings at checkout.[20]

The reduction in candy and SSB availability at checkout was responsible for most of the reduction in added sugars. SSBs were often replaced by unsweetened beverages like water, sparkling water, and coconut water.[20] Though the Berkeley HCO prohibits products with nonsugar sweeteners at checkout, previous work did not find a significant reduction in the presence of these products at checkout.[20] Future research should assess reasons for retailer noncompliance.

Though Berkeley's HCO intended to limit sodium at checkout, significant reductions were only seen in the sodium content per serving of beverage facings. This was because of a floor effect (only 9% of food facings in Berkeley checkout areas were high in sodium before implementation) and the lack of a significant decrease in noncompliant salty snacks in Berkeley checkouts.[20] Though the sodium standard set by the Berkeley HCO did not significantly decrease sodium at checkout, it did prevent the potential unintended consequence of replacing high-added-sugars products with high-sodium products.

We also examined changes in the nutrients saturated fat and fiber, which are not limited by the HCO, as well as calories. In Berkeley, relative to comparison checkouts after the HCO, there was a significant reduction in saturated fat at checkout, explained by a 38% reduction per serving of food facings, and a significant increase in fiber at checkout, explained by a 56% increase in the fiber content per serving of food facings. This increase in fiber is largely attributed to increased nuts, which are naturally high in fiber and were more frequently placed at checkout after the HCO.[20] There was also a significant relative reduction in calories, explained by a large (58%) reduction in calories per serving of beverage facings and, to a lesser extent, an 18% reduction in calories per serving of food facings. When we examined saturated fat, fiber, and calories per package (i.e., the whole product the shopper takes home), there were no significant changes. For fiber, this was explained by the high prevalence of gum and mints, and for calories, this was explained by package sizes of healthier products (e.g., nuts, seeds, whole grains) being particularly large.

The HCO nutritional standards used a hybrid approach, limiting added sugars and sodium and restricting to mostly health-promoting food groups at checkout.[15] Though we examined additional nutrients and calories as secondary outcomes, it should be noted that calorie content may not be a good indicator of the nutritional quality of some foods, such as nuts and seeds.

The earlier evaluation of the Berkeley HCO took a whole-food approach, finding a significant increase in the presence of healthy food and beverage facings and nonfood items, and a decrease in unhealthy items available at checkout.[20] The current study builds on these results, focusing on changes in specific nutrients that are overconsumed by the US population. Roughly two thirds of US adults overconsume added sugars, up to 97% overconsume sodium, three quarters overconsume saturated fat, and up to 97% underconsume fiber,[22] increasing risk of chronic diseases, including heart disease, type 2 diabetes, and certain cancers.[22,23] Fiber plays a key role in satiety, regulating blood sugar levels, and maintaining healthy cholesterol levels.[22] Promoting nutrient-dense, fiber-rich foods via HCOs may encourage healthier purchasing and consumption patterns, potentially reducing diet-related chronic disease burdens.

HCOs may be an especially helpful intervention to counteract high consumption of added sugars, which is increasing globally, particularly in the form of SSBs.[24] By limiting added sugars at checkout, HCOs could reduce the purchase and consumption of high-sugar items, though these behavioral outcomes have not yet been evaluated under a mandatory HCO. An evaluation of voluntary but meaningful healthy checkout restrictions in the United Kingdom found fewer purchases of the sweets and salty snacks previously available at checkout.[25] In the United States, no chain has voluntarily adopted meaningful healthy checkout restrictions, and incentive-based healthy retail programs are often resource-intensive and include a small number of stores.[26] By contrast, mandatory healthy checkout policies like Berkeley's HCO can have broad population reach. Future research should examine the impact of HCOs on consumer purchases and explore public perceptions of these policies. Given that public support for healthy retail initiatives varies,[27] potentially because of how they are framed, understanding how consumers respond to HCOs could help inform future policy design, adoption, and implementation strategies.

Regarding changes by store type, all store types except dollar stores significantly reduced added sugars content per serving of food and beverage facing, with the largest reductions observed in chain specialty food stores, supermarkets, and chain mass merchandisers. The overall number of food and beverage facings at checkout decreased after implementation,[20] and some remaining food and beverage products, particularly at dollar stores, remained high in added sugar. Because there were only 2 dollar stores in this study sample, further research is needed to better understand how HCO implementation differs by store type. However, previous research has documented issues in dollar stores, like understocked shelves, understaffing, and local managers with limited authority, that could pose barriers to compliance with local food policies.[28,29] In contrast to added sugars, for sodium, only chain mass merchandisers and chain supermarkets reduced sodium content per serving of food and beverage facings at checkout. Additional research[30] is needed on the Berkeley HCO implementation and enforcement process to better understand variation by store types.

Limitations and Strengths

Limitations of this study include having neither data before 2021 to test the parallel trends assumption for difference-in-differences models nor monthly data to examine fluctuations in policy impact. We also only assessed a sample (not a census) of checkouts in each store. Nonetheless, this study has several strengths, including the use of an objective and reliable tool to assess food and beverage characteristics and the inclusion of comparison cities to ensure that changes observed in Berkeley were not attributable to larger market trends. In addition, the large sample size of more than 49 000 food and beverage facings, linked with nutritional information, and the near census of stores subject to the policy provide robust data.

Public Health Implications

Healthy checkout policies can meaningfully improve the healthfulness of retail food environments at checkout. The overall healthfulness of food environments may further be improved by combining healthy checkout policies with other product placement efforts (e.g., healthy aisle endcaps and front-of-store displays), as has been done in the United Kingdom,[25] and policies like front-of-package nutrient labels and SSB taxes that have catalyzed reformulation.[16,31,32] To potentially scale healthy product placement nationally, eligibility requirements for retailers authorized to accept Supplemental Nutrition Assistance Program (SNAP) benefits could be expanded.[33,34] SNAP retailer requirements, which include stocking a variety of staple foods, could additionally require nutrition standards for prominently placed products, thus reducing promotion of and exposure to nutrients of concern in these stores.[34,35] Because the majority of food retailers are SNAP-authorized, a healthy product placement requirement could improve food environments for most households in the United States. AJPH

ABOUT THE AUTHORS

Alexandria E. Reimold, Kris Jayme G. Matas, and Jennifer Falbe are with the Department of Human Ecology, University of California, Davis. Ethan C. Wolf is with Community Health Sciences, School of Public Health, University of California, Berkeley. Samantha Marinello, Lisa M. Powell, and Rebecca M. Schermbeck are with the Institute for Health Research and Policy, School of Public Health, University of Illinois Chicago.

CORRESPONDENCE

Correspondence should be sent to Dr Alexandria E. Reimold, One Shields Ave, Davis, CA 95616 (e-mail: areimold@ucdavis.edu). Reprints can be ordered at https://ajph.org by clicking the "Reprints" link.

PUBLICATION INFORMATION

Full Citation: Reimold AE, Wolf EC, Matas KJG, et al. Impacts of a healthy checkout ordinance on added sugars, sodium, and other nutrients at checkout 1 year after implementation: Berkeley, California, 2021–2022. *Am J Public Health*. 2025; 115(10):1700–1712.

Acceptance Date: April 13, 2025.

DOI: https://doi.org/10.2105/AJPH.2025.308159

ORCID iDs:

Alexandria E. Reimold https://orcid.org/0000-0001-9777-7825

Ethan C. Wolf https://orcid.org/0009-0006-2093-0696

Kris Jayme G. Matas https://orcid.org/0000-0003-4996-7661

Jennifer Falbe https://orcid.org/0000-0002-8405-4326

CONTRIBUTORS

J. Falbe conceptualized this study, and J. Falbe and L. M. Powell designed it. A. E. Reimold and J. Falbe led the analysis and interpretation of the data and agreed to be accountable for all aspects of the work. A. E. Reimold drafted the article. All authors contributed to the acquisition, preparation, or interpretation of the data; provided critical feedback; and gave final approvals for the final version of this article.

ACKNOWLEDGMENTS

This research was supported by grant 2020-85774 from Bloomberg Philanthropies' Food Policy Program (https://www.bloomberg.org) and the National Institute of Diabetes and Digestive and Kidney Diseases (award R01DK135099).

Note. The content is solely the responsibility of the authors and does not necessarily represent the official views of Bloomberg Philanthropies or the National Institutes of Health.

CONFLICTS OF INTEREST

The authors report no conflicts of interest.

HUMAN PARTICIPANT PROTECTION

This study was determined to be not human participant research by the University of California, Davis institutional review board; thus, institutional review board review was waived (1760676).

REFERENCES

1. Karpyn A, McCallops K, Wolgast H, Glanz K. Improving consumption and purchases of healthier foods in retail environments: a systematic review. *Int J Environ Res Public Health*. 2020;17(20):7524. https://doi.org/10.3390/ijerph17207524
2. Mah CL, Luongo G, Hasdell R, Taylor NGA, Lo BK. A systematic review of the effect of retail food environment interventions on diet and health with a focus on the enabling role of public policies. *Curr Nutr Rep*. 2019;8(4):411–428. https://doi.org/10.1007/s13668-019-00295-z
3. Cameron AJ, Charlton E, Ngan WW, Sacks G. A systematic review of the effectiveness of supermarket-based interventions involving product, promotion, or place on the healthiness of consumer purchases. *Curr Nutr Rep*. 2016; 5(3):129–138. https://doi.org/10.1007/s13668-016-0172-8
4. Falbe J, White JS, Sigala DM, Grummon AH, Solar SE, Powell LM. The potential for healthy checkout policies to advance nutrition equity. *Nutrients*. 2021;13(11):4181. https://doi.org/10.3390/nu13114181
5. Falbe J, Marinello S, Wolf EC, et al. Food and beverage environments at store checkouts in California: mostly unhealthy products. *Curr Dev Nutr*. 2023;7(6):100075. https://doi.org/10.1016/j.cdnut.2023.100075
6. Houghtaling B, Holston D, Szocs C, Penn J, Qi D, Hedrick V. A rapid review of stocking and marketing practices used to sell sugar-sweetened beverages in US food stores. *Obes Rev*. 2021;22(4):e13179. https://doi.org/10.1111/obr.13179
7. Petimar J, Moran AJ, Grummon AH, et al. In-store marketing and supermarket purchases: associations overall and by transaction SNAP status. *Am J Prev Med*. 2023;65(4):587–595. https://doi.org/10.1016/j.amepre.2023.02.029
8. Cohen DA, Collins R, Hunter G, Ghosh-Dastidar B, Dubowitz T. Store impulse marketing strategies and body mass index. *Am J Public Health*. 2015; 105(7):1446–1452. https://doi.org/10.2105/AJPH.2014.302220
9. Yang Q, Zhang Z, Gregg EW, Flanders WD, Merritt R, Hu FB. Added sugar intake and cardiovascular diseases mortality among US adults. *JAMA Intern Med*. 2014;174(4):516–524. https://doi.org/10.1001/jamainternmed.2013.13563
10. Malik VS, Hu FB. Sweeteners and risk of obesity and type 2 diabetes: the role of sugar-sweetened beverages. *Curr Diab Rep*. 2012;12(2):195–203. https://doi.org/10.1007/s11892-012-0259-6
11. Malta D, Petersen KS, Johnson C, et al. High sodium intake increases blood pressure and risk of kidney disease. From the Science of Salt: a regularly updated systematic review of salt and health outcomes (August 2016 to March 2017). *J Clin Hypertens (Greenwich)*. 2018;20(12): 1654–1665. https://doi.org/10.1111/jch.13408
12. Falbe J, Cotterman C, Linchey J, Madsen KA. Ethnic disparities in trends in high BMI among California adolescents, 2003–2012. *Am J Prev Med*. 2016;51(2):e45–e55. https://doi.org/10.1016/j.amepre.2016.02.010
13. Marinello S, Powell LM, Falbe J. Neighborhood sociodemographic characteristics and healthfulness of store checkouts in Northern California. *Prev Med Rep*. 2023;35:102379. https://doi.org/10.1016/j.pmedr.2023.102379

14. Zenk SN, Powell LM, Rimkus L, et al. Relative and absolute availability of healthier food and beverage alternatives across communities in the United States. *Am J Public Health.* 2014;104(11):2170–2178. https://doi.org/10.2105/AJPH.2014.302113
15. Ch. 9.82 Healthy Checkout. Berkeley Municipal Code. Available at: https://berkeley.municipal.codes/BMC/9.82. Accessed November 11, 2024.
16. Davis JN, Goon S, Gouck J, et al. An inventory of proposed and enacted sugar-sweetened beverage policies at the state, local, and tribal levels in the United States, 2014–2023. *Am J Public Health.* 2024;114(12):1344–1353. https://doi.org/10.2105/ajph.2024.307855
17. Hawkes C, Jewell J, Allen K. A food policy package for healthy diets and the prevention of obesity and diet-related non-communicable diseases: the NOURISHING framework. *Obes Rev.* 2013;14 (suppl 2):159–168. https://doi.org/10.1111/obr.12098
18. World Cancer Research Fund. NOURISHING and MOVING policy databases. Available at: https://policydatabase.wcrf.org. Accessed February 4, 2025.
19. Scheider H. Roadmap and Tool Kit for a Healthy Checkout Ordinance. Center for Science in the Public Interest. October 2022. Available at: https://www.cspinet.org/sites/default/files/2023-01/HealthyCheckoutCaseStudy_v2_oct2022.pdf. Accessed November 18, 2024.
20. Falbe J, Marinello S, Wolf EC, Solar S, Powell LM. Food environment after implementation of a healthy checkout policy. *JAMA Netw Open.* 2024; 7(8):e2421731. https://doi.org/10.1001/jamanetworkopen.2024.21731
21. Powell LM, Li Y, Solar SE, Pipito AA, Wolf EC, Falbe J. Development and reliability testing of the Store CheckOUt Tool (SCOUT) for use in healthy checkout evaluations. Policy, Practice and Prevention Research Center, University of Illinois at Chicago. March 2022. Available at: https://p3rc.uic.edu/wp-content/uploads/sites/561/2022/04/Powell_Mar-2022_RsrchBrf-No.-125_Dvlpmnt-Rlblty-SCOUT-for-Hlthy-Chckt-Evltns.pdf. Accessed November 11, 2024.
22. US Department of Agriculture and US Department of Health and Human Services. *Dietary Guidelines for Americans, 2020–2025.* 2020. Available at: https://www.dietaryguidelines.gov. Accessed November 11, 2024.
23. Mokdad AH, Ballestros K, Echko M, US Burden of Disease Collaborators, et al. The state of US health, 1990–2016: burden of diseases, injuries, and risk factors among US states. *JAMA.* 2018;319(14): 1444–1472. https://doi.org/10.1001/jama.2018.0158
24. Lara-Castor L, Micha R, Cudhea F, Global Dietary Database, et al. Intake of sugar sweetened beverages among children and adolescents in 185 countries between 1990 and 2018: population based study. *BMJ.* 2024;386:e079234. https://doi.org/10.1136/bmj-2024-079234
25. Ejlerskov KT, Sharp SJ, Stead M, Adamson AJ, White M, Adams J. Supermarket policies on less-healthy food at checkouts: natural experimental evaluation using interrupted time series analyses of purchases. *PLoS Med.* 2018;15(12):e1002712. https://doi.org/10.1371/journal.pmed.1002712
26. Minkler M, Estrada J, Dyer S, Hennessey-Lavery S, Wakimoto P, Falbe J. Healthy retail as a strategy for improving food security and the built environment in San Francisco. *Am J Public Health.* 2019; 109(suppl 2):S137–S140. https://doi.org/10.2105/AJPH.2019.305000
27. Gómez-Donoso C, Sacks G, Vanderlee L, et al. Public support for healthy supermarket initiatives focused on product placement: a multi-country cross-sectional analysis of the 2018 International Food Policy Study. *Int J Behav Nutr Phys Act.* 2021;18(1):78. https://doi.org/10.1186/s12966-021-01149-0
28. Reimold AE, Hall MG, Ng SW, et al. "The dollar store got it going on": understanding food shopping patterns and policy preferences among dollar store shoppers with low incomes. *Curr Dev Nutr.* 2024;8(10):104457. https://doi.org/10.1016/j.cdnut.2024.104457
29. Vargas TL. Consumer redlining and the reproduction of inequality at Dollar General. *Qual Sociol.* 2021;44(2):205–229. https://doi.org/10.1007/s11133-020-09473-w
30. Smith NR, Levy DE, Falbe J, Purtle J, Chriqui JF. Design considerations for developing measures of policy implementation in quantitative evaluations of public health policy. *Front Health Serv.* 2024;4:1322702. https://doi.org/10.3389/frhs.2024.1322702
31. Roberto CA, Ng SW, Ganderats-Fuentes M, et al. The influence of front-of-package nutrition labeling on consumer behavior and product reformulation. *Annu Rev Nutr.* 2021;41:529–550. https://doi.org/10.1146/annurev-nutr-111120-094932
32. Andreyeva T, Marple K, Marinello S, Moore TE, Powell LM. Outcomes following taxation of sugar-sweetened beverages. *JAMA Netw Open.* 2022;5(6):e2215276. https://doi.org/10.1001/jamanetworkopen.2022.15276
33. Food and Nutrition Service. Food and Nutrition Service invests in SNAP integrity and modernization. Available at: https://web.archive.org/web/20241111070236/https://www.fns.usda.gov/news-item/fns-017.23. Accessed October 31, 2024.
34. John S, Johnson J, Nelms A, Bresnahan C, Tucker AC, Wolfson JA. Recommendations to Promote Healthy Retail Food Environments: Key Federal Policy Opportunities for the Farm Bill. 2023. Available at: https://www.cspinet.org/resource/report-title-recommendations-promote-healthy-retail-food-environments. Accessed October 31, 2024.
35. Thorndike AN, Sunstein CR. Obesity prevention in the supermarket—choice architecture and the Supplemental Nutrition Assistance Program. *Am J Public Health.* 2017;107(10):1582–1583. https://doi.org/10.2105/AJPH.2017.303991

Changes in Abortion Access, Travel, and Costs Since the Implementation of State Abortion Bans, 2022–2024

Nancy F. Berglas, DrPH, Jessica T. Barnes, MSW, Elizabeth Gonzalez, BA, Lisa Peters, MPH, and Diana Greene Foster, PhD

See also Hansen and Darney, p. 1564.

Objectives. To compare the experiences of people who obtained abortions before the implementation of a state abortion ban with those seeking abortion after a ban.

Methods. Using self-administered surveys (n = 855), we examined the abortion-seeking experiences of individuals recruited from clinics and call centers in 14 US states that implemented bans on abortion at all gestations, June 2022 to June 2024. We used bivariate analyses to compare differences in travel by ban status.

Results. Most people (81%) who contacted a clinic or call center after a ban reported traveling to another state for an abortion; few (3%) continued their pregnancy to birth. Compared with those who accessed abortion in their state before a ban, postban travelers were less likely to drive and more likely to travel by bus, train, or airplane. Mean travel time (2.8 vs 11.3 hours), overnight stays (5% vs 58%), and mean travel costs ($179 vs $372) increased, as did mean pregnancy duration (7.7 vs 8.8 weeks) and the proportion occurring at 13 weeks or more duration (8% vs 17%).

Conclusions. Travel burdens, costs, and delays in abortion have increased since the implementation of state abortion bans. (*Am J Public Health*. 2025;115(10):1713–1722. https://doi.org/10.2105/AJPH.2025.308191)

AJPH October 2025, Vol. 115, No. 10

Since June 2022, when the US Supreme Court ended the federally protected right to abortion in *Dobbs v Jackson Women's Health Organization* (597 US 215 [2022]; hereafter *Dobbs*), 14 states have banned abortion at all stages of pregnancy and several other states have enacted gestational duration limits before viability.[1,2] These restrictions have created considerable barriers for people seeking to end their pregnancies. With the closure of multiple abortion facilities in the South and Midwest,[3] distance and travel time to the nearest abortion facility have greatly increased.[4,5] National data indicate that substantial numbers of people have traveled across state lines to get an abortion as the number of abortions plummeted in states with bans.[6–8]

The costs, delays, and logistical challenges associated with travel place substantial burdens on those seeking an abortion outside their home state and may prevent a considerable number of people from accessing care at all.[9] These burdens are greater for those who lack access to reliable transportation, do not have the resources to pay for travel, or cannot take time off work or find childcare, as well as for minors, undocumented immigrants, and people with limited mobility (e.g., individuals with disabilities and those who are incarcerated, under court supervision, or hospitalized).[10] People who are further along in their pregnancies have fewer options for facilities that can provide abortions and thus typically travel greater distances and at greater cost.[11] Financial strain is a common reason for seeking abortion care, and three quarters of abortion patients live at or below 200% of the federal poverty level.[12] Even those with financial resources may still experience increased financial insecurity because of the costs associated with travel or delays when pursuing abortion.

Since *Dobbs* was decided, alternative modalities to having an abortion at a brick-and-mortar facility have emerged that reduce barriers associated with travel. Telehealth provision now makes up about 20% of abortions,[7] and recent shield laws allow providers to prescribe medication abortion to those living in ban states.[13] Additionally, with increased awareness of websites and online communities related to abortion, some people choose to procure medication abortion online without assistance from medical professionals.[14,15] Yet, for those who are too far along in their pregnancy for medication abortion and those who prefer or need to get an abortion in a clinical setting, travel to brick-and-mortar abortion facilities remains necessary.

In the wake of *Dobbs*, several national and regional organizations—including abortion funds, practical support organizations, patient navigators, and call centers—have emerged or expanded to offer information and practical support to pregnant people living in states with abortion bans. These organizations may provide partial or full subsidies to cover the medical costs of abortion for people with lower incomes and may offer financial or logistical support for transportation, childcare, and lodging. Although increased funding for travel assistance has become available,[16] many people may lack the knowledge and awareness of how to access and use this funding. It is not clear how abortion seekers in the post-*Dobbs* landscape cover the financial burden of out-of-state travel between their own resources and support from personal connections and outside entities such as abortion funds.

Given this shifting context of both barriers and supports, we sought to document the experiences of people seeking abortion in the 2 years after the *Dobbs* decision across multiple states. In this analysis, we compared travel, costs, and pregnancy duration of pregnant people who obtained a clinic-based abortion in their home state just before a ban on abortion at all gestations was implemented with those who traveled out of state for an abortion after a ban was implemented.

METHODS

For the End of Roe Study, we used a longitudinal cohort design to compare the experiences of individuals who were unable to obtain a legal abortion in their home state after a ban took effect with the experiences of those whose abortions were legally permitted before a ban was implemented. Using self-administered web-based surveys, we asked participants to recount their experiences seeking abortion, pregnancy outcomes, and subsequent health and economic well-being every 2 months over a 2-year period.

We began the study in June 2022 at clinics in states with bans that went into effect in the months immediately after the *Dobbs* decision. Clinics forwarded study invitations to individuals who received an abortion during the 2 weeks before ban enforcement, as well as to those whose service was canceled or who contacted the clinic but could not be scheduled because of a change in the law. In 2023, we expanded recruitment to include call centers (i.e., hotlines or referral lines affiliated with groups of clinics) that connect individuals seeking abortion to available services. These sites provided study invitations to callers from ban states who were seeking an abortion. Study recruitment is ongoing. Our analysis focused on participants who enrolled in the study and completed the baseline survey from June 2022 through June 2024 and who lived in 1 of 14 states that banned abortion at all gestations during that period (Alabama, Arkansas, Idaho, Indiana, Kentucky, Louisiana, Mississippi, Missouri, Oklahoma, South Dakota, Tennessee, Texas, West Virginia, and Wisconsin).

Participant Recruitment

For the overall study, staff at 22 clinics and 4 clinic-affiliated call centers serving people in states with abortion bans identified eligible patients and callers and informed them about the study. Participants were eligible if they lived in a state with an abortion ban, were aged 15 years or older, spoke English or Spanish, and had access to a computer or smartphone to complete surveys online. Interested participants received a link via text or e-mail to the study landing page, where they could learn about the study, provide informed consent, and complete the baseline survey. The study team subsequently contacted participants by text or e-mail to complete follow-up surveys. Participants received up to 3 reminders for each survey. Participants received a $50 gift card for completing the baseline survey and a $25 gift card for completing each follow-up survey.

Measures

On the baseline survey, we included questions about participants' demographic and socioeconomic characteristics, including age, gender identity, race, ethnicity, socioeconomic status, and reproductive history, as well as experiences with their current pregnancy. On follow-up surveys, we asked participants how their pregnancy resolved (if not previously reported) and other study outcomes, including their ongoing economic situation, physical and mental health, and aspirations (not included in this analysis).

We asked all participants about their experiences considering and seeking an abortion. When a participant reported having had an abortion, we asked about travel time, mode of transportation, need for an overnight stay, out-of-pocket medical costs, travel costs, use of health insurance, and financial support received from a personal connection (e.g., the person they became pregnant with, a friend, or family) or organizational sources (e.g., an abortion fund). Participants reported their pregnancy duration at the time of their abortion and the type of abortion received (procedure or medication) and answered 10 dichotomous items about the factors that delayed them from getting an abortion sooner. Depending on when they were able to get an abortion, participants completed these questions on the baseline, 2-month, or 4-month survey.

To explore changes in the abortion access environment since *Dobbs* was decided, we categorized postban participants based on the 6-month period of their initial abortion appointment: June to December 2022, January to June 2023, July to December 2023, or January to June 2024.

Analyses

We compared the experiences of participants who received an abortion in their home state before a ban implementation (the "preban" sample) with those traveling to another state after a ban implementation (the "postban" sample).

We assessed summary statistics for continuous measures (travel time, cost of abortion and travel, and pregnancy duration at time of abortion) and examined frequencies of categorical measures (mode of transportation, need for an overnight stay, financial support, type of abortion). We conducted bivariate tests to examine unadjusted differences between the preban and postban groups using the *t* test for continuous and the χ^2 test for categorical variables, and we present confidence intervals for each group. In post hoc exploratory analyses, we looked at postban differences in travel outcomes over time in 6-month increments, using bivariate tests to analyze differences between the immediate (June–December 2022) and most recent (January–June 2024) postban periods. We conducted the statistical analyses using Stata version 17 (StataCorp, College Station, TX).

Travel data were unavailable for 24% of the postban sample, who reported their abortion without answering travel questions because of an earlier iteration of the survey flow (Figure 1). We compared characteristics of those who were missing versus reporting postban travel data and found the groups were similar in age, ethnicity, gender identity, education, employment, income, and reproductive history; however, those who were missing travel data were more likely to be Black, less likely to be White, and more likely to have received government assistance in the previous month (data not shown).

RESULTS

We first present the pregnancy outcomes among all study participants and then compare the experiences of those who received an abortion before versus after the implementation of a state ban.

Pregnancy Outcomes

As of the end of June 2024, 855 residents of 14 states with abortion bans at all gestations enrolled in the study and completed the baseline survey. Of those, 196 participants received an abortion before a ban took effect, and 659 participants had their appointments canceled or contacted clinics or call centers after a ban implementation. Among those seeking abortion after a ban, 536 (of 659; 81%) received a clinic-based abortion in another state, 8 (1%) self-managed an abortion with medication abortion pills procured online, 26 (4%) reported a miscarriage, 1 (< 1%) reported an ectopic pregnancy, none reported a stillbirth, and 19 (3%) reported a live birth. An additional 16 (2%) reported they were no longer pregnant but did not provide details on how the pregnancy ended. Pregnancy outcomes were unavailable for 53 participants (8%). Thus, among those seeking an abortion after a state ban, between 3% and 11% (if all those with missing data carried to term) continued their pregnancies to birth (Figure 1).

Participants Who Received Abortions

Participants who received a clinic-based abortion before versus after the implementation of a state ban were demographically similar by age group, race, gender identity, education, receipt of government assistance, income, and pregnancy history. Those receiving abortions after a ban were slightly older (mean 26.3 vs 27.8 years), more likely to identify as Latina (13% vs 31%), less likely to be employed (75% vs 62%),

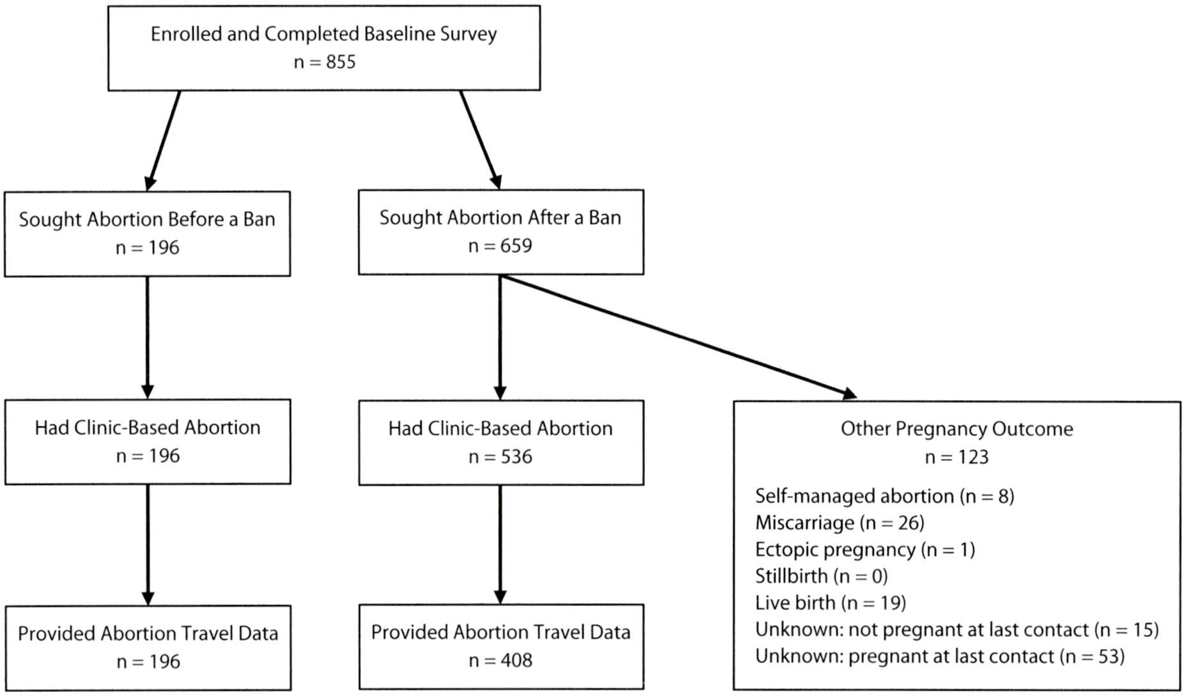

FIGURE 1— Flow Diagram of Study Enrollment, Pregnancy Outcomes, and Travel Data Completion: End of Roe Study, 14 US States, June 2022–June 2024

Note. The states studied were AL, AR, ID, IN, KY, LA, MS, MO, OK, SD, TN, TX, WV, and WI.

and more likely to report a previous abortion (28% vs 40%) than were people receiving an abortion before their state implemented a ban (Table 1).

Travel and Cost Differences

Before a state ban, all people seeking abortion traveled by car (98% personal car, 2% taxi or rideshare) to clinics in their state. After a state ban, people seeking abortion relied on a wider range of transportation options and, at times, multiple types: 76% traveled by car, 10% by taxi or rideshare, 2% by bus or train, and 20% by airplane. Mean travel time was longer, from 2.8 hours to 11.3 hours, and the proportion staying overnight was greater (5% vs 58%) after a ban (Table 2).

Average out-of-pocket medical costs for the abortion—including medications, ultrasounds, and tests—decreased ($545 before vs $377 after a ban). Similarly, the proportion who reported paying no out-of-pocket costs for the abortion increased (4% vs 37%). There were no differences in the use of health insurance. Consistent with longer travel time and greater frequency of overnight stays, the amount paid for travel and logistics was greater after a ban ($179 vs $372). Receipt of financial assistance from an organization or personal connection and the amount of support they received did not differ.

The average point in pregnancy when participants were able to get an abortion increased from 7.7 weeks before a ban to 8.8 weeks after a ban. The proportion having an abortion at 13 weeks or more of pregnancy more than doubled (8% vs 17%). There was no difference in the proportion who reported a procedural versus medication abortion.

Factors That Delayed Abortion Care

Participants who had an abortion after a state ban were more likely to report delays because of the need to raise money for the abortion or travel (40% before vs 66% after a ban). They were also more likely to report delays because of finding or getting to a clinic (33% vs 60%) and their work or school schedules (26% vs 35%), although they were less likely to report being delayed by the wait time to get an appointment (42% vs 31%). There were no differences in reports of the decision to have an abortion, recognition of pregnancy, finding childcare, interpersonal opposition, or needing parental or guardian permission as delaying factors (Table 3).

TABLE 1— Description of Sample Receiving Clinic-Based Abortions Before and After State Abortion Ban Implementation: End of Roe Study, 14 US States, June 2022–June 2024

	Had Abortion Preban, No. (%) or Mean ±SD (n = 196)	Had Abortion Postban, No. (%) or Mean ±SD (n = 536)
Age,[a] y	26.3 ±5.7	27.8 ±5.8
Age group, y		
15–19	18 (9)	31 (6)
20–24	62 (32)	145 (27)
25–29	61 (31)	164 (31)
30–34	37 (19)	119 (22)
≥ 35	18 (9)	77 (14)
Race		
White	98 (50)	253 (48)
Black/African American	72 (37)	191 (36)
Asian, Native Hawaiian, or Pacific Islander	4 (2)	9 (2)
Native American or Alaska Native	3 (2)	13 (2)
Another race	6 (3)	33 (6)
Multiracial	11 (6)	32 (6)
Hispanic/Latina ethnicity[a]	25 (13)	164 (31)
Gender identity		
Woman	193 (98)	529 (99)
Nonbinary/gender nonconforming	3 (2)	7 (1)
Transgender	0 (0)	0 (0)
Education		
Did not complete high school	13 (7)	25 (5)
High school diploma or equivalent	68 (35)	176 (33)
Some college or vocational/trade school	53 (27)	144 (27)
Associate degree or certificate/license	26 (13)	95 (18)
Bachelor's degree or beyond	36 (18)	96 (18)
Employed (full- or part-time)[a]	147 (75)	332 (62)
Government assistance in last month	73 (37)	180 (34)
Household income, % federal poverty level[b]		
< 100	79 (40)	236 (44)
100–200	42 (21)	120 (22)
≥ 200	42 (21)	93 (17)
Don't know/missing	33 (17)	87 (16)
Ever pregnant before this pregnancy	134 (68)	388 (72)
Ever given birth	121 (62)	325 (61)
Ever had a previous abortion[a]	55 (28)	215 (40)

Note. CI = confidence interval. Sample size was n = 732. Totals may not equal 100% because of rounding. The states studied were AL, AR, ID, IN, KY, LA, MS, MO, OK, SD, TN, TX, WV, and WI.
[a]The difference comparing pre- vs postban status is statistically significant, $P < .05$.
[b]As determined by the Department of Health and Human Services in 2022.

TABLE 2— Travel, Costs, and Pregnancy Duration Before and After Implementation of State Abortion Bans: End of Roe Study, 14 US States, June 2022–June 2024

	Had Abortion Preban, % or Mean (95% CI) (n = 196)	Had Abortion Postban, % or Mean (95% CI) (n = 408)
Travel		
Mode of travel		
Car[a]	98 (97, 100)	76 (72, 81)
Taxi or rideshare[a]	2 (0, 3)	10 (7, 12)
Bus or train[a]	0	2 (1, 4)
Airplane[a]	0	20 (16, 23)
Stayed overnight[a]	5 (2, 8)	58 (53, 63)
Travel time,[a] h	2.8 (1.8, 3.8)	11.3 (9.9, 12.6)
Personal costs		
Travel costs,[a] $	179 (142, 216)	372 (327, 418)
Out-of-pocket medical costs,[a] $	545 (505, 586)	377 (329, 425)
No out-of-pocket medical cost[a]	4 (1, 6)	37 (32, 41)
Financial support		
Used health insurance	4 (1, 6)	4 (2, 6)
Received financial support from an organization	35 (28, 42)	43 (39, 48)
Received financial support from a personal connection	39 (32, 46)	43 (38, 48)
Amount personal connection paid, $	416 (372, 460)	512 (428, 595)
Abortion services		
Pregnancy duration at abortion,[a] wk	7.7 (7.2, 8.1)	8.8 (8.4, 9.3)
Pregnancy duration ≥ 13,[a] wk	8 (4, 11)	17 (13, 20)
Type of abortion		
Procedural	58 (51, 65)	52 (47, 57)
Medication	42 (35, 49)	48 (43, 53)

Note. CI = confidence interval. Sample size was n = 604. The states studied were AL, AR, ID, IN, KY, LA, MS, MO, OK, SD, TN, TX, WV, and WI.
[a]The difference comparing pre- vs postban status is statistically significant, $P < .05$.

Postban Abortion Travel Over Time

Table A (available as a supplement to the online version of this article at http://www.ajph.org) shows exploratory trends over time across 6-month periods. The first 6 months after the *Dobbs* decision were marked by the greatest out-of-pocket medical costs, time and costs of travel, and delays compared with before state bans were enacted.

Travel evolved in the 2 years after *Dobbs* was decided. Compared with the immediate postban period (June–December 2022), the most recent abortion seekers (January–June 2024) were less likely to travel by car (100% vs 69%), more likely to travel by airplane (0% vs 28%), and more likely to stay overnight for their abortion (33% vs 74%). Notably, they had their abortions earlier in pregnancy (10.4 vs 8.4 weeks) but still later than those who had an abortion before state bans were enacted (7.7 weeks).

Out-of-pocket medical costs also changed over time: the proportion of participants reporting no out-of-pocket costs increased from the immediate postban period to the most recent postban period (10%–40%). Financial support from organizations increased, with more participants reporting assistance (23%–45%) in the most recent period. There was no change in financial support from a personal connection or the amount they contributed.

DISCUSSION

Our findings offer insights into the profound changes in abortion access in the wake of the *Dobbs* decision. In contrast to the early expectation that substantial numbers of abortion seekers living in ban states would be unable to

TABLE 3— Factors That Delayed Participants When Seeking an Abortion Before and After Implementation of State Abortion Bans: End of Roe Study, 14 US States, June 2022–June 2024

	Had Abortion Preban, % (95% CI) (n = 196)	Had Abortion Postban, % (95% CI) (n = 408)
Getting money for the abortion and/or travel[a]	40 (33, 47)	66 (62, 71)
Finding and/or getting to a place where I could get an abortion[a]	33 (26, 39)	60 (55, 65)
My work or school schedule[a]	26 (20, 32)	35 (30, 39)
Deciding if I wanted an abortion	33 (26, 39)	34 (29, 38)
Waiting time to get an appointment[a]	42 (35, 49)	31 (26, 35)
I didn't realize that I was pregnant	33 (26, 39)	31 (26, 35)
Finding childcare	10 (6, 14)	13 (10, 17)
Someone close to me didn't want me to have an abortion	8 (4, 11)	7 (5, 10)
Having to get parent/guardian permission	2 (0, 4)	1 (0, 2)
Another factor	3 (0, 5)	4 (2, 6)

Note. CI = confidence interval. Sample size was n = 604. The states studied were AL, AR, ID, IN, KY, LA, MS, MO, OK, SD, TN, TX, WV, and WI.
[a]The difference comparing pre- vs postban status is statistically significant, $P < .05$.

obtain care,[17,18] the majority of study participants (81%) reported being able to travel to protected access states for their abortions after contacting a clinic or call center. Only 3% to 11% of participants in ban states reported continuing their pregnancies to birth. These findings are consistent with trends identified by other national[6–8] and state-level[19–22] research undertaken since 2022 that indicate an increase in abortion numbers in protected access states.

Comparing our pre- and postban samples highlights shifts in who is able to access abortion. A large body of research has documented how the most vulnerable populations, including people of color[23] and those experiencing financial instability,[24] faced the greatest barriers to accessing abortion care under *Roe v Wade* (410 US 113 [1973]). In our sample, we found that a greater share of those receiving abortions after the *Dobbs* decision were Latina. This may reflect variation in the geographic distribution of our recruited samples (e.g., a greater proportion of the postban sample was recruited from Texas relative to the preban sample); it may also indicate improvements in abortion information and support that were not available to pregnant Latinas before *Dobbs* because of systemic inequities in the abortion delivery system.

We further found that people who reported being unemployed made up a greater proportion of those traveling out of state for abortions relative to those who received abortions before state bans. One potential explanation for this is that increased funding and practical support efforts may have particularly affected people whose socioeconomic status precluded them from receiving abortions before *Dobbs*.[25–27] Another is that employed people have less ability to travel but greater knowledge of, access to, and resources for alternatives to travel, such as ordering medication abortion pills online. Indeed, there is substantial evidence that thousands of people have been ordering medication abortion from online sellers since *Dobbs* was decided[14,15]; our sample of people seeking clinic-based care does not capture these experiences.

We found a dramatic increase in travel burdens for those who were able to access abortions after a ban in their state. Before implementation of a ban, most participants were able to get to a clinic in their state within 3 hours by car. After a ban, average travel time increased to more than 11 hours, as pregnant people traveled across state lines, sometimes requiring airplane flights and overnight stays. This increase in travel time and the associated logistical challenges substantially raised the financial costs of obtaining an abortion. The increased emotional burdens, stress, anxiety, and shame associated with such travel can be substantial.[28,29] Our findings also indicate that abortion bans delayed people from getting their abortions, reflecting the additional time required to arrange travel, secure funding, and navigate the new legal landscape. In the months after state bans, pregnancy duration was more than a week longer for those who had an abortion than before state bans, and the proportion having an abortion at 13 weeks or later more than doubled. Notably, this trend fluctuated in the 2 years since *Dobbs* was decided, with the greatest delays in the initial postban period subsiding somewhat over time.

Since *Dobbs* was decided, there have been considerable efforts by abortion funds, practical support organizations, professional associations, grantmaking entities, and health care providers to support pregnant people as they seek abortions. The observed increase in numbers of abortions after *Dobbs*[7,8] is the product of considerable organizing and fundraising. Although we found little difference in the proportion of people who reported receiving aid from organizations before versus after state bans, participants reported that their out-of-pocket medical expenses significantly decreased. Documented efforts to lower costs in protected access states[20,22,30,31] may explain the lower out-of-pocket costs reported by those having abortions after a ban. Increased donations to clinics and funds may not have been recognizable to patients as direct assistance and may instead have been experienced as a lower price of clinical care. Lower reporting of assistance may reflect a streamlining of funding whereby the provider and abortion funds worked together to lower the cost of abortion to patients.

By contrast to decreasing clinical costs, we found that overall expenses—that is, accounting for travel-related costs—were significantly greater for participants seeking abortion after a ban. The considerable financial support offered by both organizations and personal connections has not completely offset the financial burdens experienced by those who must travel to another state for an abortion. Furthermore, changes in the proportion of abortion seekers reporting organizational support across the postban periods in our exploratory analysis may be a sign of waning donations to funds.[32,33] Fluctuating levels of support suggest a need for more stable and sustained funding sources for people to be able to reliably travel across state lines.

Limitations

We note this study's limitations. First, because we were unable to obtain an accurate count of how many study invitations were received, we could not calculate a response rate. However, the overall sociodemographic similarities between the pre- and postban samples, as well as the similarities to national data on abortion patients,[12,34] suggest that we captured a sample that reflects the demographics of those seeking abortions. Second, differences in the geographic distribution of our pre- and postban samples may influence our findings about travel and result in an overestimate in the travel burden because of the change in the law.

Third, the pregnancy outcomes for a small fraction of our participants were undetermined. It is possible that participants with unknown outcomes had different experiences from those whose outcomes were captured; for example, they may have been more likely to self-manage their abortion by procuring pills online. Fourth, because of an early iteration of the survey design and flow, we lacked travel data for nearly one quarter of the postban sample; we know that they had an abortion in another state, but their specific costs and travel burdens were unknown. We identified some differences among those without travel data (i.e., they were more likely to be Black and receive government assistance than were other travelers), and we note that they may have had different travel experiences.

Finally, we note that our study design recruited people who reached out to a clinic or call center for information about clinic-based services. Our study does not reflect the experiences of people considering abortion who sought care outside the medical system or those who were unsure how to access care at all.

Public Health Implications

The legal landscape after *Dobbs* has led to significant adjustments in where and how pregnant people seek abortion care, both in the formal sector of brick-and-mortar abortion facilities and telehealth providers and through informal means outside the medical system.[14,15] Our analysis focused on clinic-based care and highlights several key areas affected by these changes. We found that the post-*Dobbs* environment has created considerable burdens for pregnant people seeking clinic-based abortion services in states that have banned abortion at all points in pregnancy. Longer travel times, higher costs, and delays in accessing services are fundamental barriers to care that exacerbate existing reproductive health inequities. Although support mechanisms have adapted to provide some relief, persistent gaps remain and may increase over time as attention and donations wane. Addressing these disparities requires public health interventions that ensure equitable access to abortion care, regardless of geographic location or financial means. AJPH

ABOUT THE AUTHORS

All authors are with Advancing New Standards in Reproductive Health, Department of Obstetrics, Gynecology & Reproductive Sciences, University of California, San Francisco.

CORRESPONDENCE

Correspondence should be sent to Nancy F. Berglas, DrPH, Advancing New Standards in Reproductive Health, University of California, San Francisco, 1330 Broadway, Suite 1100, Oakland, CA 94612 (e-mail: Nancy.Berglas@ucsf.edu).

Reprints can be ordered at https://www.ajph.org by clicking the "Reprints" link.

PUBLICATION INFORMATION

Full Citation: Berglas NF, Barnes JT, Gonzalez E, Peters L, Foster DG. Changes in abortion access, travel, and costs since the implementation of state abortion bans, 2022–2024. *Am J Public Health*. 2025;115(10):1713–1722.

Acceptance Date: May 2, 2025.

DOI: https://doi.org/10.2105/AJPH.2025.308191

ORCID iDs:
Nancy F. Berglas https://orcid.org/0000-0001-5310-4848

Jessica T. Barnes https://orcid.org/0000-0002-6550-9209

Lisa Peters https://orcid.org/0009-0006-5597-8876

CONTRIBUTORS

N. F. Berglas wrote the initial draft and analyzed the data. N. F. Berglas, J. T. Barnes, and D. G. Foster developed the study methodology. N. F. Berglas and D. G. Foster conceptualized the study. J. T. Barnes directed project administration. J. T. Barnes, E. Gonzalez, and L. Peters coordinated data acquisition and management. All authors contributed to data interpretation and reviewed, revised, and approved the final article.

ACKNOWLEDGMENTS

This work was supported by the Hewlett Foundation (award 2022-00860-GRA), an anonymous foundation, and private donors.

We are grateful to Kirsten Thompson, Molly Battistelli, Mary Beth Blasnek, and Amy Pineda for their many contributions to the initial phases of study design and implementation.

Note: The funders had no role in the study design, data collection, and analysis; the writing of the article; or the decision to submit the article for publication.

CONFLICTS OF INTEREST

The authors have no conflicts of interest to disclose.

HUMAN PARTICIPANT PROTECTION

The study protocol was approved by the University of California, San Francisco institutional review board. Participants provided digital informed consent.

REFERENCES

1. Center for Reproductive Rights. After *Roe* fell: abortion laws by state. Available at: https://reproductiverights.org/maps/abortion-laws-by-state. 2024. Accessed September 11, 2024.
2. New York Times. Tracking abortion bans across the country. 2024. Available at: https://www.nytimes.com/interactive/2024/us/abortion-laws-roe-v-wade.html. Accessed September 11, 2024.
3. Schroeder R, Kaller S, Berglas NF, Stewart C, Upadhyay UD. *Trends in Abortion Services in the United States, 2017–2023*. San Francisco: University of California, San Francisco; 2024.
4. Myers C. Forecasts for a post-*Roe* America: the effects of increased travel distance on abortions and births. *J Policy Anal Manage*. 2024;43(1): 39–62. https://doi.org/10.1002/pam.22524
5. Rader B, Upadhyay UD, Sehgal NKR, Reis BY, Brownstein JS, Hswen Y. Estimated travel time and spatial access to abortion facilities in the US before and after the *Dobbs v Jackson Women's Health* decision. *JAMA*. 2022;328(20):2041–2047. https://doi.org/10.1001/jama.2022.20424
6. Odouard I, Guadamuz JS, Chakraborty A, Alexander GC, Qato DM. Induced abortion and out-of-state travel among insured women before and after the *Dobbs v. Jackson Women's Health Organization* decision. *O&G Open*. 2024;1(2):16. https://doi.org/10.1097/og9.0000000000000016
7. Society of Family Planning. #WeCount report: April 2022 to March 2024. August 7, 2024. Available at: https://societyfp.org/wp-content/uploads/2024/07/WeCount-Report-7-Mar-2024-data.pdf. Accessed June 7, 2025.
8. Guttmacher Institute. Monthly abortion provision study. 2024. Available at: https://www.guttmacher.org/monthly-abortion-provision-study. Accessed June 7, 2025.
9. Pleasants EA, Cartwright AF, Upadhyay UD. Association between distance to an abortion facility and abortion or pregnancy outcome among a prospective cohort of people seeking abortion online. *JAMA Netw Open*. 2022;5(5):e2212065. https://doi.org/10.1001/jamanetworkopen.2022.12065
10. Kimport K. Abortion after *Dobbs*: defendants, denials, and delays. *Sci Adv*. 2022;8(36):eade5327. https://doi.org/10.1126/sciadv.ade5327
11. Barr-Walker J, Jayaweera RT, Ramirez AM, Gerdts C. Experiences of women who travel for abortion: a mixed methods systematic review. *PLoS One*. 2019;14(4):e0209991. https://doi.org/10.1371/journal.pone.0209991
12. Jerman J, Jones RK, Onda T. Characteristics of US abortion patients in 2014 and changes since 2008. May 2016. Available at: https://www.guttmacher.org/report/characteristics-us-abortion-patients-2014. Accessed June 7, 2025.
13. Cohen DS, Donley G, Rebouche R. Abortion shield laws. *NEJM Evid*. 2023;2(4):EVIDra2200280. https://doi.org/10.1056/EVIDra2200280
14. Aiken ARA, Wells ES, Gomperts R, Scott JG. Provision of medications for self-managed abortion before and after the *Dobbs v Jackson Women's Health Organization* decision. *JAMA*. 2024;331(18): 1558–1564. https://doi.org/10.1001/jama.2024.4266
15. Aiken ARA, Starling JE, Scott JG, Gomperts R. Requests for self-managed medication abortion provided using online telemedicine in 30 US states before and after the *Dobbs v Jackson Women's Health Organization* decision. *JAMA*. 2022;328(17):1768–1770. https://doi.org/10.1001/jama.2022.18865
16. Thomson-DeVeaux A. The Dobbs divide. June 15, 2023. Available at: https://fivethirtyeight.com/features/abortion-trend-after-dobbs. Accessed June 7, 2025.
17. Grossman D, Perritt J, Grady D. The impending crisis of access to safe abortion care in the US. *JAMA Intern Med*. 2022;182(8):793–795. https://doi.org/10.1001/jamainternmed.2022.2893
18. Harvey SM, Larson AE, Warren JT. The *Dobbs* decision—exacerbating US health inequity. *N Engl J Med*. 2023;388(16):1444–1447. https://doi.org/10.1056/NEJMp2216698
19. Fuerst M, Mandelbaum A, Nacev E, Rodriguez M. Trends in interstate abortion travel to Oregon following the *Dobbs* court decision. *Contraception*. 2024;138:110520. https://doi.org/10.1016/j.contraception.2024.110520
20. Keefe-Oates B, Fulcher I, Fortin J, et al. Use of abortion services in Massachusetts after the *Dobbs* decision among in-state vs out-of-state residents. *JAMA Netw Open*. 2023;6(9):e2332400. https://doi.org/10.1001/jamanetworkopen.2023.32400
21. Mandelbaum AD, Nacev EC, Fuerst MF, Colwill A, Ramanadhan S, Rodriguez M. Impact of the *Dobbs* decision on abortion services from a large tertiary center in Oregon. *Contraception*. 2024;136: 110484. https://doi.org/10.1016/j.contraception.2024.110484
22. Riley T, Fiastro AE, Benson LS, Khattar A, Prager S, Godfrey EM. Abortion provision and delays to care in a clinic network in Washington state after Dobbs. *JAMA Netw Open*. 2024;7(5):e2413847. https://doi.org/10.1001/jamanetworkopen.2024.13847
23. Fuentes L. Inequity in US abortion rights and access: the end of *Roe* is deepening existing divides. January 17, 2023. Available at: https://www.guttmacher.org/2023/01/inequity-us-abortion-rights-and-access-end-roe-deepening-existing-divides. Accessed June 7, 2025.
24. Foster DG, Biggs MA, Ralph L, Gerdts C, Roberts S, Glymour MM. Socioeconomic outcomes of women who receive and women who are denied wanted abortions in the United States. *Am J Public Health*. 2018;108(3):407–413. https://doi.org/10.2105/AJPH.2017.304247
25. Ely GE, Hales TW, Agbemenu K. An exploration of the experiences of Florida abortion fund service recipients. *Health Soc Work*. 2020;45(3):186–194. https://doi.org/10.1093/hsw/hlaa012
26. Leyser-Whalen O, Torres L, Gonzales B. Revealing economic and racial injustices: demographics of abortion fund callers on the US–Mexico border. *Womens Reprod Health (Phila)*. 2021;8(3):188–202. https://doi.org/10.1080/23293691.2021.1973845
27. Smith MH, Eggen MB, Prestrud AA, et al. Seeking financial and practical support in an abortion-hostile state: analysis of abortion fund data in Kentucky, 2014–2021: analysis of abortion fund data in Kentucky. *Perspect Sex Reprod Health*. 2024;56(3):222–227. https://doi.org/10.1111/psrh.12279
28. Kimport K, Rasidjan MP. Exploring the emotional costs of abortion travel in the United States due to legal restriction. *Contraception*. 2023;120: 109956. https://doi.org/10.1016/j.contraception.2023.109956
29. Makleff S, Blaylock R, Ruggiero S, Key K, Chandrasekaran S, Gerdts C. Travel for later abortion in the USA: lived experiences, structural contributors and abortion fund support. *Cult Health Sex*. 2023;25(12):1741–1757. https://doi.org/10.1080/13691058.2023.2179666
30. Abernathy A, Haerizadeh-Yazdi N, Sinha S, Schreiber CA, Mehta A. Strengthening the provision of abortion and sexual and reproductive health care post-*Dobbs*: an initiative of the

Philadelphia Department of Public Health. *NEJM Catal Innov Care Deliv*. 2024;5(8):10.1056/CAT.24.0105. https://doi.org/10.1056/CAT.24.0105

31. Quasebarth M, Boesche M, Turner T, et al. Patient experiences using public and private insurance coverage for abortion in Illinois: implementation successes and remaining gaps. *Perspect Sex Reprod Health*. 2024;56(3):269–281. https://doi.org/10.1111/psrh.12259
32. Goldhill O. Abortion funds run short of money as demand soars and donations fall. January 23, 2024. Available at: https://www.statnews.com/2024/01/23/abortion-fund-warning-demand-up-donations-down. Accessed June 7, 2025.
33. Stiffman E. Abortion funds face slowdown in giving a year after supreme court ruling. June 12, 2023. Available at: https://www.philanthropy.com/article/abortion-funds-face-slowdown-in-giving-a-year-after-supreme-court-ruling. Accessed June 7, 2025.
34. Jones RK, Chiu DW. Characteristics of abortion patients in protected and restricted states accessing clinic-based care 12 months prior to the elimination of the federal constitutional right to abortion in the United States. *Perspect Sex Reprod Health*. 2023;55(2):80–85. https://doi.org/10.1363/psrh.12224

The State of Sexual Education: State Laws and Regulations Mandating Sexual Education in the United States

Kimberly M. Nelson, PhD, MPH, Aaliyah Gray, PhD, Samantha Haiken, MPH, and Kristen Underhill, DPhil, JD

See also Goldfarb and Lieberman, p. 1567.

Objectives. To assess state laws and regulations mandating sexual education in US public schools in 2025.

Methods. We identified and analyzed state statutes, administrative regulations, and state court decisions that mandated sexual education in public schools in every US state and the District of Columbia. We coded content requirements, attributes (e.g., "age-appropriate"), and parental notice and consent policies.

Results. Forty-two US states required sexual education in at least 1 content area in K–12 public schools. Most required education to cover abstinence (34 states), HIV (34 states), sexually transmitted infections (32 states), and child abuse prevention (31 states). Five states required opt-in parental consent; 34 allowed parents to opt children out. Nineteen states mandated medically accurate content for any topic.

Conclusions. Although many states mandated sexual education, few required content beyond sexual abstinence, HIV, sexually transmitted infections, and child abuse prevention. Laws that make content optional or facilitate opt-outs can undermine access to this education.

Public Health Implications. This detailed accounting of the law will enable researchers and policymakers to identify opportunities to support the implementation of medically accurate, evidence-based sexual education in school settings. (*Am J Public Health*. 2025;115(10):1723–1733. https://doi.org/10.2105/AJPH.2025.308199)

AJPH October 2025, Vol. 115, No. 10

Adolescents are at greater risk of sexually transmitted infections (STIs), HIV, and unintended pregnancy compared with adults in the United States.[1–4] Sexual and gender minoritized (SGM) and racial/ethnic minoritized youths are particularly affected.[1–3,5] Because the majority of US adolescents attend public schools,[6] one intervention to address their sexual health needs is to provide evidence-based, medically accurate sexual education in public school settings.

Evidence-based sexual education is consistently associated with positive sexual health outcomes, such as delayed initiation of sexual activity, fewer unintended pregnancies, and increased use of condoms and prescription birth control.[7–10] Given this robust evidence base, medical and public health associations such as the World Health Organization, the Centers for Disease Control and Prevention, the American Public Health Association, the American Academy of Pediatrics, and the US Future of Sex Education Initiative recommend evidence-based, medically accurate approaches to school-based sexual education.[11–15] Parents overwhelmingly support comprehensive sexual education in school settings,[16–18] and increasing access to sexual education is a Healthy People 2030 goal. Despite these recommendations, however, only half of US adolescents report receiving formal sexual education by the time they graduate from high school, with little change over the past decade.[19,20]

At present, no federal laws regulate the provision of sexual education in K–12 public schools. Instead, oversight consists of state laws, state regulations, and state agency guidance. Where states lack these mandates, sexual education choices are left to local school districts. The patchwork of state sexual education laws reflects long-standing debates about school-based sexual education, which often focus on abstinence-only versus comprehensive approaches. Despite evidence that abstinence-only sexual education is not beneficial to adolescent sexual health,[21–25] federal funds continue to support abstinence-focused approaches.[22] Policy decisions about sexual education curricula, however, happen closer to home; state-level sociopolitical forces—and in turn, state policies—exert more influence on sexual education and adolescents' health outcomes.[22–26] There is, therefore, a need for rigorously coded data on statewide school-based sexual education mandates, including their content requirements, program attributes, and provisions for parental involvement.

Amendments to sexual education laws are frequent, and an updated analysis with replicable methods is important for guiding ongoing research. Organizations such as the Guttmacher Institute[27] and the Sexuality Information and Education Council of the United States[28] provide helpful state profiles for sexual education policies. These resources, however, can lack some of the methodological details that are needed to replicate the legal analysis, such as search terms and dates, information about the coding process, decisions about coding-specific language, and quality control practices. Sexual health researchers, practitioners, and policymakers would benefit from a detailed and replicable analysis of state sexual education laws.

In the current study, we used standardized legal epidemiological methods[29–31] to examine sexual education mandates in effect across all US states and the District of Columbia in 2025. The objectives were to (1) conduct a systematic search of state statutes, regulations, and relevant case law mandating sexual education in the United States as of March 2025, (2) report a replicable process, and (3) examine differences across states. This accounting can inform research and identify areas where policy changes could expand access to sexual education in school settings. The long-term goal of this work is to facilitate research, practice, and policies that increase access to evidence-based, medically accurate sexual education and, thereby, improve young people's sexual health.

METHODS

Following best practices for creating state-level public health law data sets,[29–31] we used a structured protocol to identify, code, and analyze state policies addressing sexual education. We reviewed state statutes (enacted by legislatures), administrative codes and mandatory guidance (developed by state agencies), and state court cases related to sexual education in public schools. We included laws that mandated public school education in any grade between kindergarten and 12th grade, in every US state and the District of Columbia, across a set of predetermined content areas.

We began by generating a list of state-level legal variables (e.g., is it mandatory for public schools to provide instruction on sexual abstinence at any grade level K–12?) and preparing a coding scheme with possible values for that variable (e.g., yes, no). We then developed our search strategy for identifying relevant laws in Westlaw, a legal research platform. For each state, we searched the Westlaw databases containing current state legislation, state administrative regulations, and case law. We ran searches in each of these databases in 2021 using the following search strings: ("(sex! abstinenc! pregnan! HIV STI STD venereal health)/s (educ! instruct! teach! school!)") and ((sex!/s orient!) LGBT GLBT gay lesbian (sex!/s minorit!) homosex! transgender! transsex! asex!))/s (educ! instruct! teach! school!)). We reran our searches of statutes and administrative regulations in January and March 2025 to update our findings, using the following more sensitive search string: (sex! abstinenc! pregnan! HIV STI STD venereal "health education" "family life" (sex!/s orient!) LGBT GLBT gay lesbian (sex!/s minorit!) homosex! transgender! transsex! asex! (gender/s iden!))/s (educ! instruct! teach! school!). Where sex education laws addressed parental consent, advance notice of instruction, and inspection of materials, we extracted these data. We also extracted information about mandatory sexual education content related to sexual orientation and gender identity. We did not, however, search separately for sexual orientation content, gender identity content, or parental rights outside the content areas of sexual education.

Search results were reviewed independently by 2 law student research assistants (RAs). When an RA identified a relevant state law or regulation, we obtained the full-text, current version of the law. The law student RAs also inspected subsequent citations to each law to identify cases, regulations, or administrative guidance that might affect its application. Using the full-text laws, 2 RAs worked independently to extract data on the variables of interest from the source material into an Excel spreadsheet for each state. The 2 coders met to reconcile differences in their redundant coding, resolving differences by discussion and referral to senior authors. We compared findings to existing surveys to ensure completeness.[27,28] Legal citations are provided in Table A (available as a supplement to the online version of this article at https://ajph.org). The last round of searches, as of March 2025, yielded 12 996 statutes and 4525 regulations, and we retrieved full-text versions of 864 items for detailed analysis. A comparison of our results to existing surveys[27,28] is presented in Tables B and C (available as supplements to the online version of this article at https://ajph.org).

We coded a state as "mandating sexual education" when a statute, a regulation, or mandatory administrative guidance required public schools in any grade from kindergarten to 12th grade to provide instruction in any 1 of the following prespecified content areas: sexual abstinence, HIV/AIDS, STIs/sexually transmitted diseases, condoms, contraception, "safer sex," a specific feature of state law related to sexual activity (e.g., statutory age of consent to sex, definitions of criminal sexual offenses), dating and intimate partner violence, healthy relationships, consent to sex, child sexual abuse, sexual assault, gender identity in the context of sexual education, and sexual orientation in the context of sexual education. Mandatory language included terms like "shall," "must," "will," and "required"; we classified terms like "urged to," "encouraged to," "may," "can," "voluntary," and "option" as nonmandatory. We excluded laws that created (but did not mandate) model curricula, made grant funding available, regulated the credentials of health educators, regulated the scope of school health services, prohibited discrimination based on sexual orientation or gender identity in education generally, or set procedural requirements for how districts made decisions about the content of sexual education. We also excluded mandates that did not include a sexual education content area listed above (e.g., "health education" without identifiable topic areas, "communicable diseases" without mentioning STIs, "refusal skills" without mentioning sex).

For each jurisdiction, we coded the specific mandatory content areas and key attributes. No state mandated sexual education that was exclusively focused on pregnancy; we therefore subsumed pregnancy prevention into our coding of contraception. The attributes "age-appropriate" and "developmentally appropriate" were used interchangeably across laws, so we combined them for analysis; we also combined mandates that content be "evidence-based," "evidence-informed," "research-based," or "research-informed." We restricted our "medically accurate" code to laws that specifically used the term, rather than paraphrases like "factually accurate" or "objective." Finally, we coded parental consent options and statewide mandates for parental rights specific to sex education, including the need for opt-in consent, permission to opt children out of instruction, schools' duties to notify parents in advance, and parents' rights to inspect sexual education curriculum materials. Where a state had not passed a law or regulation, we interpreted that silence as leaving discretion to local education boards.

To illustrate the reach of mandatory sexual education in US public schools, we used projected numbers of public high-school graduates for the 2024–2025 school year from the National Center for Education Statistics. These estimates included public school diploma recipients and excluded those who received a certificate of attendance or a high-school equivalency certificate.[32] We used these projections to estimate the number of public high-school graduates nationwide, the number in states that required sexual education, and the number in states that required medically accurate sexual education during K–12 instruction.

RESULTS

Mandates arose from state legislation, administrative regulations, and sometimes through administrative guidance that was incorporated by reference into statutes or the administrative code (e.g., health standards adopted by the Board of Education). Although judicial decisions sometimes cited or interpreted these laws, there were no state mandates that arose solely through judicial interpretation of a statute or state constitutional right. This is a highly active area of legislative intervention; most states have amended or enacted new sexual education laws in the past 5 years, as reflected in Table A.

Mandatory Sexual Education in Public Schools

Forty-two of the 51 jurisdictions in the United States (82%) required public school students to take a course covering at least 1 sexual education content area at any point during their K–12 instruction. Sexual education in at least 1 content area was mandatory in all 9 jurisdictions in the Northeast (100%), 15 of 17 in the South (88%), 10 of 12 in the Midwest (83%), and 8 of 13 in the West (62%; Figure 1). Approximately 89% of the 3 524 500 public high-school students who were expected to graduate during the 2024–2025 school year resided in states that required

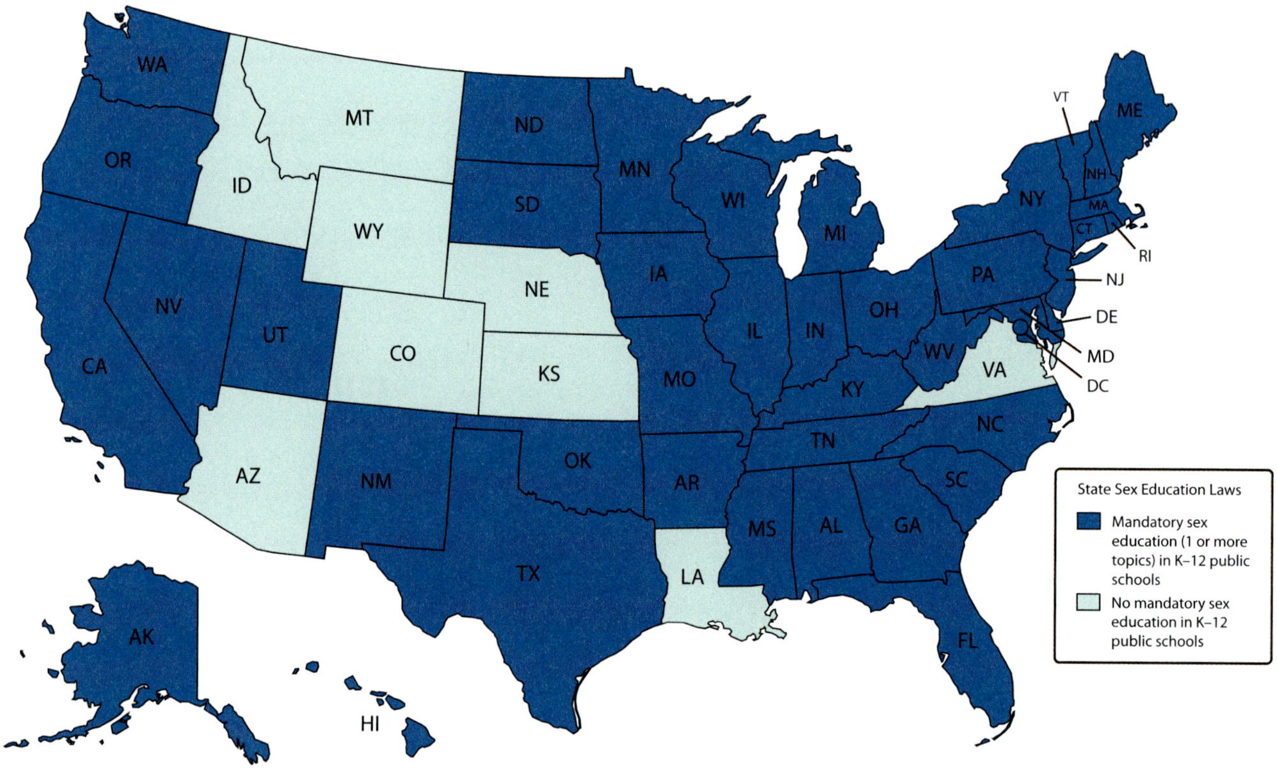

FIGURE 1— Jurisdictions Mandating Sexual Education in Any Content Area in K–12 Public Schools: United States, March 2025

AJPH October 2025, Vol. 115, No. 10

students to have instruction in at least 1 sexual education content area (Figure 2).

Required Sexual Education Content

Among the 42 jurisdictions that mandated any sexual education, the average number of mandated content areas was 7 (SD = 4; range = 1–14). The most common content mandates included sexual abstinence (n = 34), HIV/AIDS (n = 34), STIs (n = 32), prevention of child sexual abuse (n = 31), healthy relationships (n = 27), sexual assault (n = 24), and dating violence or intimate partner violence (n = 21; Table 1). Fewer than half of states required instruction about contraception (n = 20), state laws related to sex (n = 19), sexual orientation (n = 12), condoms (n = 11), consent to sex (n = 9), and gender identity (n = 7). Two of the 12 jurisdictions that mandated coverage of sexual orientation required content that was negative or stigmatizing, including messages that "engaging in homosexual activity" is "primarily responsible for contact with the AIDS virus" (Oklahoma; Okla Stat Ann tit 70, § 11-103.3; Okla Admin Code § 210:15-17-2) and that "homosexuality is not a lifestyle acceptable to the general public and . . . is a criminal offense" (Texas; Tex Health & Safety Code Ann § 163.002 [note that this criminal prohibition is no longer in effect]). The other 10 jurisdictions covering sexual orientation and 7 jurisdictions covering gender identity required instruction that was affirming or neutral in its emphasis. Although additional jurisdictions included language that stated they were "inclusive" of SGM populations, we only counted these as content mandates when they required topical instruction on SGM sexual health needs.

Required Sexual Education Attributes

Among the 42 jurisdictions that required sexual education, most (n = 35) mandated that sexual education be "age/developmentally appropriate" (Table 2). Nineteen jurisdictions required sexual education to be medically accurate in any topic area, although 5 only required medical accuracy for specific topics, such as abstinence, HIV, or contraception failure rates. Eighteen states required that sexual education be "evidence-based," "research-based," or an equivalent term; 6 required that instruction be "up to date"; and 6 required it to be "culturally appropriate." We note, however, that many states mandated discussion of culture in the

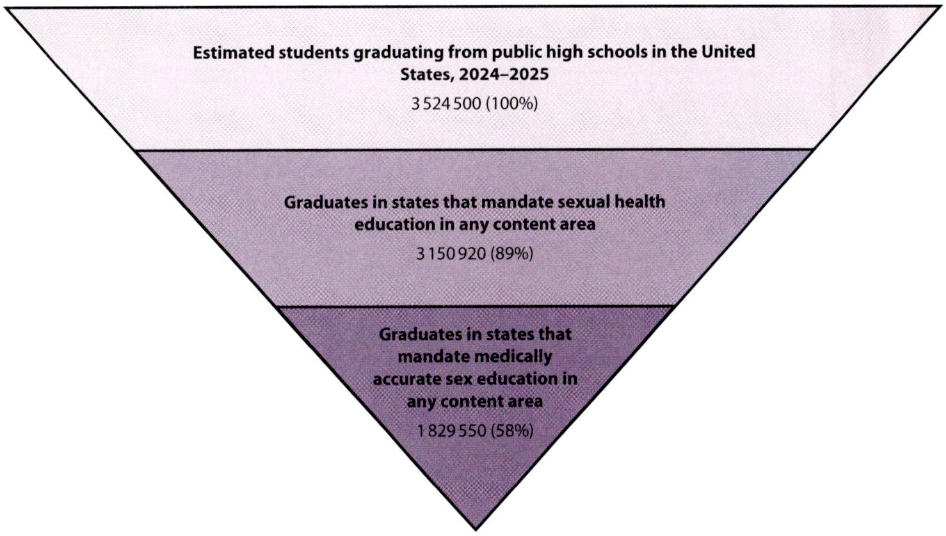

FIGURE 2— Estimated Public High-School Graduates in States Mandating Sexual Education in Any Content Area in K–12 Public Schools: United States, 2024–2025

curriculum without saying the curriculum needed to be "culturally appropriate." Using the projected numbers of high-school graduates in 2024–2025, this means that of the 3 150 920 students graduating in jurisdictions with mandatory sexual education content, 91% were in states mandating "age-appropriate" content, while 58% were in states that mandated medically accurate instruction in any content area (Figure 2). Fewer states required content that was evidence-based (43%), up to date (23%), or culturally appropriate (19%) in any topic area. Only 19% of graduating students in states with mandatory sexual education (17% of graduating students in all states) received content that was medically accurate, up-to-date, and evidence-based.

Parental Options and Requirements

Most of the 42 states with mandatory sex education had state laws addressing parental notice, consent, or inspection of materials. Thirty-four states explicitly enabled parents to opt their child out of mandatory content, generally by written request (Table D, available as a supplement to the online version of this article at https://ajph.org). Five states required parents to actively opt their children in before they received sexual education. We did not identify state laws addressing parental consent options in 5 states. Twenty-four states had statutes or regulations that required schools to provide advance notice to parents before giving sexual education instruction. In 32 of the states with mandatory sexual education, state law also gave parents the right to inspect curriculum materials that would be used for the instruction.

DISCUSSION

Receipt of evidence-based, medically accurate sexual education in school settings can help address the persistent sexual health concerns experienced by US adolescents.[7–10] Although approximately 89% of public high-school graduates must receive sexual education in at least 1 content area during their K–12 years, only 58% of these students reside in a jurisdiction that requires sexual education to be medically accurate, and many jurisdictions have content mandates that extend only to a few content areas. In jurisdictions without state-level laws on sexual education, local school districts and boards of education decide whether any sexual education will be provided—and if so, what content will be covered. These decentralized choices may leave many US adolescents at an educational deficit when it comes to their sexual health.

In the 42 states that had mandatory school-based sexual education in at least 1 content area, content mandates were most likely to include sexual abstinence, HIV, STIs, the prevention of child abuse, and healthy relationships. Programs that emphasize sexual abstinence, including "abstinence-only" approaches that exclude other methods for preventing STIs, have long received US federal funding.[22] States continue to prioritize these approaches, although consistent research demonstrates that abstinence-only sexual education is ineffective or harmful for

TABLE 1— Required Content of K–12 Public School Sex Education in States Where It is Mandatory: United States, March 2025

State	Abstinence	HIV/ AIDS	STI	Condoms	Contraception	Safer Sex[a]	State Laws	Dating Violence/ IPV	Healthy Relationships	Consent	Child Abuse	Sexual Assault	Gender Identity	Sexual Orientation
AL	✓	✓	✓								✓			
AK								✓	✓		✓	✓		
AR								✓	✓					
CA	✓	✓	✓		✓	✓	✓	✓	✓		✓	✓	✓	✓
CT		✓									✓	✓		
DC	✓	✓	✓	✓	✓		✓	✓	✓	✓	✓	✓	✓	✓
DE	✓	✓							✓	✓	✓			
FL	✓		✓					✓	✓		✓			
GA	✓	✓	✓				✓				✓	✓		
HI	✓	✓	✓		✓			✓	✓					
IL	✓	✓					✓	✓			✓	✓		
IN	✓	✓									✓			
IA			✓								✓	✓		
KY	✓	✓	✓		✓				✓			✓		
ME									✓	✓	✓			
MD	✓	✓	✓	✓	✓	✓	✓	✓	✓	✓	✓	✓	✓	✓
MA								✓	✓					
MI	✓	✓	✓									✓		
MN	✓	✓	✓											
MS	✓	✓	✓								✓			
MO	✓	✓	✓	✓	✓		✓	✓	✓	✓	✓	✓		
NV			✓											
NH	✓	✓	✓		✓		✓	✓			✓	✓		
NJ	✓	✓	✓	✓	✓	✓	✓	✓	✓	✓	✓	✓	✓	✓
NM	✓	✓	✓	✓	✓			✓	✓		✓	✓		
NY	✓	✓	✓	✓	✓		✓	✓	✓		✓	✓		✓
NC	✓	✓	✓		✓		✓		✓		✓	✓		
ND	✓	✓	✓		✓				✓					
OH	✓	✓	✓				✓	✓	✓		✓	✓		
OK	✓	✓							✓					✓[b]
OR	✓	✓	✓	✓	✓	✓	✓	✓	✓	✓	✓	✓	✓	✓
PA	✓	✓	✓											

Continued

TABLE 1— Continued

State	Abstinence	HIV/ AIDS	STI	Condoms	Contraception	Safer Sex[a]	State Laws	Dating Violence/ IPV	Healthy Relationships	Consent	Child Abuse	Sexual Assault	Gender Identity	Sexual Orientation
RI	✓	✓	✓	✓	✓	✓	✓	✓	✓	✓	✓	✓	✓	✓
SC	✓	✓	✓		✓		✓				✓	✓		
SD	✓													
TN	✓	✓	✓				✓	✓	✓		✓			
TX	✓	✓	✓	✓	✓		✓	✓	✓		✓	✓		✓[c]
UT	✓	✓	✓	✓	✓		✓	✓	✓		✓	✓		
VT	✓	✓	✓		✓		✓		✓		✓	✓		✓
WA	✓	✓	✓	✓	✓	✓	✓		✓	✓	✓	✓	✓	✓
WV	✓	✓	✓		✓	✓		✓	✓		✓			✓
WI		✓	✓								✓			

Note. IPV = intimate partner violence; STI = sexually transmitted infection.
[a]Education must include instruction on a feature of state law (e.g., age of consent to sexual activity, definition of sex trafficking, legal elements of sex offenses).
[b]Instruction must include that "engaging in homosexual activity, promiscuous sexual activity, intravenous drug use or contact with contaminated blood products is now known to be primarily responsible for contact with the AIDS virus" (Okla Stat Ann tit 70, § 11-103.3; Okla Admin Code § 210:15-17-2).
[c]Instruction must include "emphasis, provided in a factual manner and from a public health perspective, that homosexuality is not a lifestyle acceptable to the general public and that homosexual conduct is a criminal offense under Section 21.06, Penal Code" (Tex Health & Safety Code Ann § 163.002).

adolescent sexual health.[21–25] At the time of this study, 14 states required coverage of sexual abstinence but did not require coverage of condoms, contraception, or safer sex, meaning that comprehensive sexual education was allowable, but local districts could also satisfy state law by implementing abstinence-only education. Among states with mandatory sexual education, none explicitly prohibited comprehensive sexual education, which has demonstrated effectiveness for promoting adolescent sexual health.[7–10] This legal landscape is advantageous for local districts wishing to implement comprehensive sexual education approaches. State laws also reflect emerging views that public school education should cover child abuse prevention, sexual assault, dating or intimate partner violence, and healthy relationships. Many states have enacted standalone educational mandates responding to child sexual abuse or dating violence.

Few states have mandated sexual education content addressing sexual orientation and gender identity, and existing mandates include both helpful and harmful messaging. Of the 42 states that mandated sexual education content, only 10 required information about sexual orientation and gender diversity that was affirming or neutral, and 2 states mandated stigmatizing content. The lack of mandates for content that addresses SGM students' needs is at odds with growing evidence that SGM-inclusive sexual education benefits the sexual and emotional health of all adolescents, not only SGM youth.[8]

Beyond content requirements, we found that most states also regulated attributes of sexual education. Multiple public health and medical associations recommend comprehensive sexual

TABLE 2— Required Attributes of K–12 Public School Sex Education in States Where It Is Mandatory: United States, March 2025

State	Age-Appropriate	Medically Accurate	Culturally Appropriate	Up-to-Date	Evidence- or Research-Based	Other
AL	✓	✓	✓		✓	
AK	✓					
AR	✓	✓[a]			✓	✓
CA	✓	✓	✓			
CT	✓					
DC	✓		✓		✓	
DE	✓				✓	
FL	✓					
GA	✓					
HI	✓	✓			✓	
IL	✓	✓[b]			✓	
IN	✓				✓	
IA	✓	✓			✓	
KY	✓				✓	
ME	✓					
MD[c]	✓	✓				✓
MA						
MI	✓	✓				
MN		✓		✓		
MS[d]	✓					✓
MO[e]	✓	✓				✓
NV						
NH	✓					
NJ	✓	✓		✓	✓	
NM	✓				✓	
NY[f]	✓				✓	✓
NC	✓				✓	
ND						
OH	✓					
OK		✓[g]		✓		
OR[h]	✓	✓	✓	✓	✓	✓
PA	✓					
RI[i]	✓	✓	✓		✓	✓
SC[j]	✓					✓
SD						
TN	✓	✓				
TX	✓	✓[k]		✓	✓	
UT	✓	✓				
VT	✓					
WA	✓	✓	✓	✓	✓	

Continued

TABLE 2— Continued

State	Age-Appropriate	Medically Accurate	Culturally Appropriate	Up-to-Date	Evidence- or Research-Based	Other
WV	✓				✓	
WI		✓[l]				

Note. A state is listed as mandating an attribute if a state law, regulation, or mandatory guidance document requires it for any content area in Table 1. Where medical accuracy is only mandated for a specific topic area, it is noted below.
[a]Materials on preventing pregnancy must be medically accurate (ACA § 6-60-106).
[b]Materials on abstinence must be medically accurate (105 Ill Comp Stat 110/3).
[c]Materials must "reflect educational equity" (Maryland Comprehensive Health Education Framework [http://bit.ly/4l4mBI7]).
[d]"[S]ex-related education instruction may not be conducted when boys and girls are in the company of any students of the opposite gender" (Miss Code Ann § 37-13-171).
[e]Sexual abuse training must be trauma-informed (Mo Rev Stat § 170.045).
[f]AIDS education must also be "consistent with community values" (NY Comp Codes R & Regs tit 8, § 135.3). Materials must be skills-driven, learner-centered, strength-based, authentic, and integrated into the total education program (New York Guidance Document for Achieving Learning Standards [http://bit.ly/40Mdtkp]).
[g]Materials on HIV/AIDS must be medically accurate (70 Okla Stat Ann § 11-103.3).
[h]Materials must also be positive, not "fear- or shame-based," strengths-based, trauma-informed, skills-based, "complete," and "balanced." Materials must "allay fears concerning risks that are scientifically groundless," must "not devalue[e] or ignor[e] students who have had or are having sexual intercourse," and must be "sensitive to the fact that there are students who have experienced sexual abuse" (Or Rev Stat § 336.455; Or Admin R 581-021-0593; Or Admin R 581-022-2050; Oregon Health Standards 2023 [http://bit.ly/4oi3FbQ]).
[i]Materials must also be skills-based and trauma-informed (2022 RI Curriculum Framework for Health Education K–12 [http://bit.ly/3Utkldv]).
[j]"Instruction in pregnancy prevention education must be presented separately to male and female students" (SC Code Ann § 59-32-30).
[k]Materials on contraception failure rates must be medically accurate (Tex Health & Safety Code Ann § 163.002).
[l]Information about human papillomavirus and HIV must be medically accurate (Wis Stat Ann § 118.019).

education that is age-appropriate, medically accurate, evidence-based, and culturally appropriate, adaptive, or responsive.[11–15] Many states have responded by adopting some of these attributes in their sexual education laws. Although this may be helpful, adding attribute requirements can be a double-edged sword; as Santelli has noted,[33] when a state mandates a particular type of education, like "medically accurate," without specifically defining the term in the law, it allows regulators to supply their own ideas about what instruction is permissible. Some of these descriptors have predictable or widely recognized definitions, such as "medically accurate" or "up to date." But others, such as "age-appropriate," can be unpredictable and grounds for challenging programming. Different parents, students, teachers, administrators, and regulators may hold different views about what content is "age-appropriate." Laws requiring attributes that are vague, subject to varying or politicized interpretations, or lacking in statutory definitions may deter educators from implementing sexual education programming.

Most states that require sexual education allow parents to opt children out of the requirement. This likely reflects a pragmatic compromise: although most parents support school-based sexual education,[16–18] it may be politically difficult to pass a sexual education mandate without providing for parental opt-out. But where sexual education mandates exist, opt-out policies can limit their impact. States further weaken sexual education mandates if they require parents to actively opt their children in, a policy used by 5 states. Research is needed to understand how opt-in requirements, opt-out opportunities, rights to inspect educational materials, and advance notice requirements mediate the impacts of sexual education laws.

Strengths and Limitations

Our study has many strengths, including a replicable search strategy; a detailed coding scheme; a systematic search for state statutes, regulations, and judicial opinions; and a rigorous approach to redundant coding and reconciliation of discrepancies. This study also has limitations. We did not assess municipal laws, and cities have their own sexual education ordinances. In the 9 jurisdictions that did not mandate sexual education content in K–12 public schools, local school districts and boards of education made all such decisions. In the 42 jurisdictions with mandates, local schools could add content areas of their own choosing (if they did not conflict with prohibitions). We only assessed laws affecting public schools, which did not extend to other educational settings. We also made analytic choices to focus on mandates at any time before high-school graduation, which collapses many years of education into a single time frame. Future research might seek to examine mandates at particular educational levels (e.g., kindergarten, middle school).

Although we aimed for sensitivity in our search design, we may have missed laws if they did not use terminology from our search string. Some laws that address education generally (e.g., laws prohibiting content on sexual orientation and gender identity across all subjects) may affect sexual education but may not have reliably been identified as part of our search. Similarly, we did not search for laws that allowed parents to inspect instructional materials generally, outside the sexual education setting. Legislators are currently advocating or passing "parents' rights" laws at the state and federal levels,[34,35] so future research should consider how these new provisions affect sexual education and adolescents' health outcomes. We did not extract data on mandatory education regarding "sexting," sharing, or posting sexual content, but we suggest doing so in future research. Finally, this article does not report laws that "conditionally" regulate sexual education—that is, laws that do not mandate sexual education but that establish rules for school districts that voluntarily choose to provide it.

Public Health Implications

Adolescents in the United States continue to experience substantial sexual health concerns. School-based sexual education is an essential public health intervention with the potential to reach most youths, and public health and medical organizations recommend instruction on a wide range of sexual health topics.[11–15] Although most US states require public schools to provide some sexual education content in the K–12 years, most mandates are limited to a combination of abstinence, HIV, STIs, child abuse prevention, and healthy relationships. Few states require that this content be medically accurate or evidence-based. Policy features like vaguely defined or unpredictable attribute mandates and expansive parental rights protections may also complicate the impacts of sexual education programming.

Recent, frequent, and ongoing legislative activity in this area suggests that there will be many opportunities to revisit sexual education mandates. Most states have enacted or amended parts of their sexual education laws in the past 5 to 10 years, suggesting that policymakers have the motivation and opportunity to revisit these policies over time. Policy studies that identify differences across state laws can advance research on how these policy choices affect adolescents' health during and after their school years. Alongside recommendations by medical and educational organizations, this research base will provide information for policymakers, funders, and researchers to advocate state laws that promote adolescent sexual health. State laws that mandate sexual education play an important role in the sexual health of young people in the United States, but there is still a long way to go. AJPH

ABOUT THE AUTHORS

Kimberly M. Nelson is with the School of Public Health and the Chobanian & Avedisian School of Medicine, Boston University, Boston, MA. Aaliyah Gray is with the Center for Women's and Gender Studies, Florida International University, Miami. Samantha Haiken is with the School of Public Health, Boston University, Boston, MA. Kristen Underhill is with the Cornell Law School, Ithaca, NY, and the Weill Cornell Medical College, New York, NY.

CORRESPONDENCE

Correspondence should be sent to Kimberly Nelson, PhD, MPH, 801 Massachusetts Ave, 4th Floor, Boston, MA 02118 (e-mail: knel@bu.edu). Reprints can be ordered at https://ajph.org by clicking the "Reprints" link.

PUBLICATION INFORMATION

Full Citation: Nelson KM, Gray A, Haiken S, Underhill K. The state of sexual education: state laws and regulations mandating sexual education in the United States. *Am J Public Health*. 2025; 115(10):1723–1733.

Acceptance Date: May 11, 2025.

DOI: https://doi.org/10.2105/AJPH.2025.308199

ORCID iDs:

Kimberly M. Nelson https://orcid.org/0000-0001-8893-5764

Aaliyah Gray https://orcid.org/0000-0003-1788-1791

Samantha Haiken https://orcid.org/0009-0004-6916-3913

Kristen Underhill https://orcid.org/0009-0000-0349-2846

CONTRIBUTORS

All authors made substantial contributions to this article. K. Nelson and K. Underhill conceptualized the study. K. Nelson acquired the funding. K. Underhill led the legal coding, cleaning, and updating process. A. Gray and S. Haiken conducted data coding, cleaning, and initial analyses. K. Underhill finalized the data set and analyses. All authors wrote, reviewed, and edited the article.

ACKNOWLEDGMENTS

We would like to thank the Youth Advisory Board and the law student research assistants who helped collect and code the initial legal citations. This work is supported by the National Institutes of Mental Health (R01MH119892, PI: Nelson; R01MH119892-01A1S1, PI: Nelson).

Note. The content of this publication is solely the responsibility of the authors and does not represent the official views of the National Institutes of Health. The National Institutes of Health had no role in the design and conduct of the study; collection, management, analysis, and interpretation of the data; preparation, review, or approval of the article; or decision to submit the article for publication.

CONFLICTS OF INTEREST

The authors have no conflicts of interest to report.

HUMAN PARTICIPANT PROTECTION

This study did not include human participants and was exempted by the Boston University Medical Campus institutional review board.

REFERENCES

1. Centers for Disease Control and Prevention. Sexually Transmitted Disease Surveillance, 2023. 2024. Available at: https://www.cdc.gov/sti-statistics/annual/summary.html. Accessed December 19, 2024.
2. Centers for Disease Control and Prevention. *HIV Surveillance Report: Diagnoses, Deaths, and Prevalence of HIV in the United States and 6 Territories and Freely Associated States, 2022.* 2024. Available at: https://stacks.cdc.gov/view/cdc/156509. Accessed December 19, 2024.
3. Centers for Disease Control and Prevention. Unintended pregnancy. 2021. Available at: https://www.cdc.gov/reproductivehealth/contraception/unintendedpregnancy/index.htm. Accessed September 10, 2022.
4. The Lancet Child & Adolescent Health. Youth STIs: an epidemic fuelled by shame. *Lancet Child Adolesc Health.* 2022;6(6):353. https://doi.org/10.1016/S2352-4642(22)00128-6
5. Centers for Disease Control and Prevention. Youth Risk Behavior Surveillance System—United States, 2021 Supplementary Tables. 2024. Available at: https://www.cdc.gov/yrbs/results/2021-supplementary-tables.html. Accessed January 2, 2025.
6. National Center for Education Statistics. National Center for Education Statistics fast facts. US Department of Education. 2024. Available at: https://nces.ed.gov/fastfacts/display.asp?id=372#PK12-enrollment. Accessed December 19, 2024.
7. Denford S, Abraham C, Campbell R, Busse H. A comprehensive review of reviews of school-based interventions to improve sexual-health. *Health Psychol Rev.* 2017;11(1):33–52. https://doi.org/10.1080/17437199.2016.1240625
8. Goldfarb ES, Lieberman LD. Three decades of research: the case for comprehensive sex education. *J Adolesc Health.* 2021;68(1):13–27. https://doi.org/10.1016/j.jadohealth.2020.07.036
9. Coyle K, Anderson P, Laris BA, Barrett M, Unti T, Baumler E. A group randomized trial evaluating High School FLASH, a comprehensive sexual health curriculum. *J Adolesc Health.* 2021;68(4):686–695. https://doi.org/10.1016/j.jadohealth.2020.12.005
10. Banerjee D, Rao TSS. Comprehensive sex education—why should we care? *J Psychosexual Health.* 2022;4(2):73–75. https://doi.org/10.1177/26318318221092076
11. American Public Health Association. Sexuality Education as Part of a Comprehensive Health Education Program in K to 12 Schools. 2014. Available at: https://www.apha.org/policies-and-advocacy/public-health-policy-statements/policy-database/2015/01/23/09/37/sexuality-education-as-part-of-a-comprehensive-health-education-program-in-k-to-12-schools. Accessed March 6, 2025.
12. United Nations Educational, Scientific, and Cultural Organization. *International Technical Guidance on Sexuality Education: An Evidence-Informed Approach.* World Health Organization. 2018. Available at: https://cdn.who.int/media/docs/default-source/reproductive-health/sexual-health/international-technical-guidance-on-sexuality-education.pdf?sfvrsn=10113efc_29&download=true. Accessed December 20, 2024.
13. Centers for Disease Control and Prevention. Sexual health education. 2024. Available at: https://www.cdc.gov/healthy-youth/what-works-in-schools/sexual-health-education.html. Accessed December 20, 2024.
14. American Academy of Pediatrics. The importance of access to comprehensive sex education. 2024. Available at: https://web.archive.org/web/20250614033542/https://www.aap.org/en/patient-care/adolescent-sexual-health/equitable-access-to-sexual-and-reproductive-health-care-for-all-youth/the-importance-of-access-to-comprehensive-sex-education. Accessed December 20, 2024.
15. Future of Sex Education Initiative. *National Sex Education Standards: Core Content and Skills, K-12.* 2020. Available at: https://siecus.org/wp-content/uploads/2020/03/NSES-2020-2.pdf. Accessed May 22, 2023.
16. Szucs LE, Harper CR, Andrzejewski J, Barrios LC, Robin L, Hunt P. Overwhelming support for sexual health education in US schools: a meta-analysis of 23 surveys conducted between 2000 and 2016. *J Adolesc Health.* 2022;70(4):598–606. https://doi.org/10.1016/j.jadohealth.2021.05.016
17. Hurst JL, Widman L, Brasileiro J, Maheux AJ, Evans-Paulson R, Choukas-Bradley S. Parents' attitudes towards the content of sex education in the USA: associations with religiosity and political orientation. *Sex Educ.* 2024;24(1):108–124. https://doi.org/10.1080/14681811.2022.2162871
18. Kantor L, Levitz N. Parents' views on sex education in schools: how much do Democrats and Republicans agree? *PLoS ONE.* 2017;12(7):e0180250. https://doi.org/10.1371/journal.pone.0180250
19. Office of Disease Prevention and Health Promotion. Increase the proportion of adolescents who get formal sex education before age 18 years — FP-08. US Department of Health and Human Services. 2020. Available at: https://web.archive.org/web/20250423020637/https://odphp.health.gov/healthypeople/objectives-and-data/browse-objectives/family-planning/increase-proportion-adolescents-who-get-formal-sex-education-age-18-years-fp-08. Accessed November 5, 2024.
20. Lindberg LD, Kantor LM. Adolescents' receipt of sex education in a nationally representative sample, 2011–2019. *J Adolesc Health.* 2022;70(2):290–297. https://doi.org/10.1016/j.jadohealth.2021.08.027
21. Stanger-Hall KF, Hall DW. Abstinence-only education and teen pregnancy rates: why we need comprehensive sex education in the US. *PLoS ONE.* 2011;6(10):e24658. https://doi.org/10.1371/journal.pone.0024658
22. Santelli JS, Kantor LM, Grilo SA, et al. Abstinence-only-until-marriage: an updated review of US policies and programs and their impact. *J Adolesc Health.* 2017;61(3):273–280. https://doi.org/10.1016/j.jadohealth.2017.05.031
23. Fox AM, Himmelstein G, Khalid H, Howell EA. Funding for abstinence-only education and adolescent pregnancy prevention: does state ideology affect outcomes? *Am J Public Health.* 2019;109(3):497–504. https://doi.org/10.2105/AJPH.2018.304896
24. Mark NDE, Wu LL. More comprehensive sex education reduced teen births: quasi-experimental evidence. *Proc Natl Acad Sci USA.* 2022;119(8):e2113144119. https://doi.org/10.1073/pnas.2113144119
25. Atkins DN, Bradford WD. The effect of state-level sex education policies on youth sexual behaviors. *Arch Sex Behav.* 2021;50(6):2321–2333. https://doi.org/10.1007/s10508-020-01867-9
26. Landry DJ, Darroch JE, Singh S, Higgins J. Factors associated with the content of sex education in US public secondary schools. *Perspect Sex Reprod Health.* 2003;35(05):261–269. https://doi.org/10.1363/3526103
27. Guttmacher Institute. Sex and HIV education as of March 1, 2025. 2025. Available at: https://www.guttmacher.org/state-policy/explore/sex-and-hiv-education. Accessed March 10, 2025.
28. Sexuality Information and Education Council of the United States. Sex ed state law and policy chart: SEICUS state profiles, July 2022. 2022. Available at: https://siecus.org/resource/2022-sex-ed-state-law-and-policy-chart. Accessed March 10, 2025.
29. Anderson E, Tremper C, Thomas S, Wagenaar A. Measuring statutory law and regulations for empirical research. In: Wagenaar A, Burris S, eds. *Public Health Law Research: Theory and Method.* San Francisco, CA: Wiley; 2013.
30. Hall M. Coding case law for public health law evaluation. In: Wagenaar A, Burris S, eds. *Public Health Law Research: Theory and Method.* San Francisco, CA: Wiley; 2013.
31. Burris S, Hitchcock L, Ibrahim J, Penn M, Ramanathan T. Policy surveillance: a vital public health practice comes of age. *J Health Polit Policy Law.* 2016;41(6):1151–1173. https://doi.org/10.1215/03616878-3665931
32. National Center for Education Statistics. Public high school graduates, by region, state, and jurisdiction: selected school years, 1980–81 through 2031–32. US Department of Education. 2023. Available at: https://nces.ed.gov/programs/digest/d23/tables/dt23_219.20.asp. Accessed December 20, 2024.
33. Santelli JS. Medical accuracy in sexuality education: ideology and the scientific process. *Am J Public Health.* 2008;98(10):1786–1792. https://doi.org/10.2105/AJPH.2007.119602
34. Letlow J. H.R.5 - Parents Bill of Rights Act. 2023. Available at: https://www.congress.gov/bill/118th-congress/house-bill/5/text. Accessed January 3, 2025.
35. DiMarco B. Legislative Tracker: 2023 Parent-Rights Bills in the States. Georgetown University's McCourt School of Public Policy. 2023. Available at: https://www.future-ed.org/legislative-tracker-2023-parent-rights-bills-in-the-states. Accessed January 3, 2025.

Self-Managed Medication Abortion: History, Evidence, Models of Care, and Policy Considerations

Laura E. Jacobson, PhD, MPH, and Caitlin Gerdts, PhD, MHS

Self-managed abortion (SMA) represents a significant shift in the abortion landscape, offering an alternative to facility-based care via the medication misoprostol with or without mifepristone. The World Health Organization recommends SMA with medications as safe and effective up to 12 weeks' gestation and with access to information and health system referrals. Increasing prevalence of SMA can be attributed to a range of factors, including legal and logistical barriers to facility-based care as well as a social movement advocating autonomy and demedicalized practices in the United States, particularly after the US Supreme Court decided *Dobbs v Jackson Women's Health Org.*, 597 US (2022).

We document the history, safety and effectiveness, measurement challenges, and models of SMA care and review ongoing legal and policy challenges. Despite its clinical and practical advantages, SMA exists in a complex policy environment that hinders access to safe abortion. Evidence from diverse regions demonstrates the potential for SMA to expand access, especially where care is limited or restricted.

As research affirms the safety of SMA, including later in pregnancy, it remains vital to protect and expand access to abortion medications, without threat of criminalization, to ensure that individuals can exercise their reproductive rights and autonomy. (*Am J Public Health.* 2025;115(10):1734–1741. https://doi.org/10.2105/AJPH.2025.308133)

AJPH October 2025, Vol. 115, No. 10

People capable of pregnancy have always sought to regulate their fertility.[1] Self-managed abortion (SMA) is broadly understood as actions or activities undertaken by an individual to terminate their pregnancy without formal clinician management[2] using a range of methods that vary in safety and efficacy.[3] Since the late 1980s, 2 widely recognized medication abortion regimens—misoprostol alone or in combination with mifepristone—have significantly increased the safety and effectiveness of SMA.[4,5] Although many people choose SMA because of barriers to facility-based care, others prefer it for its convenience, accessibility, and privacy.[2] Over the past 50 years, the development of networks supporting individuals in SMA has transformed the abortion landscape.[6]

Strategies to facilitate access to medication abortion encompass a variety of approaches, including hotlines for information, medication-by-mail services, clinics staffed with trained medical personnel or lay activists, online sources offering detailed instructions, and mobile apps. Greater access to medication abortion has not only expanded access[7] but also contributed to the reduction of maternal morbidity and mortality in several countries.[8,9] In 2022, SMA was incorporated into the World Health Organization's (WHO's) guidelines as a recommended model of abortion care at less than 12 weeks of gestation and when the pregnant person has access to quality medications and health system referrals if needed or wanted.[10] SMA has also created much legal ambiguity,[11] muddied the boundaries of health systems,[12] and sparked debate on its definition and scope.[13–15]

In addition to being part of a model of abortion care, SMA is supported by a social movement built on the belief that people can, and should, have the ability to legally terminate a pregnancy safely in the community, without medical supervision.[6] This sentiment is sometimes at odds with clinician-managed organizations or health service delivery systems,[16,17] whose goal is also to provide abortion care but who benefit from legal protections in some settings.[18] Because *Dobbs v Jackson Women's Health Org.*, 597 US (hereafter *Dobbs*) eliminated the constitutional right to abortion in the United States in 2022, the legality of abortion now depends on one's geographic residence—with some states having moved to ban abortion entirely and others having expanded access.[19]

With nationwide access to facility-based abortion care significantly reduced, interest in abortion care by telehealth has grown. Several states have enacted "shield laws" in an attempt to offer legal protection to providers seeking to offer abortion care to patients who live in restrictive states.[18] Abortions provided through shield law services are clinically indistinguishable from other telehealth abortion services, yet it is critical to note that while providers operating under shield laws do so with some legal protection, people seeking abortions from such services (and the people in their communities who support them) remain vulnerable to criminalization. While it is important to acknowledge that people obtaining abortion services through telehealth shield (including shield law providers) may experience and describe their abortions in ways that resemble self-managed abortion, and that people can and do self-manage abortion using a range of methods,including herbs, massage, and invasive practices, within the scope of this essay we focus solely on SMA with medications (misoprostol alone or with mifepristone) and without clinical supervision. We aimed to encapsulate the history, safety, and effectiveness; measurement challenges; models of care; and ongoing legal and policy challenges of self-managed medication abortion.

HISTORY OF MEDICATION ABORTION

Although misoprostol was initially developed in the United States for treating gastric ulcers, its repurposing as an abortifacient occurred serendipitously in Brazil during the 1980s. In a legally restricted environment, people seeking pregnancy termination options discovered the off-label use of misoprostol—sold for ulcer treatment under the brand name Cytotec—as a safe and effective abortifacient. This discovery was based on the information provided on the drug's label.[20] Following this discovery, the widespread use of misoprostol for inducing abortions outside the health care system in Brazil led to a measurable decrease in complications from unsafe abortion.[20] However, the publicity of misoprostol's widespread use sparked a heated debate, leading to tightened regulations. The self-use of misoprostol in Brazil eventually led to more research documenting its safety and effectiveness[20] and a diffusion of this practice throughout Latin America in countries (e.g., Chile, Mexico, and Colombia) with similar legal restrictions that spurred the need for safe and accessible abortion methods.[21]

Although the United States played a pivotal role in the initial development and regulatory approval of misoprostol, it was the innovative, self-managed use in Brazil that redefined the drug's potential in reproductive health—a process that has since influenced both clinical practices and global reproductive health policies.[10] Misoprostol was developed by Searle (now Pfizer) in the United States in the 1970s for the prevention of gastric ulcers. Misoprostol causes uterine contractions and found widespread off-label use in reproductive medicine particularly in labor induction, postpartum hemorrhage, and abortion care.[22] Despite the drug's beneficial applications, Searle faced controversy and issued warnings against its use in pregnancy,[23] even as the American College of Obstetricians and Gynecologists actively promoted its use in reproductive medicine.[24,25] Misoprostol's use and scope have since been expanded and refined based on extensive research, and it is now among the WHO's essential medicines.[26] Together, these histories illustrate how misoprostol's evolution—from a US-developed medication to a grassroots tool in Brazil—has reshaped abortion care in legally restrictive settings across Latin America and beyond.

A second abortion medication, mifepristone (first known as RU-486), was developed by French scientists in the 1980s. It works by inhibiting the hormone progesterone, which is crucial for maintaining pregnancy. Although it was approved for use in France in 1988, mifepristone faced intense political opposition in the United States, leading to a significant delay in availability.[27] The US Food and Drug Administration (FDA) did not approve mifepristone for up to 7 weeks of gestation until September 2000. Over the next decade and a half, accumulating evidence and advocacy pushed for updated regulations. In 2016, the FDA revised mifepristone's label, extending its approved use to up to 70 days (10 weeks) of gestation and demonstrating significant safety and effectiveness.[28]

Unlike misoprostol, mifepristone is specifically approved in the United States and elsewhere as an abortifacient, which has subjected it to heightened scrutiny, barriers, and restrictions that continue to exist today.[29,30] The FDA's Risk Evaluation and Mitigation

Strategy Program oversees distribution of mifepristone in the United States, even though the imposed precautions are inconsistent with the evidence of this drug's safety profile.[31] Under the current risk evaluation and mitigation strategy, mifepristone must be prescribed by certified providers or dispensed through certified pharmacies, although in-person dispensing requirements have been removed, allowing telehealth consultations where state laws permit.[32]

SAFETY AND EFFECTIVENESS

Decades of clinical evidence have demonstrated that medication abortion (misoprostol alone or in combination with mifepristone) is a safe and effective method of terminating a pregnancy.[33,34] However, most studies were conducted in clinical settings, where procedural intervention was easily accessible and may have been used preemptively, possibly leading to overestimates of failed abortion—which were already low.[35–37] Although political, legal, and social factors significantly influence abortion decision-making and care seeking, the consistency with which medication abortion's safety and effectiveness has been demonstrated across diverse regions, contexts, and both in and outside formal health care settings[5,38–41] remains an essential consideration.

A noninferiority analysis compared SMA with accompaniment group support in Nigeria and Argentina to historical controls of clinician-managed medication abortion conducted as a part of the SAFE (Studying Accompaniment model Feasibility and Effectiveness) study, a prospective, observational cohort study of SMA in Argentina, Nigeria, and a Southeast Asian country. The results revealed that 97% of 951 users had a complete abortion without intervention after 4 weeks, and 87% reported no warning signs of a complication.[5] Most of the pregnancies (95%) in the study were of 12 weeks or less duration. This study also found that SMA using misoprostol alone is as effective as using misoprostol in combination with mifepristone[5]—an important finding given that misoprostol is less regulated and more accessible than mifepristone.[42] Additional studies in Bangladesh,[43,44] India,[40] Nigeria,[45] and Pakistan[39] and along the Thailand–Myanmar border[38] demonstrated similar evidence of safety, effectiveness, and acceptability. A cross-sectional study using data from India's National Family Health Survey found that SMA was associated with lower odds of complications than clinician-managed abortion.[40]

The WHO currently recommends medication abortion up to 12 weeks of gestation, after which they advise that procedural backup and proper infrastructure be available to address incomplete abortion or potential complications.[10] During later stages of pregnancy, the process of medication abortion tends to take longer and has a higher chance of complications or needing additional medical intervention.[46–48] However, recent studies indicate that SMA can be safe and effective after 12 weeks of gestation.[41,48–50] In the SAFE study, people who self-managed with medication between 9 and 16 weeks of gestation had high levels of abortion completion, with follow-up care primarily accessed to confirm completion.[48]

A retrospective analysis of client records from a safe abortion hotline in Indonesia found that 91.2% (83/91) of people who were 13 to 22 weeks' pregnant successfully terminated their pregnancies with medications without seeking medical care; only 6% (6/91) sought care for potential complications or failed abortion.[41] Similarly, a retrospective analysis of client records from accompaniment groups in Argentina, Chile, and Ecuador supporting abortions between 13 and 24 weeks showed 95% (302/318) of SMA attempts were complete.[50] Some studies on SMA have limitations, including the reliance of self-report for gestational duration and self-report, often in consultation with trained counselors, of abortion outcomes as well as small sample sizes for studies of abortion after 12 weeks' gestation. Self-managed medication abortion, with support and linkages to the formal health system if needed or wanted, may be an effective and safe option for abortion later in pregnancy—particularly in legally restrictive settings, where it can provide a safe alternative to clandestine procedures.

Measuring Self-Managed Abortion

Accurate estimates of abortion incidence, outcomes, and safety are important for informing public health strategies and resource allocation. However, making these measurements, particularly in SMA, poses significant challenges because of legal restrictions, privacy concerns, and stigma.[51] The decentralized distribution of medication complicates data collection on SMA users, most of whom do not seek facility-based care and thus evade research recruitment. Reliable data collection is hindered by several factors, including the difficulty of quantifying total SMA users, challenges in studying outcomes, and users' legitimate fears of legal repercussions.[52]

Direct measurement using official statistics and surveys of SMA is infeasible because people are not coming in for care, so their records cannot be analyzed, and people notoriously underreport abortion when asked directly, even in legal settings.[53] Common indirect estimation methodologies for abortion incidence, such as the abortion incidence complications method,[51] rely on a range of data sources, assumptions, and adjustments to facility-based measures and proxies that are unavailable or irrelevant for SMA. However, documenting trends in the incidence and prevalence of SMA is needed to inform interventions that support people who cannot or may not want to access abortion in formal health systems to reduce the risks of criminalization and to identify where information needs and barriers may exist.[54]

Because of these measurement challenges, robust national-level incidence measures of SMA are scarce. However, researchers in India and the United States have been able to produce estimates using indirect methods or data sources not readily available elsewhere. For example, in India, Singh et al. estimated that of the 15.6 million abortions that occurred in 2015, 73% were likely self-managed medication abortions taking place outside facilities.[55] To make this estimation, Singh et al. used pharmaceutical sales data and information from hotlines that provide accompaniment for medication abortions and made several adjustments for incomplete data, drug waste, cross-border exports, and the use of nonpharmaceutical methods to induce abortions,[55] all factors that complicate the accuracy of such estimates.

More recently, in the United States, Ralph et al. conducted a series of national surveys and documented that 1.4% of respondents ever attempted SMA and that 7.0% of US women will attempt SMA at some point in their lives.[56] Ralph et al. followed up on this to capture estimates just before and after the *Dobbs* decision. They showed a rise in reported SMA attempts from 2.4% in 2021 (before) to 3.4% in 2023 (after the *Dobbs* decision). This translated to a projected lifetime experience with SMA of 10.7%.[57] As legal constraints on abortion continue across the United States, the prevalence of SMA is expected to rise. This trend underscores the urgent need for health care systems to adapt by providing comprehensive and nonstigmatizing support for individuals considering SMA. Moreover, higher SMA attempts reported among marginalized groups such as Black, LGBTQ+ (lesbian, gay, bisexual, transgender, queer or questioning, and all subsects), and adolescent individuals[57] highlight significant access and equity issues in health systems,[58,59] necessitating targeted interventions to address these inequities.

Models of Care and Points of Access

The increasing use of abortion medications has enabled safer self-management practices that center autonomy, privacy, confidentiality, and harm reduction.[11] A pregnant person's SMA trajectories are influenced by various actors at different points. SMA can occur on a continuum: at 1 end, someone may self-manage with minimal external support or information; in the middle, they may be supported by activists known as *acompañantes*, most commonly occurring in Latin America,[60] or safe abortion hotline counselors; and at the more medicalized end, they may receive assistance from lay health workers, midwives, or pharmacists or pharmacy workers.[61]

Before the advent of medication abortion and *Roe v Wade* (410 US 113 [1973]) in the United States, physicians, nurses, midwives, and lay persons with varying levels of skill provided procedural abortion discreetly, often outside health facilities.[62] For example, the Jane Collective in Chicago, Illinois, provided illegal but safe abortions before federal legalization in 1973.[63] During the *Roe* era (1973–2022), the use of misoprostol outside formal health systems increased the demand for accessible, accurate information and support to self-administer abortion medications effectively. This demand has grown significantly since the 2022 *Dobbs* decision.[64]

Feminist activism for SMA began outside traditional health systems and spread globally, promoting demedicalized practices.[6,60] Activists have created many avenues for accurate information and support to self-administer abortion medications effectively, such as feminist websites, safe abortion hotlines, and accompaniment groups.[6] Several websites have emerged that allow abortion seekers to easily find evidence-based information about timing, dosing schedules, side effects, complications, expected outcomes, when to seek medical attention, and how to procure medications; some even offer pills to order by mail. Some such established platforms with detailed information are available in Table A (available as a supplement to the online version of this article at http://www.ajph.org). Globally, findings on the experiences and outcomes of SMA in which information from websites was used are consistent with facility-managed medication abortion via telemedicine, for which complication rates are low and the process is acceptable to users.[65,66] However, depending on the country and context, studies have also shown variability in the quality of medications available by mail order from websites.[67,68]

Safe abortion hotlines provide interactive information and support for safely self-managing an abortion. These hotlines typically provide evidence-based guidance on pregnancy termination, covering topics such as dosage, symptoms, and potential side effects.[69,70] Hotlines also offer broader support, including a sense of community, particularly in restricted settings.[71,72] Some hotlines function as community-based models developed by activists,[73] whereas others are part of formal health systems.[74] Studies show that hotlines in legally restricted settings are particularly effective in engaging hard-to-reach populations and ensuring safer conditions for abortion[75] as well as fostering high levels of preparedness, confidence, and feelings of support among callers.[76]

The groups often seen in Latin American settings known as *acompañantes*—whose work is grounded in feminist praxis—accompany people who have a medication abortion outside clinical settings.[60] They offer support through various means, including in person, online, or on mobile platforms, and, as with safe abortion hotlines, they provide protocols for how to use medication to safely induce abortion.[77] Some organizations provide information on where to obtain quality medications, how the drugs function, what to expect, how to manage pain, how to recognize signs of complication, how to interact with medical personnel if needed, how to confirm a complete abortion, and how to prevent a future unwanted pregnancy.[77] Many *acompañantes* go beyond describing and coordinating logistical matters to also providing social and emotional support.[72,78,79] Interviews with *acompañantes* in Mexico revealed a holistic model of care that involved trusting clients, not asking for the reasons for their abortion, preventing criminalization, providing economic support, respecting autonomy, offering emotional support, and being flexible.[72]

Socorristas en Red in Argentina is a nationwide accompaniment network that provides access and information by telephone, in-person accompaniment, and group meetings as well as partnerships with clinicians.[80] In a prospective study of client experience with accompaniment support in Argentina, clients highlighted continual emotional support, empathy, and understanding from *acompañantes* and described open communication, comprehensive information, and nonjudgmental care as key components of a positive abortion experience.[79]

Pharmacy provision of medication abortion outside the United States offers an option that is more medicalized than unsupported SMA but less medicalized than facility-based abortion. Pharmacy or drugstore provision of medication abortion is often preferred in low- and middle- income countries because of their convenience, privacy, anonymity, and affordability.[81] However, studies indicate that the quality of pharmaceutical products can vary and that the accuracy and completeness of information supplied by pharmacy workers is lacking.[44,81–83] A study in India showed that the quality of information provided to clients purchasing medications at pharmacies was low, especially information related to timing and dosing of misoprostol, where only 18% (51/283) of pharmacists knew correct timing and 31% (88/283) offered no information on expected or concerning side effects.[82]

LEGAL AND POLICY CONSIDERATIONS

Despite the robust evidence supporting the safety and effectiveness of self-managed medication abortion, restrictive abortion laws and policies in many settings contradict clinical evidence and global care standards.[13] Current clinical guidelines do not require preabortion testing or routine follow-up visits for medication abortions, provided there is access to health system referrals if necessary.[10,28] Mandating follow-up care can perpetuate misconceptions about the safety and effectiveness of self-managed abortions, contrary to existing evidence.[84] Although the medical risks of SMA are few, the legal risks may be significant. In the United States, individuals who self-manage abortions can and have been criminalized under a range of charges, including those related to fetal harm, practicing medicine without a license, aiding an illegal abortion, and even homicide or manslaughter.[85]

However, these laws are often applied inconsistently, leading to legal ambiguity that can result in the misapplication of statutes not directly related to abortion—such as those designed to penalize physical assault or drug use—or can affect immigration status or child custody disputes. The United States has a long history of criminalizing reproductive behaviors,[85] and punitive policies have historically targeted communities of color, immigrant communities, people with low incomes, and young people.[86,87] For example, between 2000 and 2020, at least 61 people across 26 US states were criminally investigated or arrested for allegedly ending their own pregnancy or assisting someone else to do so.[85] These cases were overrepresented by people of color and most involved were living in poverty.

Globally, legal challenges to abortion reflect patterns of discrimination and marginalization similar to those seen in the United States. For example, in Poland, following a near-total ban on abortion in 2020, authorities have increasingly initiated investigations on dubious legal grounds against people who seek medical attention for miscarriages or following legal medication abortions and against the providers and activists who support them.[88,89] Restrictive laws and judicial decisions not only limit access to safe and legal abortion but compound social stigma, increase financial burdens, and discourage individuals from accessing future health care services.[90]

CONCLUSIONS

The discovery of abortifacient medications revolutionized safe abortion access worldwide. The self-management of these medications has been proven safe and effective in both clinical settings and outside formal health systems, a practice that centers autonomy. Evidence from diverse regions demonstrates the potential for SMA to expand access to reproductive health care, especially where access to care is limited or restricted. As research continues to affirm the safety of medication abortion, including later in pregnancy, it remains crucial that access to these medicines be protected and expanded, without threat of criminalization, to ensure that all individuals can exercise their reproductive rights and autonomy. AJPH

ABOUT THE AUTHORS

Laura E. Jacobson is with the Oregon Health & Science University–Portland State University School of Public Health, Portland. Caitlin Gerdts is with Ibis Reproductive Health, Oakland, CA.

CORRESPONDENCE

Correspondence should be sent to Laura E. Jacobson, OHSU-PSU School of Public Health, 1810 SW 5th Ave, Portland, OR 97201 (e-mail: jacobsonlaura@gmail.com). Reprints can be ordered at https://www.ajph.org by clicking the "Reprints" link.

PUBLICATION INFORMATION

Full Citation: Jacobson LE, Gerdts C. Self-managed medication abortion: history, evidence, models of care, and policy considerations. *Am J Public Health*. 2025;115(10):1734–1741.

Acceptance Date: March 17, 2025.

DOI: https://doi.org/10.2105/AJPH.2025.308133

ORCID iD:
Laura E. Jacobson https://orcid.org/0000-0002-0996-7408

CONTRIBUTORS

L. E. Jacobson prepared the original draft of the essay. C. Gerdts reviewed and edited the essay and supervised its writing. Both authors conceptualized the essay and approved its final form.

ACKNOWLEDGMENTS

L. E. Jacobson held an American Dissertation Fellowship from the American Association of University Women at the time this essay was conceptualized.

CONFLICTS OF INTEREST

The authors have no conflicts of interest to disclose.

HUMAN PARTICIPANT PROTECTION

No protocol approval was necessary because no human participants were involved in the writing of this essay.

REFERENCES

1. Riddle JM. *Contraception and Abortion From the Ancient World to the Renaissance*. Cambridge, MA: Harvard University Press; 1994.
2. Moseson H, Herold S, Filippa S, Barr-Walker J, Baum SE, Gerdts C. Self-managed abortion: a systematic scoping review. *Best Pract Res Clin Obstet Gynaecol*. 2020;63:87–110. https://doi.org/10.1016/j.bpobgyn.2019.08.002
3. Harris LH, Grossman D. Complications of unsafe and self-managed abortion. *N Engl J Med*. 2020;382(11):1029–1040. https://doi.org/10.1056/NEJMra1908412
4. Kapp N, Lohr PA. Modern methods to induce abortion: safety, efficacy and choice. *Best Pract Res Clin Obstet Gynaecol*. 2020;63:37–44. https://doi.org/10.1016/j.bpobgyn.2019.11.008
5. Moseson H, Jayaweera RT, Egwuatu I, et al. Effectiveness of self-managed medication abortion with accompaniment support in Argentina and Nigeria (SAFE): a prospective, observational cohort study and non-inferiority analysis with historical controls. *Lancet Glob Health*. 2022;10(21):1–9. https://doi.org/10.1016/S2214-109X(21)00461-7
6. Braine N, Velarde M. Self-managed abortion: strategies for support by a global feminist movement. *Womens Reprod Health*. 2022;9(3):183–202. https://doi.org/10.1080/23293691.2022.2016142
7. Gerdts C, Bell SO, Shankar M, Jayaweera RT, Owolabi O. Beyond safety: the 2022 WHO abortion guidelines and the future of abortion safety measurement. *BMJ Glob Health*. 2022;7(6):e009557. https://doi.org/10.1136/bmjgh-2022-009557
8. Briozzo L. From risk and harm reduction to decriminalizing abortion: the Uruguayan model for women's rights. *Int J Gynaecol Obstet*. 2016;134(suppl 1):S3–S6. https://doi.org/10.1016/j.ijgo.2016.06.003
9. Singh S, Maddow-Zimet I. Facility-based treatment for medical complications resulting from unsafe pregnancy termination in the developing world, 2012: a review of evidence from 26 countries. *BJOG*. 2016;123(9):1489–1498. https://doi.org/10.1111/1471-0528.13552
10. World Health Organization. *Abortion Care Guideline*. 2022. Available at: https://iris.who.int/bitstream/handle/10665/349316/9789240039483-eng.pdf?sequence=1. Accessed June 2, 2025.
11. Pizzarossa LB, Nandagiri R. Self-managed abortion: a constellation of actors, a cacophony of laws? *Sex Reprod Health Matters*. 2021;29(1):23–30. https://doi.org/10.1080/26410397.2021.1899764
12. Yanow S, Pizzarossa LB, Jelinska K. Self-managed abortion: exploring synergies between institutional medical systems and autonomous health movements. *Contraception*. 2021;104(3):219–221. https://doi.org/10.1016/j.contraception.2021.06.006
13. Skuster P, Moseson H, Perritt J. Self-managed abortion: aligning law and policy with medical evidence. *Int J Gynaecol Obstet*. 2023;160(2):720–725. https://doi.org/10.1002/ijgo.14607
14. Aiken ARA, Wells ES, Gomperts R, Scott JG. Provision of medications for self-managed abortion before and after the *Dobbs v Jackson Women's Health Organization* decision. *JAMA*. 2024;331(18):1558–1564. https://doi.org/10.1001/jama.2024.4266
15. Jelinska K, Yanow S. Putting abortion pills into women's hands: realizing the full potential of medical abortion. *Contraception*. 2018;97(2):86–89. https://doi.org/10.1016/j.contraception.2017.05.019
16. Karlin J, Novaes J, Sarnaik S, Holt K, Steinauer J, Dehlendorf C. "It's a reality that we in medicine should catch up with": physician's attitudes about self-sourced and managed abortion in the United States. *Soc Sci Med*. Epub ahead of print. https://doi.org/10.1016/j.socscimed.2025.117708
17. Baldwin A, Johnson DM, Broussard K, et al. US abortion care providers' perspectives on self-managed abortion. *Qual Health Res*. 2022;32(5):788–799. https://doi.org/10.1177/10497323221077296

18. Cohen DS, Donley G, Rebouché R. Abortion shield laws. *NEJM Evid.* 2023;2(4): EVIDra2200280. https://doi.org/10.1056/EVIDra2200280
19. Guttmacher Institute. Interactive map: US abortion policies and access after *Roe*. May 28, 2025. Available at: https://states.guttmacher.org/policies. Accessed June 2, 2025.
20. Costa SH. Commercial availability of misoprostol and induced abortion in Brazil. *Int J Gynaecol Obstet*. 1998;63(suppl 1):131–139. https://doi.org/10.1016/S0020-7292(98)00195-7
21. Zamberlin N, Romero M, Ramos S. Latin American women's experiences with medical abortion in settings where abortion is legally restricted. *Reprod Health.* 2012;9(1):34. https://doi.org/10.1186/1742-4755-9-34
22. Creinin MD. Medical abortion regimens: historical context and overview. *Am J Obstet Gynecol*. 2000; 183(2 suppl):S3–S9. https://doi.org/10.1067/mob.2000.107948
23. Cullen M. Important drug warning concerning unapproved use of intravaginal or oral misoprostol in pregnant women for induction or labor or abortion. *AIMS Journal.* 2000;13(3). Available at: https://www.aims.org.uk/journal/item/misoprostol-cytotec. Accessed June 2, 2025.
24. Hale R, Zingberg S. Use of misoprostol in pregnancy. *N Engl J Med.* 2001;344(1):59–60. https://doi.org/10.1056/NEJM200101043440112
25. Goldberg AB, Greenburg MB, Darney PD. Misoprostol and pregnancy. *N Engl J Med.* 2001; 344(1):38–47. https://doi.org/10.1056/NEJM200101043440107
26. World Health Organization. World Health Organization model list of essential medicines. 2019. Available at: https://iris.who.int/bitstream/handle/10665/325771/WHO-MVP-EMP-IAU-2019.06-eng.pdf?sequence=1. Accessed June 2, 2025.
27. Ulmann A. The development of mifepristone: a pharmaceutical drama in three acts. *J Am Med Womens Assoc.* 2000;55(3, suppl):117–120.
28. American College of Obstetricians and Gynecologists' Committee on Practice Bulletins–Gynecology, Society of Family Planning. Medication abortion up to 70 days of gestation: ACOG Practice Bulletin, number 225. *Obstet Gynecol.* 2020;136(4):e31–e47. https://doi.org/10.1097/AOG.0000000000004082
29. Espey E, Hailstorks T, Hofler L. Understanding the impacts of the Supreme Court case *FDA v Alliance for Hippocratic Medicine*. *JAMA.* 2024;331(18): 1529–1530. https://doi.org/10.1001/jama.2024.5376
30. Thompson A, Singh D, Ghorashi AR, Donovan MK, Ma J, Rikelman J. The disproportionate burdens of the mifepristone REMS. *Contraception.* 2021;104(1):16–19. https://doi.org/10.1016/j.contraception.2021.05.001
31. Mifeprex REMS Study Group. Sixteen years of overregulation: time to unburden Mifeprex. *N Engl J Med.* 2017;376(8):790–793. https://doi.org/10.1056/NEJMsb1612526
32. American College of Obstetricians and Gynecologists. Updated mifepristone REMS requirement. 2023. Available at: https://www.acog.org/clinical/clinical-guidance/practice-advisory/articles/2023/01/updated-mifepristone-rems-requirements. Accessed February 11, 2024.
33. Chen MJ, Creinin MD. Mifepristone with buccal misoprostol for medical abortion: a systematic review. *Obstet Gynecol.* 2015;126(1):12–21. https://doi.org/10.1097/AOG.0000000000000897
34. Raymond EG, Shannon C, Weaver MA, Winikoff B. First-trimester medical abortion with mifepristone 200 mg and misoprostol: a systematic review. *Contraception*. 2013;87(1):26–37. https://doi.org/10.1016/j.contraception.2012.06.011
35. Sharvit M, Yagur Y, Shams R, Daykan Y, Klein Z, Schonman R. Outcomes of incomplete abortion related to treatment modality. *Arch Gynecol Obstet*. 2023;308(5):1543–1548. https://doi.org/10.1007/s00404-023-07182-7
36. Schmidt-Hansen M, Cameron S, Lohr PA, Hasler E. Follow-up strategies to confirm the success of medical abortion of pregnancies up to 10 weeks' gestation: a systematic review with meta-analyses. *Am J Obstet Gynecol.* 2020;222(6):551–563.e13. https://doi.org/10.1016/j.ajog.2019.11.1244
37. Von Hertzen H, Huong NTM, Piaggio G, et al. Misoprostol dose and route after mifepristone for early medical abortion: a randomised controlled noninferiority trial. *BJOG.* 2010;117(10):1186–1196. https://doi.org/10.1111/j.1471-0528.2010.02636.x
38. Foster AM, Arnott G, Hobstetter M. Community-based distribution of misoprostol for early abortion: evaluation of a program along the Thailand–Burma border. *Contraception*. 2017; 96(4):242–247. https://doi.org/10.1016/j.contraception.2017.06.006
39. Foster AM, Messier K, Aslam M, Shabir N. Community-based distribution of misoprostol for early abortion: outcomes from a program in Sindh, Pakistan. *Contraception*. 2022;(109):49–51. https://doi.org/10.1016/j.contraception.2022.01.005
40. Goemans S, Singh A, Yadav AK, McDougal L, Raj A, Averbach SH. The association between self-managed versus clinician-managed abortion and self-reported abortion complications: a cross-sectional analysis in India. *Int J Womens Health*. 2023;15:1467–1473. https://doi.org/10.2147/IJWH.S414599
41. Gerdts C, Jayaweera RT, Baum SE, Hudaya I. Second-trimester medication abortion outside the clinic setting: an analysis of electronic client records from a safe abortion hotline in Indonesia. *BMJ Sex Reprod Health*. 2018;44(4):286–291. https://doi.org/10.1136/bmjsrh-2018-200102
42. Jayaweera RT, Moseson H, Gerdts C. Misoprostol in the era of COVID-19: a love letter to the original medical abortion pill. *Sex Reprod Health Matters*. 2020;28(1):1829406. https://doi.org/10.1080/26410397.2020.1829406
43. Footman K, Scott R, Taleb F, et al. Feasibility of assessing the safety and effectiveness of menstrual regulation medications purchased from pharmacies in Bangladesh: a prospective cohort study. *Contraception*. 2018;97(2):152–159. https://doi.org/10.1016/j.contraception.2017.08.002
44. Jacobson LE, Baum SE, Pearson E, et al. Client-reported quality of facility-managed medication abortion compared with pharmacy-sourced self-managed abortion in Bangladesh. *BMJ Sex Reprod Health*. 2024;50(1):33–42. https://doi.org/10.1136/bmjsrh-2023-201931
45. Stillman M, Owolabi O, Fatusi AO, et al. Women's self-reported experiences using misoprostol obtained from drug sellers: a prospective cohort study in Lagos State, Nigeria. *BMJ Open.* 2020; 10(5):e034670. https://doi.org/10.1136/bmjopen-2019-034670
46. Autry AM, Hayes EC, Jacobson GF, Kirby RS. A comparison of medical induction and dilation and evacuation for second-trimester abortion. *Am J Obstet Gynecol*. 2002;187(2):393–397. https://doi.org/10.1067/mob.2002.123887
47. Grossman D, Constant D, Lince N, Alblas M, Blanchard K, Harries J. Surgical and medical second trimester abortion in South Africa: a cross-sectional study. *BMC Health Serv Res.* 2011;11:224. https://doi.org/10.1186/1472-6963-11-224
48. Moseson H, Jayaweera R, Egwuatu I, et al. Effectiveness of self-managed medication abortion between 9 and 16 weeks of gestation. *Obstet Gynecol*. 2023;142(2):330–338. https://doi.org/10.1097/AOG.0000000000005266
49. Kapp N, Andersen K, Griffin R, Handayani AP, Schellekens M, Gomperts R. Medical abortion at 13 or more weeks gestation provided through telemedicine: a retrospective review of services. *Contracept X.* 2021;3:100057. https://doi.org/10.1016/j.conx.2021.100057
50. Moseson H, Bullard KA, Cisternas C, Grosso B, Vera V, Gerdts C. Effectiveness of self-managed medication abortion between 13 and 24 weeks gestation: a retrospective review of case records from accompaniment groups in Argentina, Chile, and Ecuador. *Contraception*. 2020;102(2):91–98. https://doi.org/10.1016/j.contraception.2020.04.015
51. Singh S, Juarez F, Prada E, Bankole A. Estimating abortion incidence: assessment of a widely used indirect method. *Popul Res Policy Rev.* 2019;38(3): 429–458. https://doi.org/10.1007/s11113-019-09517-2
52. Kristianingrum IA, Nmezi S, Zurbriggen R, Gerdts C, Jayaweera R, Moseson H. Overcoming challenges in research on self-managed medication abortion: lessons from a collaborative activist–researcher partnership. *Sex Reprod Health Matters.* 2022;30(1):2077282. https://doi.org/10.1080/26410397.2022.2077282
53. Rossier C. Estimating induced abortion rates: a review. *Stud Fam Plann*. 2003;34(2):87–102. https://doi.org/10.1111/j.1728-4465.2003.00087.x
54. Gerdts C, Sunderlin K, Cárdenas-Peña N. Self-managed abortion and criminalization in the post-*Dobbs* US. *JAMA Netw Open*. 2024;7(7): e2424298. https://doi.org/10.1001/jamanetworkopen.2024.24298
55. Singh SC, Shekhar C, Acharya R, et al. The incidence of abortion and unintended pregnancy in India, 2015. *Lancet Glob Health.* 2018;6(1): e111–e120. https://doi.org/10.1016/S2214-109X(17)30453-9
56. Ralph L, Foster DG, Raifman S, et al. Prevalence of self-managed abortion among women of reproductive age in the United States. *JAMA Netw Open*. 2020;3(12):1–15. https://doi.org/10.1001/jamanetworkopen.2020.29245
57. Ralph L, Schroeder R, Kaller S, Grossman D, Biggs MA. Self-managed abortion attempts before vs after changes in federal abortion protections in the US. *JAMA Netw Open*. 2024;7(7): e2424310. https://doi.org/10.1001/jamanetworkopen.2024.24310
58. Crear-Perry J, Correa-De-Araujo R, Lewis Johnson T, Mclemore MR, Neilson E, Wallace M. Social and structural determinants of health inequities in maternal health. *J Womens Health (Larchmt)*. 2021;30(2):230–235. https://doi.org/10.1089/jwh.2020.8882
59. Treder KM, Amutah-Onukagha N, White KO. Abortion bans will exacerbate already severe racial inequities in maternal mortality. *Womens Health Issues.* 2023;33(4):328–332. https://doi.org/10.1016/j.whi.2023.04.007

60. McReynolds-Pérez J, Kimport K, Bercu C, et al. Ethics of care born in intersectional praxis: a feminist abortion accompaniment model. *Signs.* 2023;49(1):63–87. https://doi.org/10.1086/725843

61. Veldhuis S, Sánchez-Ramírez G, Darney BG. Locating autonomous abortion accompanied by feminist activists in the spectrum of self-managed medication abortion. *Stud Fam Plann.* 2022;53(2):377–387. https://doi.org/10.1111/sifp.12194

62. Joffe C. Physician provision of abortion before *Roe v Wade. Res Sociol Health Care.* 1991;9:21–32.

63. O'Donnell KS. Reproducing Jane: abortion stories and women's political histories. *Signs.* 2017;43(1): 77–96. https://doi.org/10.1086/692444

64. Aiken ARA, Starling JE, Scott JG, Gomperts R. Requests for self-managed medication abortion provided using online telemedicine in 30 US states before and after the *Dobbs v Jackson Women's Health Organization* decision. *JAMA.* 2022;70(6):922–927. https://doi.org/10.1001/jama.2022.18865

65. Gomperts R, Jelinska K, Davies S, Gemzell-Danielsson K, Kleiverda G. Using telemedicine for termination of pregnancy with mifepristone and misoprostol in settings where there is no access to safe services. *BJOG.* 2008;115(9):1171–1178. https://doi.org/10.1111/j.1471-0528.2008.01787.x

66. Endler M, Lavelanet A, Cleeve A, Ganatra B, Gomperts R, Gemzell-Danielsson K. Telemedicine for medical abortion: a systematic review. *BJOG.* 2019;126(9):1094–1102. https://doi.org/10.1111/1471-0528.15684

67. Endler CA, Gemzell-Danielsson K. Online access to abortion medications: a review of utilization and clinical outcomes. *Best Pract Res Clin Obstet Gynaecol.* 2020;63:74–86. https://doi.org/10.1016/j.bpobgyn.2019.06.009

68. Moore AM, Philbin J, Ariawan I, et al. Online abortion drug sales in Indonesia: a quality of care assessment. *Stud Fam Plann.* 2020;51(4):295–308. https://doi.org/10.1111/sifp.12138

69. Gill RK, Cleeve A, Lavelanet AF. Abortion hotlines around the world: a mixed-methods systematic and descriptive review. *Sex Reprod Health Matters.* 2021;29(1):1907027. https://doi.org/10.1080/26410397.2021.1907027

70. Drovetta RI. Safe abortion information hotlines: an effective strategy for increasing women's access to safe abortions in Latin America. *Reprod Health Matters.* 2015;23(45):47–57. https://doi.org/10.1016/j.rhm.2015.06.004

71. Baum SE, Ramirez AM, Larrea S, et al. "It's not a seven-headed beast": abortion experience among women that received support from helplines for medication abortion in restrictive settings. *Health Care Women Int.* 2020;41(10): 1128–1146. https://doi.org/10.1080/07399332.2020.1823981

72. Veldhuis S, Sánchez-Ramírez G, Darney BG. "Becoming the woman she wishes you to be": a qualitative study exploring the experiences of medication abortion acompañantes in three regions in Mexico. *Contraception.* 2022;106: 39–44. https://doi.org/10.1016/j.contraception.2021.10.005

73. Walsh A. Feminist networks facilitating access to misoprostol in Mesoamerica. *Fem Rev.* 2020; 124(1):175–182. https://doi.org/10.1177/0141778919888070

74. Ahmed NU, Rahman MH, Roy SS, Chowdhury SA, Chowdhury R. Telemedicine services of "Shasthyo batayon 16263" during COVID-19 pandemic: opportunities and challenges. *Bangladesh Med Res Counc Bull.* 2020;46(3):240–244. https://doi.org/10.3329/bmrcb.v46i3.52259

75. Casas L, Vivaldi L. Abortion in Chile: the practice under a restrictive regime. *Reprod Health Matters.* 2014;22(44):70–81. https://doi.org/10.1016/S0968-8080(14)44811-0

76. Gerdts C, Jayaweera RT, Kristianingrum IA, Khan Z, Hudaya I. Effect of a smartphone intervention on self-managed medication abortion experiences among safe-abortion hotline clients in Indonesia: a randomized controlled trial. *Int J Gynaecol Obstet.* 2020;149(1):48–55. https://doi.org/10.1002/ijgo.13086

77. Zurbriggen R, Keefe-Oates B, Gerdts C. Accompaniment of second-trimester abortions: the model of the feminist Socorrista network of Argentina. *Contraception.* 2018;97(2):108–115. https://doi.org/10.1016/j.contraception.2017.07.170

78. Wollum A, Huerta SG, Uribe OL, et al. The influence of feminist abortion accompaniment on emotions related to abortion: a longitudinal observational study in Mexico. *SSM Popul Health.* 2022;19:101259. https://doi.org/10.1016/j.ssmph.2022.101259

79. Bercu C, Fillipa S, Ramirez AM, et al. Perspectives on interpersonal care among people who obtain abortions through clinical and accompaniment models in Argentina. *Reprod Health.* 2022;19(107): 1–16.

80. Burton J, Peralta G. Redes en torno al aborto clandestino: vínculos de Socorristas y sistema de salud en Neuquén, Argentina [Networks surrounding clandestine abortion: connections between Socorristas and the health system in Neuquén, Argentina]. *Clivajes Revista de Ciencias Sociales.* 2016;(6):159. Available at: http://revistas.uv.mx/index.php/Clivajes/article/view/2156. Accessed June 2, 2025.

81. Footman K, Keenan K, Reiss K, Reichwein B, Biswas P, Church K. Medical abortion provision by pharmacies and drug sellers in low- and middle-income countries: a systematic review. *Stud Fam Plann.* 2018;49(1):57–70. https://doi.org/10.1111/sifp.12049

82. Diamond-Smith N, Percher J, Saxena M, Dwivedi P, Srivastava A. Knowledge, provision of information and barriers to high quality medication abortion provision by pharmacists in Uttar Pradesh, India. *BMC Health Serv Res.* 2019;19(1):476. https://doi.org/10.1186/s12913-019-4318-4

83. Huda FA, Ngo TD, Ahmed A, Alam A, Reichenbach L. Availability and provision of misoprostol and other medicines for menstrual regulation among pharmacies in Bangladesh via mystery client survey. *Int J Gynaecol Obstet.* 2014;124(2):164–168. https://doi.org/10.1016/j.ijgo.2013.07.037

84. Jacobson LE, Jayaweera R, Footman K, Goodman JM, Gerdts C, Darney BG. Self-reported follow-up care needs can be met in both facility and self-managed abortion: evidence from low- and middle-income countries. *Contraception.* 2025;141:110700. https://doi.org/10.1016/j.contraception.2024.110700

85. Huss L, Diaz-Tello F, Samari G. Self-care, criminalized. the criminalization of self-managed abortion from 2000 to 2020. 2023. Available at: https://www.ifwhenhow.org/wp-content/uploads/2023/10/Self-Care-Criminalized-2023-Report.pdf. Accessed June 2, 2025.

86. Perritt J. #WhiteCoatsForBlackLives—addressing physicians' complicity in criminalizing communities. *N Engl J Med.* 2020;383(19):1801–1804. https://doi.org/10.1056/NEJMp2023305

87. Riley T, Zia Y, Samari G, Sharif MZ. Abortion criminalization: a public health crisis rooted in White supremacy. *Am J Public Health.* 2022;112(11): 1662–1667. https://doi.org/10.2105/AJPH.2022.307014

88. United Nations. Poland violated women's rights by unduly restricting access to abortion, UN committee finds. August 26, 2024. Available at: https://www.ohchr.org/en/press-releases/2024/08/poland-violated-womens-rights-unduly-restricting-access-abortion-un. Accessed October 28, 2024.

89. Amnesty International. Poland: prosecuting activist accused of aiding abortion "sets a dangerous precedent." January 10, 2023. Available at: https://www.amnesty.org/en/latest/news/2023/01/poland-prosecuting-activist-accused-of-aiding-abortion-sets-a-dangerous-precedent. Accessed October 28, 2024.

90. Center for Reproductive Rights. Available at: https://reproductiverights.org. Accessed October 27, 2024.

Suicide Prevention Training Among Occupational Groups: A Cross-Sectional Study of State-Level Policies as of July 2022

Anne E. Massey, PhD, MPH, Avery K. Druyon, JD, Sandra Roettgering, JD, Janessa M. Graves, PhD, MPH, Jennifer Stuber, PhD, Paul R. Borghesani, MD, PhD, Anna M. Ratzliff, MD, PhD, Frederick P. Rivara, MD, MPH, and Ali Rowhani-Rahbar, MD, PhD, MPH

We systematically assessed the presence and distribution of state-level policies, specifically statutes and regulations that were in effect as of July 1, 2022, related to training any occupational groups in suicide prevention.

Utilizing legal epidemiology methods, we conducted a cross-sectional assessment of all 50 states and the District of Columbia. We identified 824 policies in our initial search and retained 477 in our final policy database. Policies were distributed across 5 occupational settings: educational (n = 142), behavioral health (n = 130), carceral (n = 111), primary and specialty care (n = 60), and other (n = 58). Fourteen policies pertained to multiple settings. On average, each state had 9.4 policies and covered 3 occupational settings. All states had at least 1 policy (minimum: 1; maximum: 42).

Training occupational groups in suicide prevention is a widespread strategy, but significant variation exists across states, occupational settings, and specific occupational groups. Further research is necessary to determine whether this is an effective suicide prevention strategy at the population level.
(*Am J Public Health*. 2025;115(10):1742–1752. https://doi.org/10.2105/AJPH.2025.308193)

AJPH October 2025, Vol. 115, No. 10

Suicide is a leading cause of death in the United States.[1] Over the past 2 decades, suicide rates increased by 36%, and in 2022, more than 49 000 people died by suicide.[1,2] Suicide occurs across the lifespan and is consistently the second or third leading cause of death among people aged 10 to 34 years.[3] Impacts also extend to family, friends, and community. For each suicide death, there are an estimated 6 loss survivors (i.e., loved ones of the decedent) and 135 people who are exposed (i.e., personally knew the individual who died).[4–6] The economic toll associated with suicide is also significant, with lifetime medical and work-loss costs estimated to be $70 billion annually.[7]

Given these substantial impacts, there is widespread momentum to develop more robust suicide prevention infrastructure. The US Department of Health and Human Services' 2024 National Strategy for Suicide Prevention emphasizes the importance of workplaces—both generally and in specific settings such as education and health care—in expanding such infrastructure and includes a goal to integrate suicide prevention into workplace culture through activities such as staff training.[8] Legislation may offer a key mechanism to operationalize these efforts. The Suicide Prevention Resource Center describes state laws' potential to impact suicide prevention and highlights mandated training for specific occupational groups as a key example.[9] Several studies have described such policies within specific occupational groups, such as individuals working in educational or health care settings.[10–11] However, to our knowledge, there has yet to be an investigation that includes all occupational groups.

Training specific groups in suicide prevention, sometimes referred to as gatekeeper training, involves teaching individuals who have regular contact with populations who may be at increased risk of suicide how to identify warning signs and connect those with identified risk to relevant services.[12] These trainings can have an impact on participants' knowledge, beliefs and attitudes, reluctance and stigma, and self-efficacy.[13] In turn, well-equipped training participants can intervene effectively, which, when scaled, may decrease suicide rates overall. Though we are unaware of any evidence that demonstrates that such trainings have a population-level impact, existing studies show promising increases in participant knowledge, attitudes, confidence, self-efficacy, and skills.[14–16]

Despite calls to train a variety of professionals in suicide prevention—and the recommendation and precedent to do so via state legislation—to our knowledge, no studies have assessed these policies collectively (i.e., not restricted to a specific occupational setting). Determining whether this strategy has an impact at the population level will require understanding which occupational groups existing policies apply to and where such policies are in effect. To address this gap, we investigated the presence and distribution of state-level policies (i.e., statutes and regulations) related to suicide prevention training for any occupational group. By using methods designed for public health policy research and an occupation-agnostic approach, our results can serve as a resource for policymakers, suicide prevention advocates, and researchers seeking to better understand, improve upon, and evaluate occupational awareness and knowledge as a suicide prevention strategy. In doing so, we may be better equipped to both intervene effectively and allocate resources strategically, to decrease suicide rates overall.

METHODS

We used legal epidemiology methods[17] to conduct a cross-sectional study of state-level policies, specifically statutes and regulations, related to suicide prevention training among occupational groups. Our data collection team included 2 Juris Doctor candidates (A. K. D. and S. R.) and 1 epidemiologist (A. E. M.). We developed a study protocol and search strategy in consultation with 3 subject-matter experts: a law librarian, a law professor, and a nursing professor with legal epidemiology experience. We then used the legal research platform, Westlaw, to search for and identify relevant policies that were in effect as of July 1, 2022 (i.e., had an effective date on or before July 1, 2022) using the following terms: "suicide prevention," "training," and "+suicide & prevention." The 2 Juris Doctor candidates conducted independent Westlaw searches for relevant statutes and regulations in all 50 states and the District of Columbia. Each researcher recorded their findings in a master sheet (i.e., a document specific to that jurisdiction and researcher) using a standardized template to document key elements of each unique policy (i.e., citation, title, enacted and effective dates, and relevant legal text).

Determining Our Final Policy Set

We conducted data collection from summer 2022 through fall 2023 (i.e., identified policies across all 51 jurisdictions that were in effect as of July 1, 2022) and met regularly to review our findings, discuss questions and divergences, and refine our inclusion and exclusion criteria. After data collection was complete for a given jurisdiction, the epidemiologist populated the components of the master sheet template (e.g., citation, title, effective dates) into a reconciliation spreadsheet. We then used consensus-based decision-making to review each unique policy and determine whether to include it in our final set. Recognizing that we would refine our policy set in this final step, we erred toward being overly inclusive during data collection. This 2-step process allowed us to (1) maximize sensitivity when collecting policies (i.e., increase the proportion of policies that we accurately identified among all potentially relevant policies that exist), (2) develop increasingly precise inclusion and exclusion criteria in response to the wide range of policies we encountered, and (3) apply our final, most restrictive inclusion and exclusion criteria when selecting our final policy set, thus improving the positive predictive value of our sample.

Inclusion and Exclusion Criteria

We included enacted statutes and regulations that were promulgated at the state level and were (1) in effect as of July 1, 2022, and (2) required or encouraged suicide prevention training for any occupational group. To be included, a policy needed to be specific to either a distinct occupational group (e.g., dentists) or employees of a distinct occupational setting (e.g., staff in juvenile detention facilities). Policies that did not specify an audience or related solely to training students, parents, or community members were excluded.

Included policies also needed to specify training of some kind (e.g., instruction,

AJPH October 2025, Vol. 115, No. 10

education) and suicide prevention–related content. For example, if a policy required physicians to complete a mental health training, but suicide prevention—or some related aspect (e.g., suicide risk assessment)—was not specified as a component of that training, we excluded the policy. Training could occur in any format (e.g., training on a facility's suicide prevention protocol during orientation, annual web-based training as a condition of employment) to account for the wide range of potential training approaches. Lastly, we only included policies in which training was the immediate mechanism (i.e., directly required or encouraged) and excluded policies that focused solely on creating capacity for hypothetical or more broadly defined suicide prevention efforts (e.g., establishing a suicide prevention program, creating funds one could apply for that may support training if received). We considered training to be encouraged if completion was either optional (e.g., training was available but not mandatory) or possible but not guaranteed (e.g., suicide prevention was 1 of several content areas that would satisfy a broader training requirement).

Coding Policies

All policies in our final set were coded in MonQcle, an online platform developed specifically for public health law research. To build our policy set, we used (1) the previously collected citation, title, and effective dates; (2) Westlaw Campus Research, a version of the Westlaw database described previously; and (3) state legislature websites. We reviewed and coded each policy to determine (1) which occupational settings it applied to (i.e., behavioral health, primary and specialty care, educational, carceral, or other) and (2) which occupational groups were specified (e.g., psychologists, nurses, teachers). We used 5 primary coding questions, 1 for each occupational setting in our study (e.g., "Does this state have one or more laws that apply to occupational groups in educational settings?"). Each primary coding question had a corresponding child question (e.g., "Which educational occupations are included?").

We generated preliminary versions of our primary coding questions before data collection, then refined them after data collection and before coding. We generated the corresponding child questions after data collection by reviewing policies from a 20% sample (n = 10 jurisdictions) with differing degrees of potentially relevant state-level characteristics (i.e., high and low suicide rates; West Coast, Midwest, East Coast, and Southern geographic regions; historically Democratic and Republican populations; and high and low urbanicity). Within each jurisdiction, we reviewed all policies and documented every named occupational group. The groups mentioned most frequently formed the categories that we used to code the entire sample. We organized specific occupational groups (e.g., psychologists) by the larger occupational settings (e.g., behavioral health). In instances in which a policy applied to more than 1 setting (e.g., both behavioral health and primary and specialty care), we coded both settings accordingly.

The epidemiologist completed all coding. When questions arose, the epidemiologist consulted with the Juris Doctor candidates or other members of the study team. All variables were coded at the jurisdiction level. We summarized our findings by both jurisdiction (i.e., how many unique statutes and regulations in each jurisdiction) and occupational setting (i.e., among the unique statutes and regulations within a jurisdiction, how many applied to each occupational setting).

RESULTS

We identified 824 policies across 51 jurisdictions (i.e., all 50 states and the District of Columbia). After de-duplicating, 626 unique policies remained. We then retained 477 total policies in our final database after using consensus-based decision-making to review each unique policy and determine whether it met our final inclusion and exclusion criteria.

Occupational Settings

The 477 policies in our final database were distributed across 5 distinct occupational settings: (1) behavioral health, (2) primary and specialty care, (3) educational, (4) carceral, and (5) other (i.e., did not belong to one of the other categories). We combined behavioral health with primary and specialty care in some analyses to represent all health care professionals, aligning with the approach used by Graves et al. in 2017.[11] Most policies applied to only 1 setting, but several (n = 14) pertained to 2 or more settings (e.g., a policy might apply to both carceral and primary and specialty care settings). Accordingly, the distribution across the 5 settings totals slightly over 100: 38% (n = 182) in health care settings, with 27% (n = 130) in behavioral health and 13% (n = 60) in primary and specialty care), 30% (n = 142) in educational settings, 23% (n = 111) in carceral settings, and 12% (n = 58) in other settings (e.g., child welfare, veterans' services).

Each of the 51 jurisdictions had at least 1 policy related to suicide prevention training for some occupational group that was in effect as of July 1, 2022 (Table 1). On average, there were 9.4 policies per jurisdiction, with a minimum of 1 policy in Michigan and a maximum of 42 policies in Washington. The distribution of policies across jurisdictions varied by occupational setting (Figure A, available as a supplement to the online version of this article at https://ajph.org). Jurisdictions were most likely to have at least 1 policy related to educational settings (90% of jurisdictions; n = 46), followed by carceral settings (65% of jurisdictions; n = 33), health care settings (63% of jurisdictions; n = 32), with 55% of jurisdictions (n = 28) having policies related to behavioral health settings and 33% of jurisdictions (n = 17) having policies related to primary and specialty care settings, and other settings (59% of jurisdictions; n = 30).

The number of occupational settings covered within each jurisdiction also varied (Figure 1). Eight jurisdictions had at least 1 policy pertaining to each of the 5 occupational settings (e.g., Connecticut had policies related to behavioral health, primary and specialty care, educational, carceral, and other settings). On average, policies within a given jurisdiction applied to 3 of the 5 occupational settings. Eight jurisdictions had policies that only applied to 1 occupational setting.

Specific Occupational Groups

In the 20% sample that we reviewed to develop our coding categories, we identified more than 100 specific occupations. By occupational setting, the specific professions most frequently required or encouraged to complete suicide prevention training were marriage and family therapists, physicians, teachers and educators, carceral staff who work with children or youths, and people associated with the foster care system (Table 2). Occupations in the "other" setting varied widely and included professions such as community health workers and employees in residential group homes.

DISCUSSION

We identified state-level suicide prevention training policies in every jurisdiction across the United States (i.e., all 50 states and the District of Columbia). Collectively, policies were distributed across 5 distinct occupational settings. Though we are aware of previous investigations in health care and educational settings, to our knowledge, this is the first study to include carceral and other settings (e.g., foster care). The potential for this suicide prevention strategy to have a meaningful impact on population-level suicide rates likely depends on collective enactment, implementation, and enforcement across occupational settings. Accordingly, occupation-agnostic approaches are necessary to characterize the degree to which this strategy is being leveraged. In this study, such an approach allowed us to (1) incorporate previously unstudied settings, (2) create a comprehensive, cross-sectional data set that could be leveraged to evaluate population-level effectiveness, and (3) generate data and methods that could be used, updated, or adapted by others.

Policy Implementation and Enforcement

Meaningful implementation and enforcement are critical to the success of enacted suicide prevention training policies and require (1) thoughtful planning, (2) evaluation, and (3) typically some level of dedicated resources to both build effective training (e.g., tailored to specific jurisdictions or occupational settings) and offset training costs for participants. Because most health care occupations require professional certification or licensure, a common, cost-effective, and efficient strategy is to include suicide prevention training in existing continuing education requirements and license application or renewal cycles (e.g., RCW 43.70.442 in Washington).[18] In the absence of comparable preestablished infrastructure, alternate systems will likely need to be developed. For example, a suicide prevention program in Michigan, with workforce training for child welfare staff, includes relevant activities at 3 specific milestones: preservice, new-hire, and ongoing continuing education.[8] Given that any new infrastructure development will usually require additional resources, adopted but unfunded policies may face significant, potentially insurmountable challenges.

Very few policies specified mandatory training content or required that training be evaluated, enforced, or evidence based. These factors may contribute to uneven skill uptake, creating significant barriers to our ability to assess the collective impact of occupational training as a mechanism for reducing suicide. Participants may also face confusion navigating complex systems while attempting to satisfy their requirements (e.g., determining which training to complete). These challenges could be mitigated by ensuring that all trainings align with a minimum set of standards (e.g., the 4 competencies proposed by Hawgood et al.),[19] leveraging previously developed and evaluated trainings where applicable,[12,14–16] updating

TABLE 1— Distribution of Suicide Prevention Training Policies by Jurisdiction and Occupational Setting: United States, July 2022

Jurisdiction	Behavioral Health	Primary and Specialty Care	Education	Carceral	Other	Multiple[a]	Total
Alabama	2	0	2	2	4	0	10
Alaska	0	0	3	3	1	0	7
Arizona	0	0	2	0	0	0	2
Arkansas	0	0	12	0	1	0	13
California	12	0	3	7	0	1	23
Colorado	2	0	0	0	0	0	2
Connecticut	6	9	3	1	2	0	21
Delaware	1	0	2	0	0	0	3
District of Columbia	0	0	0	0	3	1	4
Florida	0	0	1	2	1	0	4
Georgia	1	0	3	0	0	0	4
Hawaii	0	0	2	0	0	0	2
Idaho	0	0	1	3	0	0	4
Illinois	1	0	2	4	1	0	8
Indiana	0	1	5	3	0	1	10
Iowa	1	0	2	5	0	0	8
Kansas	0	0	2	1	1	0	4
Kentucky	11	3	2	1	0	1	18
Louisiana	0	0	6	3	0	0	9
Maine	0	0	1	1	0	0	2
Maryland	2	0	4	0	1	0	7
Massachusetts	0	1	1	6	0	0	8
Michigan	0	0	0	0	1	0	1
Minnesota	1	1	4	5	2	1	14
Mississippi	2	0	3	4	1	0	10
Missouri	6	0	2	2	1	1	12
Montana	7	0	1	2	0	2	12
Nebraska	0	0	2	4	0	0	6
Nevada	13	5	4	3	2	0	27
New Hampshire	10	0	1	0	0	0	11
New Jersey	3	0	2	2	4	0	11
New Mexico	0	0	0	2	0	0	2
New York	0	0	0	4	2	0	6
North Carolina	0	0	5	1	0	1	7
North Dakota	3	0	1	0	3	0	7
Ohio	0	1	1	5	0	0	7
Oklahoma	1	0	2	5	0	1	9
Oregon	4	3	4	1	4	1	17
Pennsylvania	1	1	1	1	1	0	5
Rhode Island	0	0	2	0	0	0	2
South Carolina	2	0	1	0	0	0	3
South Dakota	0	0	22	0	0	0	22
Tennessee	2	1	2	2	1	1	9

Continued

TABLE 1— Continued

Jurisdiction	Behavioral Health	Primary and Specialty Care	Education	Carceral	Other	Multiple[a]	Total
Texas	1	0	5	10	1	0	17
Utah	8	2	1	0	1	0	12
Vermont	0	0	0	2	0	0	2
Virginia	0	0	2	7	2	0	11
Washington	11	20	6	0	3	2	42
West Virginia	4	0	1	0	1	0	6
Wisconsin	3	0	1	3	3	0	10
Wyoming	0	0	1	0	3	0	4
Total	121	48	136	107	51	14	477

[a]Includes policies that applied to more than one setting (e.g., a single policy that applied to both behavioral health and primary and specialty care would be counted once in this column and zero times in the other 2 relevant columns. All cells are mutually exclusive.)

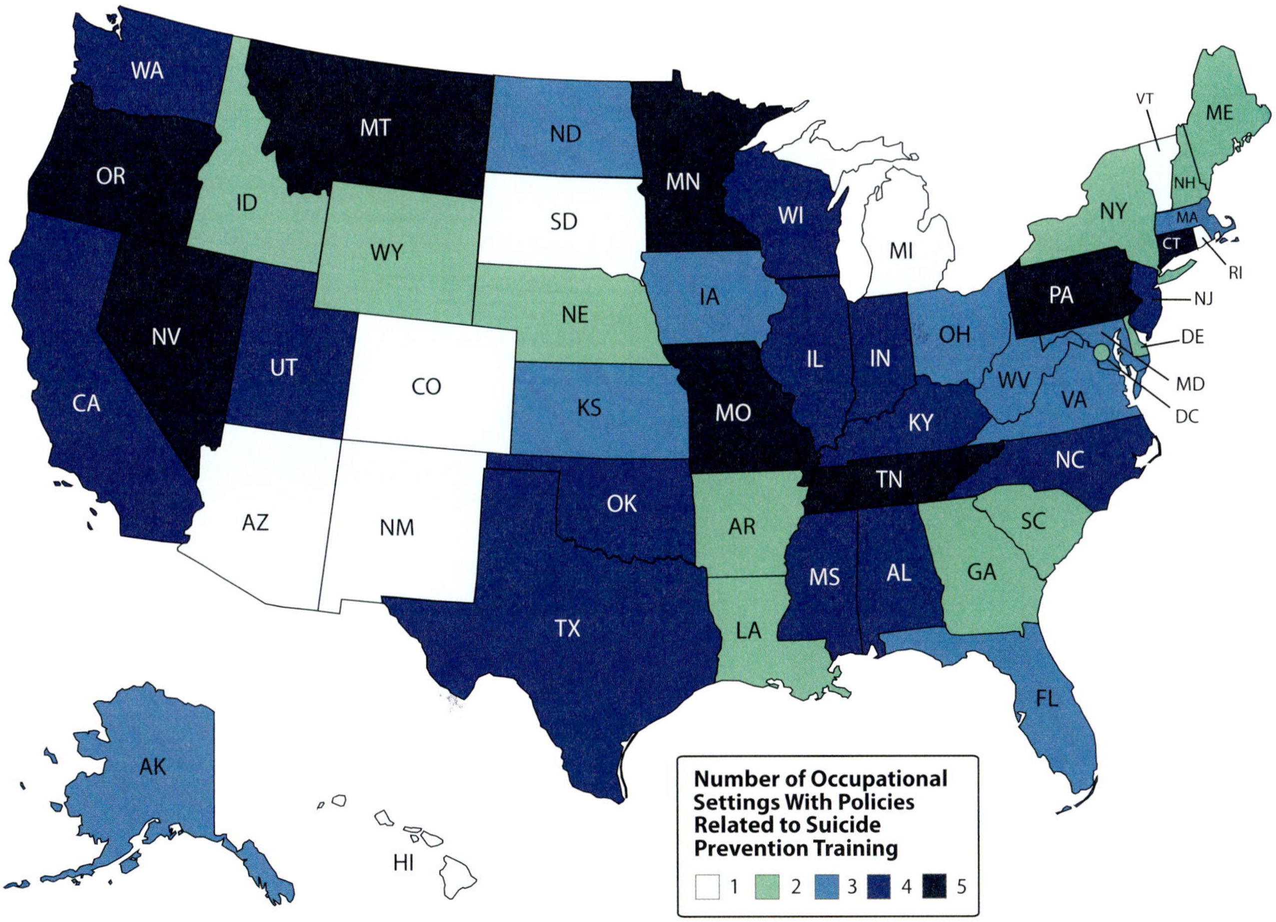

FIGURE 1— Number of Occupational Settings With Policies Requiring or Encouraging Suicide Prevention Training for Specific Occupational Groups in That Setting, by Jurisdiction: United States, July 2022

Note. Occupational settings = behavioral health, primary and specialty care, educational, carceral, or other. For example, Alaska had policies requiring or encouraging suicide prevention training for specific occupational groups in 3 of the 5 occupational settings: educational, carceral, and other.

TABLE 2— Specific Occupations Required or Encouraged to Complete Suicide Prevention Training, by Occupational Setting: United States, July 2022

Specific Occupations by Occupational Setting	No. of Jurisdictions[a] (%)
Behavioral health	
Marriage and family therapists (e.g., LMFT)	14 (27.5)
Social workers	13 (25.5)
Addiction professionals (e.g., alcohol and drug counselors, chemical dependency professionals)	12 (23.5)
Non-MHC counselors (e.g., LPC)	11 (21.6)
Psychologists	9 (17.6)
Broadly defined (e.g., "mental health professionals")	6 (11.8)
Spiritual care workers (e.g., pastoral counselors)	4 (7.8)
Mental health counselors (e.g., LMHC)	3 (5.9)
Other (e.g., peer support specialists, behavioral analysts, outdoor behavioral program staff)	22 (43.1)
Primary and specialty care	
Physicians (i.e., MD)	7 (13.7)
Emergency medical services personnel (e.g., EMT, firefighters)	6 (11.8)
Nurse practitioners (i.e., ARNP)	6 (11.8)
Nurses (e.g., RN, LPN)	5 (9.8)
Physician assistants (i.e., PA)	5 (9.8)
Occupational therapy practitioners (e.g., OT)	4 (7.8)
Chiropractors (i.e., DC)	3 (5.9)
Osteopathic doctors (i.e., DO)	3 (5.9)
Broadly defined (e.g., "medical professionals")	2 (3.9)
Physical therapy practitioners (e.g., PT)	2 (3.9)
Other (e.g., pharmacists)	7 (13.7)
Educational	
Broadly defined (e.g., "all school personnel")	38 (74.5)
Teachers/educators	29 (56.9)
School administrators (e.g., principals)	21 (41.2)
School counselors	17 (33.3)
Other (e.g., cafeteria staff)	23 (45.1)
Carceral	
Staff who work with children or youths (e.g., in juvenile detention facilities)	24 (47.1)
Broadly defined (e.g., "jail staff")	21 (41.2)
Police or peace officers	6 (11.8)
Staff involved with intake/booking	3 (5.9)
Other (e.g., staff working on a specific unit)	9 (17.6)
Other	
Those associated with the foster care system (e.g., employees, foster families)	5 (9.8)
Other (e.g., youth shelter staff)	28 (54.9)

Note. ARNP = advanced registered nurse practitioner; DC = doctor of chiropractic, DO = doctor of osteopathic medicine; EMT = emergency medical technician; LMFT = licensed marriage and family therapist; LMHC = licensed mental health counselor; LPC = licensed professional counselor; LPN = licensed practical nurse; MD = medical doctor; MHC = mental health counselor; OT = occupational therapist; PA = physician assistant; PT = physical therapist; RN = registered nurse.
[a]Jurisdictions include all 50 states and the District of Columbia (n = 51).

existing policies as needed (e.g., providing guidance on implementation and enforcement), and coordinating efforts within and between jurisdictions whenever possible.

Training Content

In addition to the minimum set of standards noted previously, there are other topics that may be worth incorporating across trainings. For example, lethal means safety refers to an intentional, voluntary process to limit one's access to potentially lethal means (i.e., items such as medications, bridges, sharp objects, or firearms that could be used to inflict self-directed violence) while one is experiencing suicide risk.[20] Putting time and distance between a person at risk and potentially lethal means saves lives and is one of the goals of the 2024 National Strategy for Suicide Prevention.[8,21–23] Accordingly, it may be advantageous to integrate lethal means safety education into training curricula, and it may be useful to leverage statutes and regulations to require such content.

Impacting training participants' reluctance and stigma are key mechanisms of suicide prevention training.[13] One potential source of reluctance might be concerns about liability. Interestingly, we identified several policies that included liability clauses (e.g., descriptions of the conditions in which an employee may be immune from civil liability). It may be beneficial to directly address such topics in trainings, particularly because liability is likely to vary by occupation.[24] Similarly, it might also be valuable to expand the use of curricula that address stigma. Promising examples, with potential for wider applicability, include a training that demonstrated a reduction in suicide-related stigma among participants[15] and the STAND Up campaign, which normalizes discussions about suicide and mental health among people working in the construction industry.[25]

Efforts to standardize training content should be balanced with thoughtful tailoring. It is unlikely that a single approach will be effective for all participants in all settings, and overstandardization may even cause harm. For example, when a widely used suicide prevention training was evaluated among a group of Canadian First Nations participants, it lacked efficacy, and there was even a trend toward increased suicidal ideation among participants.[26] By contrast, Australia now has an Indigenous-specific adaptation of the original training that was codesigned with Indigenous communities.[27,28] The former example underscores the risks of overstandardization and the importance of evaluation, and the latter offers a framework for meaningfully scaling trainings.

Occupation-Specific Considerations

Although many specific occupations were mentioned in our sample, there were several notable omissions. The 2012 National Strategy for Suicide Prevention recommended training for 13 occupational groups who have high contact with populations who may have elevated suicide risk.[29] Ten years later, only 8 of those groups were identified in our sample. Should this strategy prove to be effective on the population level, policymakers might consider expanding training requirements to the remaining 5 occupations.[29] However, it is possible that the impact of training may be differential by occupational group (e.g., particularly effective among some groups and not effective, or even potentially harmful, among others). Accordingly, subsequent policy expansion efforts should be informed by evaluation data whenever possible, and future research efforts might benefit from stratifying findings by profession.

Most policies focused on preventing suicide among the general public (e.g., patients, students). By contrast, only a few policies focused on preventing suicide within specific occupational groups themselves (e.g., firefighters). This is surprising given the high suicide rates among some of the occupational groups in our study, such as individuals who work in carceral settings and first responders.[30–33] Future efforts to evaluate the overall effectiveness of this strategy would benefit from specifically assessing the impact of suicide prevention training on those who work within these occupational settings, as well as the populations with whom they work.

Study Limitations

New statutes and regulations are consistently being passed, and bills move through multiple phases; therefore, the inherently fluid nature of the legislative process poses challenges to policy research. To address this constantly changing landscape, and in alignment with legal epidemiology best practices, we selected a specific point in time (i.e., July 1, 2022) and collected policies that were in effect as of that date (i.e., had an effective date on or before July 1, 2022). To increase the usefulness and stability of our findings, we leveraged the seasonality of the legislative cycle and selected a summer date when most legislatures are not in session. Though new laws have passed, and will continue to do so, this study provides an important update on how this overall strategy is evolving over time (e.g., it is useful to compare this distribution of policies pertaining to health care professionals against the Graves et al. study from 5 years before[11]). Our findings can also serve as exposure data for effectiveness evaluations.

It is possible that our approach was less sensitive (i.e., the proportion of policies that we accurately identified out of all potentially relevant policies that exist was lower) than we had anticipated, despite using an evidence-based search strategy that was vetted by colleagues with expertise in legal epidemiology, suicide prevention, and law. To mitigate this, each jurisdiction was searched by 2 researchers, and we erred toward being overly inclusive during data collection. We also cross-checked our findings with relevant previous studies[10,11,34] (i.e., those in health care and education) to gauge how comprehensive our findings might be in novel settings (i.e., carceral and other areas). Our final set maps closely to previous findings. Divergences between our findings and previous studies, where identified, are likely attributable to differences in search strategy, legislative platforms used, and study timing. The level of concordance between our findings and those of previous studies is reassuring in terms of overall sensitivity. In addition, the higher policy volume in our study relative to comparable previous studies among specific occupational groups (e.g., health care professionals) suggests that policies related to suicide prevention training are increasing over time.

Many training components (e.g., whether training was required or encouraged, training frequency, training duration, mechanism of training) varied widely within and across policies, occupations, and jurisdictions. In some policies, training was mandatory for some professions and encouraged or available for others. In addition, training frequency, duration, and mechanism were often unspecified. Given the volume, variability, and complexity of the statutes and regulations in our sample—and that our primary goal was to characterize the presence and distribution of this approach at the jurisdiction level, not the individual policy level—we opted to not code these policy-level components. Future evaluation efforts might consider incorporating these policy-level components to determine whether, and to what degree, such features may impact overall population-level effectiveness.

Research Priorities

It is important to better understand the effectiveness of this suicide prevention strategy. Several studies of specific trainings found improvements in participant knowledge, attitudes, confidence, self-efficacy, and skills.[14–16] While important, this overall approach will only be meaningful if these intrapersonal improvements consistently occur across trainings and participants, such improvements then translate into relevant interpersonal behaviors (e.g., with the training participants' patients), and when scaled, these interpersonal behaviors collectively decrease suicide rates overall. To our knowledge, only 1 study has assessed the relationship between suicide prevention training requirements (i.e., for state school personnel) and specific suicide outcomes (i.e., changes in youth suicide rates), and the authors found no association.[34] Evaluating the population-level impact of this strategy will require comprehensive characterization of the policy landscape (i.e., across all occupational groups) and linking to multiple suicide outcomes (e.g., attempts and death). Evaluation efforts should also determine the direction and magnitude of any potential intervention impact (i.e., if it is beneficial, harmful, or neutral).

Although we assessed cross-sectional policy enactment using an occupation-agnostic approach, additional research is needed to examine

1. these efforts longitudinally,
2. geographic patterns and regional variability,
3. policy implementation and enforcement,
4. the population-level impact on suicide outcomes,
5. whether population-level impacts differ by which occupational groups are trained,
6. whether population-level impacts differ by the presence of various policy-level training components, and
7. the impact on suicide outcomes among professionals themselves.

It will also be important to better understand training participant outcomes, including whether any initial training effects decay over time. The latter will be particularly relevant to policies in which training only occurs once. In keeping with legal epidemiology best practices, we produced a policy index to accompany this article (available as a supplement to the online version of this article at https://ajph.org).

Public Health Implications

To our knowledge, this study is the first comprehensive, systematic assessment of state-level policies on suicide prevention training across all occupational groups in the United States. The findings serve as a resource for policymakers, suicide-prevention advocates, and researchers seeking to further evaluate this strategy. A substantial amount of time and resources are being invested in this approach, both on the part of those creating and administering policies and among the individual professionals completing training. Given the often-limited funds available for public health interventions and the countless competing demands for professionals' time, increased understanding about the short- and long-term effectiveness of suicide prevention training programs is needed. If this approach proves to be effective at the population level, is used and scaled thoughtfully, and is leveraged in conjunction with other evidence-based approaches, it stands to be a critical suicide prevention strategy. AJPH

ABOUT THE AUTHORS

Anne E. Massey and Ali Rowhani-Rahbar are with the Department of Epidemiology, School of Public Health, University of Washington, Seattle, WA. Avery K. Druyon and Sandra Roettgering were with the School of Law, Seattle University, Seattle, WA, at the time of this study. Janessa M. Graves is with the Department of Family Medicine, School of Medicine, University of Washington. Jennifer Stuber is with the School of Social Work, University of Washington. Paul R. Borghesani and Anna M. Ratzliff are with the Department of Psychiatry & Behavioral Sciences, School of Medicine, University of Washington. Frederick P. Rivara is with the Department of Pediatrics, School of Medicine, University of Washington.

CORRESPONDENCE

Correspondence should be sent to Anne E. Massey, PhD, MPH, 3980 15th Ave NE, Seattle, WA 98195 (e-mail: aemassey@uw.edu). Reprints can be ordered at https://ajph.org by clicking the "Reprints" link.

PUBLICATION INFORMATION

Full Citation: Massey AE, Druyon AK, Roettgering S, et al. Suicide prevention training among occupational groups: a cross-sectional study of state-level policies as of July 2022. *Am J Public Health*. 2025; 115(10):1742–1752.

Acceptance Date: May 7, 2025.

DOI: https://doi.org/10.2105/AJPH.2025.308193

ORCID iDs:

Anne E. Massey https://orcid.org/0000-0001-9764-4627

Sandra Roettgering https://orcid.org/0009-0007-8684-9011

Anna M. Ratzliff https://orcid.org/0000-0002-6654-8007

Ali Rowhani-Rahbar https://orcid.org/0000-0002-2705-4485

CONTRIBUTORS

A. E. Massey contributed to the design of the study; acquisition, analysis, and interpretation of the data; and drafting the article. A. K. Druyon and S. Roettgering contributed to the design of the study, acquisition and interpretation of the data, and revising the article critically for important intellectual content. J. M. Graves, J. Stuber, P. R. Borghesani, A. M. Ratzliff, F. P. Rivara, and A. Rowhani-Rahbar contributed to the conceptualization and design of the study, interpretation of the data, and revising the article critically for important intellectual content. All authors contributed to final approval of the version to be published.

ACKNOWLEDGMENTS

This study was supported by a grant from the Centers for Disease Control and Prevention (R49CE003087).

Early findings were presented at the 2024 Society for Epidemiologic Research Annual Meeting.

CONFLICTS OF INTEREST

We have no conflicts of interest to report.

HUMAN PARTICIPANT PROTECTION

This study did not involve human participants, and, thus, institutional review board approval was not required.

REFERENCES

1. Centers for Disease Control and Prevention. WONDER. Underlying cause of death, 2018–2022, single race results form. Available at: https://wonder.cdc.gov/controller/datarequest/D158;jsessionid=2A10FA4DF37D0925C45B124558D9. Accessed July 14, 2024.
2. Centers for Disease Control and Prevention. Facts about suicide. May 13, 2024. Available at: https://www.cdc.gov/suicide/facts/index.html. Accessed July 14, 2024.
3. Centers for Disease Control and Prevention. WISQARS Leading Causes of Death Visualization Tool. Available at: https://wisqars.cdc.gov/lcd. Accessed July 14, 2024.
4. Cerel J, Brown MM, Maple M, et al. How many people are exposed to suicide? Not six. *Suicide Life Threat Behav*. 2019;49(2):529–534. https://doi.org/10.1111/sltb.12450
5. Drapeau CW, McIntosh JL. USA suicide 2017: official final data. December 10, 2018. American Association of Suicidology. Available at: https://neusha.org/wp-content/uploads/2022/01/U.S.A.-SUICIDE-2019-OFFICIAL-FINAL-DATA.pdf. Accessed July 14, 2024.
6. Maryland Department of Health. What survivors of suicide want you to know. Available at: https://health.maryland.gov/bha/suicideprevention/Documents/What%20Survivors%20of%20Suicide%20Want%20You%20to%20Know.pdf. Accessed July 14, 2024.
7. Centers for Disease Control and Prevention. Suicide prevention. Polaris. ADP for Policy and Strategy. April 26, 2023. Available at: https://www.cdc.gov/policy/polaris/healthtopics/suicide/index.html. Accessed July 14, 2024.
8. US Department of Health and Human Services. 2024 National Strategy for Suicide Prevention. April 15, 2024. Available at: https://www.hhs.gov/programs/prevention-and-wellness/mental-health-substance-abuse/national-strategy-suicide-prevention/index.html. Accessed July 24, 2024.
9. Suicide Prevention Resource Center. Suicide prevention policy and legislation. Available at: https://sprc.org/wp-content/uploads/2022/12/FromthefieldLegislation.pdf. Accessed July 15, 2024.
10. Rosenblum K, Dunphy C, Wang J, Frantz K, Hulkower R, Wong S. Changes in state laws on suicide prevention training for school staff, 2002–2022. *Public Health Rep*. May 2024; 139(6):750–759. https://doi.org/10.1177/00333549241249922
11. Graves JM, Mackelprang JL, Van Natta SE, Holliday C. Suicide prevention training: policies for health care professionals across the United States as of October 2017. *Am J Public Health*. 2018;108(6):760–768. https://doi.org/10.2105/AJPH.2018.304373
12. Suicide Prevention Resource Center. Choosing a suicide prevention gatekeeper training program: a comparison table of trainings available online. 2020. Available at: https://sprc.org/online-library/choosing-a-suicide-prevention-gatekeeper-training-program-a-comparison-table-of-trainings-available-online. Accessed July 16, 2024.
13. Burnette C, Ramchand R, Ayer L. Gatekeeper training for suicide prevention. *Rand Health Q*. 2015;5(1):16. Available at: https://pmc.ncbi.nlm.nih.gov/articles/PMC5158249/. Accessed July 16, 2024.
14. Isaac M, Elias B, Katz LY, Swampy Cree Suicide Prevention Team, et al. Gatekeeper training as a preventative intervention for suicide: a systematic review. *Can J Psychiatry*. 2009;54(4):260–268. https://doi.org/10.1177/070674370905400407
15. Hill RM, Picou P, Hussain Z, Vieyra BA, Perkins KM. Randomized controlled trial of an online suicide prevention gatekeeper training program: impacts on college student knowledge, gatekeeper skills, and suicide stigma. *Crisis*. 2024;45(1):57–64. https://doi.org/10.1027/0227-5910/a000917
16. Stuber J, Massey A, Payn B, Porter S, Ratzliff A. Training health care professionals in suicide assessment, management, and treatment. *Psychiatr Serv*. 2023;74(1):88–91. https://doi.org/10.1176/appi.ps.202100571
17. Center for Public Health Law Research. Defining legal epidemiology. Available at: https://phlr.org/content/defining-legal-epidemiology. Accessed July 28, 2024.
18. Washington State Legislature. RCW 43.70.442: Suicide assessment, treatment, and management training—Requirement for certain professionals—Exemptions—Model list of programs—Rules—Health profession training

standards provided to the professional educator standards board. Available at: https://app.leg.wa.gov/rcw/default.aspx?cite=43.70.442. Accessed July 17, 2024.

19. Hawgood J, Woodward A, Quinnett P, De Leo D. Gatekeeper training and minimum standards of competency. *Crisis.* 2022;43(6):516–522. https://doi.org/10.1027/0227-5910/a000794

20. US Department of Veterans Affairs. Lethal means safety and suicide prevention. Available at: https://www.mirecc.va.gov/visn19/lethalmeanssafety. Accessed September 24, 2024.

21. Harvard T. H. Chan School of Public Health. Means Matter. Available at: https://means-matter.hsph.harvard.edu/means-matter. Accessed September 24, 2024.

22. Boggs JM, Beck A, Ritzwoller DP, Battaglia C, Anderson HD, Lindrooth RC. A quasi-experimental analysis of lethal means assessment and risk for subsequent suicide attempts and deaths. *J Gen Intern Med.* 2020;35(6):1709–1714. https://doi.org/10.1007/s11606-020-05641-4

23. Barber CW, Miller MJ. Reducing a suicidal person's access to lethal means of suicide: a research agenda. *Am J Prev Med.* 2014;47(3 suppl 2):S264–S272. https://doi.org/10.1016/j.amepre.2014.05.028

24. Pinals DA. Liability and patient suicide. *Focus (Am Psychiatr Publ).* 2019;17(4):349–354. https://doi.org/10.1176/appi.focus.20190023

25. Construction Industry Alliance for Suicide Prevention. Take the Stand Up Pledge. Available at: https://www.preventconstructionsuicide.com/copy-of-pledge-to-stand-up33be6691. Accessed September 15, 2024.

26. Sareen J, Isaak C, Bolton SL, et al. Gatekeeper training for suicide prevention in First Nations community members: a randomized controlled trial. *Depress Anxiety.* 2013;30(10):1021–1029. https://doi.org/10.1002/da.22141

27. Nasir BF, Kisely S, Hides L, et al. Translating research into action: the design and development of an Indigenous specific suicide intervention skills training program (I-ASIST). *Aust J Rural Health.* 2022;30(6):870–875. https://doi.org/10.1111/ajr.12903

28. Mental Health Association of Central Australia. I-ASIST (Indigenous Applied Suicide Intervention Skills Training)-Alice Springs. Mental Health Association of Central Australia. Available at: https://www.mhaca.org.au/event/i-asist-alice-springs-2-2/. Accessed July 18, 2025.

29. US Office of the Surgeon General, National Action Alliance for Suicide Prevention. *2012 National Strategy for Suicide Prevention: Goals and Objectives for Action: A Report of the US Surgeon General and of the National Action Alliance for Suicide Prevention.* US Department of Health and Human Services. 2012. Available at: http://www.ncbi.nlm.nih.gov/books/NBK109917. Accessed July 17, 2024.

30. Stack SJ, Tsoudis O. Suicide risk among correctional officers: a logistic regression analysis. *Arch Suicide Res.* 1997;3(3):183–186. https://doi.org/10.1080/13811119708258270

31. Sussell A, Peterson C, Li J, Miniño A, Scott KA, Stone DM. Suicide rates by industry and occupation—National Vital Statistics System, United States, 2021. *MMWR Morb Mortal Wkly Rep.* 2023;72(50):1346–1350. https://doi.org/10.15585/mmwr.mm7250a2

32. Tiesman HM, Elkins KL, Brown M, Marsh S, Carson LM. Suicides among first responders: a call to action. April 6, 2021. Centers for Disease Control and Prevention. Available at: https://blogs.cdc.gov/niosh-science-blog/2021/04/06/suicides-first-responders. Accessed September 15, 2024.

33. Vigil NH, Grant AR, Perez O, et al. Death by suicide—the EMS profession compared to the general public. *Prehosp Emerg Care.* 2019;23(3):340–345. https://doi.org/10.1080/10903127.2018.1514090

34. Shah-Hartman ML, Greenawalt KE, Schaefer EW, Sekhar DL. Associations between youth suicide rates and state school personnel suicide prevention training requirements. *Prev Med Rep.* 2024;43:102768. https://doi.org/10.1016/j.pmedr.2024.102768

Erratum In: "Collecting Data Is Just the First Step: The Importance of Training Providers for Patient Encounters"

In: Chang S, Kano M. Collecting data is just the first step: the importance of training providers for patient encounters. *Am J Public Health*. 2025;115(8):1327–1328.

When originally published, an author was listed incorrectly in the Acknowledgments section and in reference 1.

The Acknowledgments section should read:

We are grateful for the thoughtful insights provided by Irene Tamí-Maury and Mary-Louise E. Millett.

Reference 1 should read:

Tamí-Maury I, Millett ME. Recommendations and implementation considerations for the routine collection of sexual orientation and gender identity data in research and practice. *Am J Public Health*. 2024;114(8):777–781. https://doi.org/10.2105/AJPH.2024.307695 AJPH

https://doi.org/10.2105/AJPH.2025.308106e

Erratum In: "Association of the COVID-19 Pandemic with Women, Infants, and Children (WIC) Receipt among Pregnant Individuals"

In: Busch S, Andersen JA, Willis DE, et al. Association of the COVID-19 pandemic with Women, Infants, and Children (WIC) receipt among pregnant individuals: United States, 2016–2022. *Am J Public Health*. 2023;113(S3):S240–S247.

When originally published, one of the grant funding numbers in the acknowledgments was incorrect. The grant number should read:

OT2HL158287. AJPH

https://doi.org/10.2105/AJPH.2023.307525e

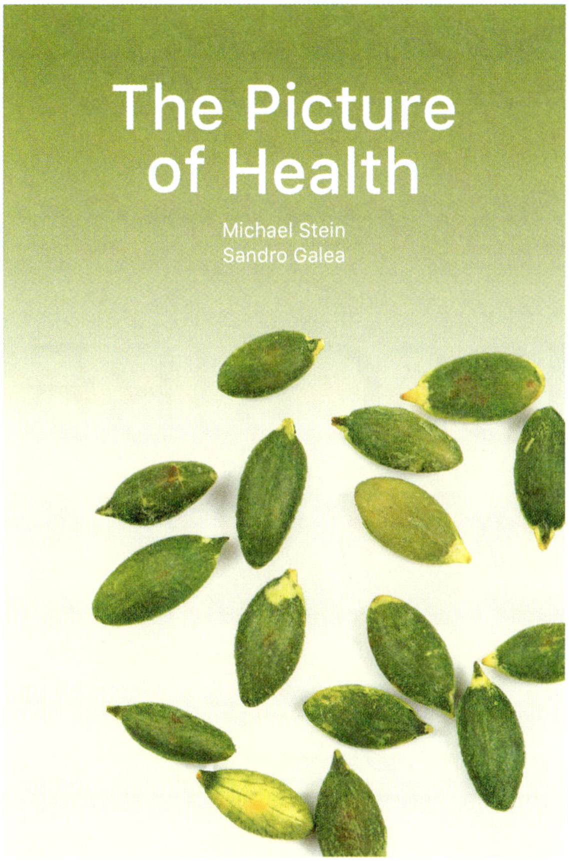

2023, SOFTCOVER, 230 PP, 9780875533247

The Picture of Health

By Sandro Galea and Michael Stein

The Picture of Health is an essential resource for student and early-career professionals learning the importance of visuals in public health storytelling. This introductory book breaks down public health issues through 100 compelling, "databytes" of pictures and text that can stand alone as research summaries compared to table and chart-heavy journals and papers. Through curating these databytes, *The Picture of Health* shows how public health workers can merge visuals with data to create a larger storyline about the issues, conditions and pressures that shape the health of the population.

APHABOOKSTORE.ORG

APHA PRESS

AN IMPRINT OF **AMERICAN PUBLIC HEALTH ASSOCIATION**